DATE DUE			

ANNUAL REVIEW OF NURSING RESEARCH

Volume 6, 1988

ANNUAL REVIEW OF NURSING RESEARCH

Volume 6

Joyce J. Fitzpatrick, Ph.D.
Roma Lee Taunton, Ph.D.
Jeanne Quint Benoliel, D.N.Sc.
Editors

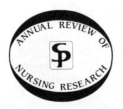

SPRINGER PUBLISHING COMPANY
New York

Order ANNUAL REVIEW OF NURSING RESEARCH, Volume 7, 1989, prior to publication and receive a 10% discount. An order coupon can be found at the back of this volume.

Copyright © 1988 by Springer Publishing Company, Inc.
All rights reserved

Springer Publishing Company, Inc.
536 Broadway
New York, NY 10012

88 89 90 91 92 / 5 4 3 2 1

ISBN 0-8261-4355-5
ISSN 0739-6686

ANNUAL REVIEW OF NURSING RESEARCH is indexed in *Cumulative Index to Nursing and Allied Health Literature* and *Index Medicus*.

Printed in the United States of America

Contents

Preface

We have received much positive feedback regarding the contribution of the first five volumes of the *Annual Review of Nursing Research* series to the development of nursing knowledge for the discipline. One of the most gratifying affirmations came this past year in the form of an *American Journal of Nursing (AJN)* Book of the Year Award for Volume 4. We were honored and encouraged by it. With the series now well established, there is a firm foundation for future volumes. We hope that the scientists and professional practitioners in nursing will continue to use these volumes to strengthen research and its applications in practice.

As in previous volumes, research reviewed for Volume 6 follows the established format of five major parts: Nursing Practice, Nursing Care Delivery, Nursing Education, the Profession of Nursing, and Other Research. In each of these areas we identify experts to review the research in a defined topic area.

The chapters under Nursing Practice for the present Volume are focused on specific nursing interventions. Sandra J. Weiss reviews research on touch, Carol A. Lindeman examines patient education research, Margaret A. Williams reviews research on the physical environment and patient care, Jane S. Norbeck examines research on social support, and Mariah Snyder reviews the research on relaxation. Chapters in this area in Volumes 1 and 4 were focused on human development along the life span, chapters in Volume 2 on the family, chapters in Volume 3 on the community, and chapters in Volume 5 on human responses to actual and potential health problems. Authors in Volumes 7 and 8 will address physiological aspects of care.

In the area of nursing care delivery, Margaret D. Sovie analyzes the research on variable costs of nursing care in hospitals. In the section on nursing education, there is a focus on areas of specialized clinical education. Maxine E. Loomis reviews research on psychiatric-mental health nursing education and Beverly C. Flynn reviews community health nursing education. Research on the profession of nursing includes a chapter by Luther P. Christman on men in nursing.

In the area of other research, three chapters are included. Nancy Fugate Woods examines women's health research, and Sister Callista Roy reviews research on human information processing. Also in the area of other research, we have continued our efforts to include a focus on international nursing research. Phoebe Dauz Williams examines nursing research in the Philippines. We are interested particularly in continuing this effort and have targeted chapters in future volumes that will be focused on nursing research in other countries.

The success of the Review over the past six years has been enhanced in many ways by the contributions of the distinguished Advisory Board. We express our appreciation to them; their advice and support have been invaluable. With sorrow, we report the death of Rosemary Ellis. Another Advisory Board member, Lucille Notter, is retiring for health reasons. We acknowledge the contributions of these two esteemed scholars.

We welcome Jeanne Quint Benoliel as an editor for Volumes 6 through 8. She has been involved in the Review since the first volume as an Advisory Board member and a contributing author. We shall benefit from her expertise in this new role.

We also most gratefully acknowledge the critiques of anonymous reviewers, and the editorial and clerical assistance provided by support staff at Case Western Reserve University, the University of Kansas, and the University of Washington. We are particularly indebted to Nikki S. Polis, Ph.D. candidate at Case Western Reserve University, for her editorial assistance throughout the production of this and previous volumes.

As always, we welcome readers' comments and suggestions for shaping the upcoming volumes, including identifying potential chapter contributors. Please let us know your interests in contributing to the series and your comments on this volume.

Contributors

Luther P. Christman, Ph.D.
College of Nursing
Rush University
Chicago, Illinois

Beverly C. Flynn, Ph.D.
School of Nursing
Indiana University
Indianapolis, Indiana

Carol A. Lindeman, Ph.D.
School of Nursing
Oregon Health Sciences University
Portland, Oregon

Maxine E. Loomis, Ph.D.
College of Nursing
University of South Carolina
Columbia, South Carolina

Jane S. Norbeck, D.N.Sc.
School of Nursing
University of California,
   San Francisco
San Francisco, California

Sister Callista Roy, Ph.D.
School of Nursing
Boston College
Chestnut Hill, Massachusetts

Mariah Snyder, Ph.D.
School of Nursing
University of Minnesota
Minneapolis, Minnesota

Margaret D. Sovie, Ph.D.
School of Nursing
University of Rochester
Strong Memorial Hospital
Rochester, New York

Sandra J. Weiss, D.N.Sc.
School of Nursing
University of California, San Francisco
San Francisco, California

Margaret A. Williams, Ph.D.
School of Nursing
University of Wisconsin–Madison
Madison, Wisconsin

Phoebe Dauz Williams, Ph.D.
College of Nursing
University of Florida
Gainesville, Florida

Nancy Fugate Woods, Ph.D.
School of Nursing
University of Washington
Seattle, Washington

Forthcoming

ANNUAL REVIEW OF
NURSING RESEARCH, Volume 7

Tentative Contents

PART I

Research on Nursing Practice

Chapter 1

Touch

SANDRA J. WEISS
SCHOOL OF NURSING
UNIVERSITY OF CALIFORNIA, SAN FRANCISCO

CONTENTS

In this review of research, published studies are examined in which physical contact between persons is a major phenomenon of interest. Excluded from the review is research (a) that involves contact using intermediary objects or equipment, such as in nursing procedures, (b) in which the effects of touch are not examined specifically even though its influence may be readily apparent in the treatment or con-

3

text for study, or (c) in which the term *touch* is used to describe movement of the hand above the actual surface of the body, as in the work of Krieger (1975) and others. In addition, only studies where nurses assumed a major role as investigators have been included, even though the content of research in other fields might have been related closely to nursing research. These limitations reflect an attempt to examine a body of congruent research with direct implications for the discipline of nursing.

All studies from 1960 to 1985 have been included, at least those that could be identified through computer search, review of nursing research journals, follow-up of citations from references, and personal contacts with those known to be studying the phenomenon. Key words used in the search were *touch, tactile experience, tactile sensation, physical contact*, and *physical interaction*. Tactile research in nursing falls nicely into three major areas: descriptive studies about either the properties or patterns of touch, and predictive studies about human responses associated with touch.

PROPERTIES OF TOUCH

Three classes of tactile properties have been examined: the meaning of touch, types of touch, and qualities of touch. In each of these classes, definitions are included for common attributes of touch that need to be considered in its conceptualization or clinical use.

Meaning of Touch

The meaning of touch has been examined from the perspective of both nurses and patients. Farrah (1971) conducted a study to determine the reported use of touch by medical–surgical nurses. She reported that nurses saw touch as capable of conveying many positive meanings to patients such as security, understanding, support, warmth, caring, reassurance, empathy, closeness, and willingness to be involved.

Two observational studies were conducted to examine meanings of touch between hospitalized psychiatric patients and staff.

De Augustinis, Isani, and Kumler (1969) indicated that a majority of observed touches were interpreted by both personnel and patients as expression of tender feelings. Instigating action, gaining attention, punishment or restraint, aggression, and reality testing or orienting also were identified purposes. Cashar and Dixson (1967) identified reality orientation, support, and physical protection as the three main purposes for which they observed touch being used. De Augustinis et al. (1969) found that only 50% of the interpretations by recipients and initiators of touch were similar. In contrast to personnel, patients described touch less positively, viewing it as the staff's attempt to get the patient's attention or to have the patient do something that was being requested. The investigators concluded that touch gestures do not have universal meaning but are influenced by the patient's diagnosis, the nurse's idea of what is appropriate, and the patient's developmental level and previous experience.

Penny (1979) studied perceptions of postpartum patients about the touch they received during labor. In her interview data, touch perceived as positive by patients came primarily from the spouse rather than from health professionals. The majority of touches seen as negative involved physicians. The meanings identified for positive touch included reassurance, caring, someone to be with them, security, pain relief, and comfort. Negative touch usually occurred when procedures were being done or when attempts to be supportive had become annoying or irritating. In conclusion, Penny indicated that the meaning of touch appeared to depend on the specific relationship in question as well as culture, age, and part of the body touched.

Although diverse in their approaches, these four studies lead to the conclusion that the meaning of touch is not always positive to patients. Rather than having universal meaning, the meaning of touch gestures may be context-dependent and person-specific.

Types of Touch

Two studies were found in which the properties of touch were considered from a typological perspective. Dunbar (1977) observed the touch of mothers with their full-term newborns during early postpartum feeding periods. There were two modes of contact in the mothers' touching: direct touching involving use of the fingertips, face, or palm of hand; and indirect touching involving contact through intermediary objects such as a paper napkin or a bottle. Two modes of holding also were identified: proximate and distant. Lastly, two types of functional touch were described: instrumental and expressive.

Chamorro, Davis, Green, and Kramer (1973) made a contribution to understanding the properties of touch by the development and testing of an observational instrument to measure the amount and type of handling received by premature infants in the neonatal intensive care unit. The two touch categories within the measure specified social and instrumental caretaking activities and therapeutic activities. Some of the interobserver reliabilities for various tactile behaviors were as low as 40 to 43%. The independence of behaviors was also in question. Because only some of the categories in the tool were tested, the reliability and validity of the entire measure is unknown.

Qualities of Touch

The final study contributing to a definition of tactile properties involved the development and testing of an instrument to differentiate various qualities of physical touch (Weiss, 1985, in press). This instrument included both a series of videotapes and an observational coding system for microanalysis of videotaped or filmed tactile interactions.

The first version of Weiss's measure included categories for coding location, duration, intensity, and comfort or discomfort sensation of touch. After initial testing, the instrument was revised by deleting the sensation indicator and adding a new category that measured the specific type of action or gesture used in touch, for example, stroking, rubbing, and patting. Testing gave evidence of significant validity based on judgments of experts and prediction to established criteria, as well as intercoder and test–retest reliability (Weiss, 1985).

Although much work remains to understand types and qualities of touch, a common knowledge base was emerging in the work of Chamorro et al. (1973) and Dunbar (1977) in differentiating instrumental and expressive types. Similarly, some of the Chamorro et al. (1973) caretaking subcategories parallelled those of the Weiss (1985) 28 subcategories of tactile action. The value in analyzing the properties of touch lay in the increased capacity to measure and understand the specific characteristics that may have been responsible for any behavioral responses observed.

PATTERNS OF TOUCH

Research on patterns of touch covers three areas of investigation: (a) attitudinal and behavioral patterns of touch between nurses and patients, (b) patterns of tactile sensitivity in selected patient populations, and (c) patterns of maternal touch with newborns.

Nurse–Patient Touch

Attitudes of Nurses. The first set of investigations sheds light on attitudes of nursing students and nurses toward touching patients. Ellis, Taylor, and Walts (1979) surveyed associate degree students and found that nearly all students felt comfortable being touched and using touch. Only a few students feared that their use of touch would be misinterpreted by patients.

Tobiason (1981) found that baccalaureate students used more positive words to describe touching of newborns than of elderly. However, her classification of words as positive or negative seemed somewhat biased and arbitrary, as did her interpretation of their relationship to student anxiety about touching.

Through a questionnaire submitted to medical–surgical nurses, Farrah (1971) found that touch accompanied by a verbal intervention was the most preferred intervention for use in patient care. Verbal behavior alone ranked second, and touch alone ranked third. Many of the nurses believed that touch alone could be misinterpreted, whereas words prevented any misunderstanding. Nurses identified misinterpretation of meaning, social mores and taboos, and both the nurse's and patient's comfort with touch as major considerations in its use. Nurses seemed more comfortable touching older patients than younger ones, and females more than males. The more highly educated and experienced nurses were most favorable toward use of touch.

Attitudes of Clients. Three studies have been conducted to examine client attitudes toward touch. Penny (1979) found that only 62% of the labor patients she interviewed described the touch they received during their labor as completely positive. Evaluations were not related to the amount of touch received. Adolescents and nonwhites saw touch as much less positive than did other women.

Using assessment of photographed situations, DeWever (1977) found that elderly patients in a nursing home were most likely to perceive discomfort when an older male nurse was pictured touching a person, especially if he held the person's hand. Discomfort also was indicated when the staff member had his or her arm placed around the patient's shoulder. Female subjects were more likely than males to perceive discomfort with being touched by a male nurse.

Morse (1983) found that the appropriateness of touch was distinguished according to the amount of trust and intimacy in a relationship. Considering possible combinations of touch and talking, touching was seen as appropriate only with a spouse or child who was feeling afraid or unloved. Touching with a little talking was viewed as appropriate for situations in which a person was in pain; and talking with a little touch was seen as most appropriate when an individual was insecure, in a new situation, depressed, or feeling loss.

Use of Touch. Four investigators looked at patterns of use of touch between health personnel and patients. Barnett (1972) suggested that registered nurses touched more frequently than any other health personnel, and that white, younger, female personnel touched more than any other staff group. She also indicated that young adult female patients were touched most, followed by infants, with 6- to 17-year-olds not being touched at all. Severely ill patients were touched the least, whereas patients in good condition were touched the most. The hand, forehead, and shoulder, in that order, were touched most frequently. Mexican-Americans touched the least as personnel and received the least touching as patients.

De Augustinis et al. (1969) found that psychiatric personnel initiated touching between patients and staff most of the time. The staff stated that they were always aware if any touching had occurred with the patient, regardless of who had initiated the touch, whereas patients were often not aware that a touch had occurred between themselves and staff. A majority of the personnel described their touching as automatic or spontaneous touching, whereas one third said they had thought about it before deciding to touch.

Copstead (1980) found that two thirds of nursing home patients received some touch from the medication nurse as she made rounds. Touch was usually light contact on the wrist or hand. For females, the back and neck were also touched. Patients who received no touch were older than those who were touched, but equal percentages of males and females were touched. All touches were described as helping the patient receive medication rather than as expressive gestures.

Blackburn and Barnard (1985) analyzed four types of caregiving activities for premature infants, using time lapse video recordings over a 24-hour period. The most frequent type was handling related to miscellaneous/technical procedures, and the least frequent was stroking. Each episode of handling within the incubator was $3^1/2$ minutes or less. The investigators found tremendous variation in amount of handling across infants, ranging from as little as 5% of a day to 38%.

These various studies on the attitudes toward and actual uses of touch in nurse–patient relationships yielded little that could be merged into a cohesive body of knowledge. One convergent finding was the indication from both Copstead's (1980) and Blackburn and Barnard's (1985) research that procedural or instrumental touch seems to be used by caregivers much more frequently than expressive or affective touching. This fact could be related to the expressed concern by nurses that their touching may be misinterpreted (Ellis et al., 1979; Farrah, 1971), but it also may reflect the task-oriented nature of nurses' work.

There was disparity across studies regarding age and sex as predictors of attitudes toward touch and its actual use; the role of ethnicity was also unclear. The only apparent commonality in the research was that very diverse views existed concerning whether or when touch was appropriate. This outcome clearly supported the previously cited studies on meaning of touch, reinforcing individual differences in evaluation of tactile experiences.

Thresholds for Touch

Different degrees of tactile sensitivity across individuals have been identified that may help to explain why touch is evaluated and experienced differentially. Using a pressure aesthesiometer, Thornbury and Mistretta (1981) found that thresholds for tactile sensitivity decreased with age although a number of individuals over 60 retained high tactile acuity. The investigators also found lower thresholds (greater acuity) in females, but because they did not report the number of younger and older subjects who were male or female, it was difficult to distinguish the effects of age and sex.

McBride and Mistretta (1982) demonstrated that thresholds for touch of persons with diabetes were higher than those of non-diabetics. For diabetics, both the duration of having the disease and the use of insulin treatment were related to higher tactile thresholds (lower acuity). There were no differences in tactile acuity between those diabetics with neurological symptoms and those without such symptoms. The same measurement problem occurred in both of these studies in that many of the subjects appeared to have been able to discriminate thresholds lower than the testing device allowed; thus, the full variance among subjects was not examined.

Mother-Infant Touch

Three researchers have examined the patterns of touch used by mothers in handling newborns. Tulman (1985) found that mothers handled newborn infants more than female nursing students did. Mothers also demonstrated a common pattern of touching their infants, whereas no common pattern was observed for students. Tulman found no differences in pattern for race, parity, handedness, or amount of recent experience with infants.

In a study of the first postpartum contact Cannon (1977) showed that mothers of undressed infants began to touch the trunk of the baby sooner than those with dressed infants. In contrast to the differences in progression for trunk contact, fewer mothers with undressed babies completely enfolded the infant against the body with their arms surrounding him or her. Cannon (1977) found that the majority of mothers completed the same stages of contact as defined by previous research (Rubin, 1963), although at a faster rate than proposed. No significant differences were observed for multiparas and primiparas in their patterns of touching.

Dunbar (1977) examined the pattern of maternal touch over the first 4 days postpartum. She found that most of a mother's touch was direct touching of the infant rather than through use of intermediary objects, that proximate versus distant holding was used the majority of the time, and that the majority of touches were instrumental (caretaking) rather than expressive of affect. Frequency of these tactile approaches was fairly constant across the first 3 days, with an increase in instrumental touching of the infant observed on the fourth postpartum day.

This cluster of studies on maternal touch provided conflicting evidence regarding the nature of any patterns that may have existed during the first few days postpartum. For instance, Cannon's (1977) research supported the previous theories of Klaus and Kennell (1976) and Rubin (1963) regarding patterns of maternal touch, but Tulman's (1985) research did not. Differences in the situational context must be considered as an intervening variable; Tulman's observational method was quite intrusive, but Cannon attended to needs for privacy between mother and infant. One common outcome from these studies was the lack of any differences in patterns of maternal touch based on whether the infant was the mother's first child.

HUMAN RESPONSES ASSOCIATED WITH TOUCH

Developmental Responses

A large number of studies have been conducted to examine the relationship between touch and developmental responses, mostly in infancy. Studies can be grouped into three clusters: those in which researchers examined the relationship of touch to behavioral phenomena, physical phenomena, and psychological phenomena.

Behavioral Phenomena. Blackburn and Barnard (1985) examined the relationship between handling of infants and infant activity levels in the intensive care nursery. Primarily, they found that infant activity levels peaked at different times than caregiving peaks. However, increased infant motor activity prior to certain caregiving events may have reflected the responsiveness of caregivers to handling infants, in that they were more likely to provide care when they observed the infants to be active and awake rather than sleeping. In addition, an infant's activity level decreased after the child was diapered or fed; but it remained high following technical procedures, perhaps because of the arousing nature of the procedural stimuli.

Hasselmeyer (1963) conducted a study to determine the behavioral effects of extra handling of premature infants. She showed that infants receiving more handling demonstrated less crying and more quiescent states both in general and before feedings than infants who were handled less.

Jay (1982) found that the incidence of both startle and nonstartle responses across mechanically ventilated premature infants decreased substantially as a result of planned intermittent touch. Also, observations of tightly clenched fists in infants decreased, while observations of relaxed, open hands and grasping behavior increased slightly. The investigator postulated that infants were more relaxed over time as a result of the touch; however, the changes could have reflected development.

Kramer, Chamorro, Green, and Knudtson (1975) found a significantly greater rate of social development for preterm infants receiving extra nonrhythmic stroking than for a group who did not. However, this finding showed no convergent validity based on two different measures of development. In addition, there were no differences in levels of eventual development between the experimental and matched groups.

Blackburn and Barnard (1985), Hasselmeyer (1963), and Jay (1982) all gave evidence that certain types of touch were effective in enhancing behavioral organization of the infant, resulting in states of relaxation or calm. However, it was impossible to identify the common types of touch used across these studies because all investigators did not control for the quality of touch used. The size of Kramer et al.'s (1975) sample combined with the multiple staff administering the interventions raised serious questions regarding the generalizability of their findings.

Physical Phenomena.   Three studies have been conducted to examine the effects of placing the nude neonate on the mother's bare chest immediately after birth on maintenance of the infant's body temperature (Gardner, 1979; Hill & Shronk, 1979; Phillips, 1974). In each study, it was hypothesized that infants who had been dried well and adequately covered could retain their body temperature if held by their mothers equally as well as infants who were placed in a heated crib. All investigators found no significant differences in the mean rectal temperatures of the two groups of infants at 15 minutes.

Although the Phillips (1974) study was the most comprehensively described of the three, all had similar methodological limitations. For instance, sex, ethnicity, weight, and other important variables were not considered for their potential moderating effects. There was no apparent standardization of approach for the nurses to use in determining such matters as the nature of touch by mothers or the method of taking temperatures. In spite of any resulting extraneous variance, the validity of the findings was supported by their consistency across three separately studied samples.

A second cluster of researchers studied the effects of tactile intervention programs on the physical responses of preterm infants. Rausch (1981) examined effects of gentle rubbing as well as limb flexion and extension to preterm infants. There were no statistically significant differences in weight between the group receiving the intervention and a control group over a 10-day period. The mean feeding intake of the treatment group was significantly greater, as was the frequency of stooling.

As a result of her intervention program, Hasselmeyer (1963) found that a group of premature infants receiving extra handling passed significantly less feces than their controls. She found no differences between the groups in incidence of morbidity or weight gain.

In comparing a group of premature infants who received a program of touch to a control group, Jay (1982) found no differences between groups in weight gain, need for mechanical ventilation, apnea and bradycardia, blood pH, or tolerance of oral nutrients. She did find a significantly higher hematocrit for the intervention group and a shorter length of hospitalization.

Kramer et al. (1975) presented data on physical development that showed no significant differences between the infants receiving extra touch and a control group. Neither weight gain nor amount of cortisol production of infants differed.

In general, investigators in this latter cluster of studies gave evidence that brief programs of tactile intervention were not particularly effective in enhancing the physical development of preterm infants. Although in two of the studies infant stooling patterns seemed to be affected significantly by touch, the investigators reported opposite effects (Hasselmeyer, 1963; Rausch, 1981).

Psychological Phenomena.   Only one study could be found on developmental responses from a psychological perspective. Weiss (1984, in press) conducted an investigation to examine differential qualities of parental touch and their relationship to the body image of children ranging from 8 to 11 years old. Data were collected using videotapes of parent–child interaction in a laboratory playroom.

She found no differences in the pattern of touch by mothers and fathers, either in the intensity, duration, or degree of comfort observed in their touching. However, mothers did touch a greater diversity of the child's body parts and touched more frequently than fathers. For boys and girls alike, the qualities of touch associated with a sophisticated body concept and positive body sentiment involved the touching of highly innervated body areas, longer duration of touch, greater frequency of touch, and more active, assertive patterns of touch by parents. However, there were very different patterns of relationships observed depending on the sex of parent and sex of child involved in the interaction. Weiss suggested that the results indicated different types of sensory reactivity for boys and girls or different interpretations of various qualities of touch based on the gender of parent and child.

Interpersonal Responses

Two clusters of nursing research were centered around touch as it influences responses within interpersonal relationships. Several studies were reviewed on parent–infant attachment and on the efficacy of the nurse–patient interaction.

Parent–Infant Attachment. Curry (1982) examined the effect of skin-to-skin contact between mothers and their infants during the first hour following delivery on later maternal attachment to the infant. Results showed no differences between mothers of the experimental group and a control group on observed attachment behaviors at either 36 hours or 3 months after delivery.

Three investigators studied the effects of early tactile contact between father and infant on the father's attachment to the infant. Pannabecker and Emde (1977) demonstrated no significant differences in behaviors toward infants at 4 weeks postpartum for fathers who had received a tactile experience with their newborns and those who had not. Jones (1981) also showed no differences between fathers who held their infant during the first hour after delivery and a control group who did not in their perceptions of their infant at one month of age. There were no differences in frequency of caregiving or play with the infant at one month. The only behavioral difference was that fathers who had early physical contact interacted nonverbally with their infants to a greater degree than did other fathers.

Similarly, Toney (1982) found no consistent differences in the interactions of fathers who held their infants during the first hour after delivery and a control group who did not, although fathers in the experimental group did smile more at their infants and display more whole hand touching. Considering both groups as a whole, fathers showed more fingertip touching with male infants than female infants.

In these studies investigators provided evidence that brief physical contact with the infant during the first few hours or even days of life may not be critical to attachment or bonding to the infant. There were implications within each study that other variables, which the investigators did not control, may have been influential to the infant-parent relationship. Standardization was needed of the interactions experienced by the experimental and control groups during and immediately after delivery as well as more comprehensive assessment of mediating factors. In addition, there were problems in each study with the validity and reliability of self-report and observational measures of attachment, a factor that could enhance the potential for a Type II error.

Efficacy of Nurse–Patient Interaction.   Six studies have been conducted to examine the effects of touch by nurses on various aspects of observed patient response to the interaction. Four of these studies had very similar designs. Ellis et al. (1979) studied the effects of touch such as pulse-taking or patting patients' arm or hand on their positive or negative nonverbal responses during the interaction. McCoy (1977) conducted a study with emergency room patients to determine whether periodic touching of the patient's wrist or arm during an assessment interview would increase rapport with the nurse. McCorkle (1974) conducted a similar study with seriously ill patients to examine whether patients who had their wrists touched "gently" throughout an interview would demonstrate more positive verbal and nonverbal responses to the interaction. Lastly, Knable (1981) studied the effect on critically ill patients' nonverbal responses of having their regular nurse hold their hands at two times during a 4-hour period.

In each of these studies, almost identical outcomes were observed. In general, patients who received some form of touch responded positively to the interaction with the nurse as defined by arbitrary classifications of verbal or nonverbal behaviors. In contrast, patients not receiving touch during the interaction showed more negative behaviors. Facial expression, eye contact, and body movement were assessed across all studies. McCorkle (1974) also examined verbal responses and found that more of the subjects who were touched had positive verbal responses. In addition, McCoy (1977) and McCorkle asked patients their perception of the nurse's interest in them as a person. Patients who were touched in McCoy's study responded much more positively about the nurse's interest in them than those not touched, whereas McCorkle found no differences in the evaluations of the two groups. One other fascinating outcome from McCorkle's research was that only 2 of the 30 patients touched were aware that they had been touched, even though the investigator touched their wrists throughout the interview.

In these four studies, similar observational measures of the dependent variables were used to examine the effects of nursing touch on patient response to the interaction. As a result, they had some common methodological limitations. The major problem was the validity of the way in which certain nonverbal responses were coded as positive or negative. A further problem was that positive responses were interpreted frequently as indicating that the touch should be considered beneficial or therapeutic for the patient when no evidence was provided that the touch influenced the individual's health in any way. In addition, none of the investigators reported any validity testing or test–retest reliability with the observational method used. Two of the investigators did assess interobserver agreement. Lastly, lack of standardization of the touching and absence of any controls for other types of communication were significant oversights that could have influenced outcomes. McCorkle's (1974) work is the exception here as she did build in some standardized words and touch.

In a different approach to looking at the effects of touch on efficacy of the interaction, Aguilera (1967, p. 7) found that use of "simple, appropriate touch gestures" by nurses along with their verbal communication resulted in increased verbal interaction, rapport, and approach behavior by psychiatric patients. How those conclusions were reached from the data remained unknown because the measures specific to the variables were not described. The investigator also stated that, over a 2-week period of using touch, positive attitude changes toward the nurse were greater than negative changes.

Langland and Panicucci (1982) conducted a study to determine the effects of touching an elderly, confused patient's arm on the patient's attention and response to a verbal request. Patients who were touched showed greater evidence of attention during the request than the control group, but no differences were observed in appropriateness of verbal or behavioral responses to the request. Because there were no controls for certain moderating variables, such as the fact that baseline mental status scores for controls were not as good as for those who were touched, the difference in attention may have been influenced by factors other than touch.

In spite of the validity and reliability issues associated with the first four studies on the nurse–patient relationship, there were consistent indications that touch may enhance the patient's positive response to the interaction. In contrast, the impact of touch on patients' behavioral competence was difficult to assess since the designs of the two studies in this area were so different.

Psychological Responses

Studies in the last major category of nursing research regarding touch were clustered around its effects on psychological responses. The specific phenomena studied were self-image and emotional arousal.

Self-Image.   There were only two studies on self-image. Their distinct samples and focus did not allow for any synthesis of outcomes. Curry (1982) found no effect of skin-to-skin contact between mothers and infants during the first hour following delivery on the mother's self-concept 3 months after delivery. The investigator acknowledged that the self-concept measure had not been pretested for normative data with pregnant women and new mothers, so its validity with these groups was unknown. There also were multiple variables that could have influenced self-concept over which the investigator had no control.

Copstead (1980) found a correlation between the number of times an elderly patient was touched by a medication nurse during rounds and his or her score on a self-esteem scale immediately after the interaction. The investigator interpreted the findings to suggest that touch had affected self-appraisal. Rather than assuming that a brief tactile encounter could modify a lifetime of feelings toward the self, it would seem more logical that a person's self-esteem would influence the likelihood of him or her being perceived as touchable by others.

Emotional Arousal.   The research on emotional arousal included studies of behavioral, cognitive, and physiological parameters of the phenomenon. From a behavioral perspective, Triplett and Arneson (1979) demonstrated that verbal comfort measures were rarely successful in quieting emotionally distressed infants and children from a pediatric unit within 5 minutes, whereas interventions using a combined tactile and verbal approach were usually successful within that time period. However, verbal interventions were more successful in retaining a quiet state once achieved. Combined tactile–verbal interventions were most effective with infants younger than 6 months and least effective with children ages 13 to 18 months. The investigators stated that there were no gender differences in effectiveness of the two interventions; however, the 7 children who responded successfully to verbal intervention alone were all girls.

Although the investigators suggested that tactile comfort appeared to be the method of choice in relieving emotional distress, the intervention using touch also involved verbal comfort, so the effect of touch alone was not known. In fact, because the tactile–verbal intervention involved any combination of touch and sounds that the nurse chose to use, some interventions may have included primarily touch and others primarily words or sounds. Thus, it was difficult to assess whether touch played any key role in reducing distress.

Heidt (1981) compared anxiety responses of three groups of cardiovascular patients receiving (a) physical touch that involved apical, radial, and pedal pulse-taking, (b) "therapeutic touch," which involved some physical touch but primarily moving the hands above the surface of the body with the intent to help the patient, and (c) no touch. Findings showed that the no-touch and physical touch groups had higher anxiety scores after the intervention than did the therapeutic touch group. Only the therapeutic touch group had a significant decrease in anxiety from pretest to posttest. Based on other research, it would seem feasible that the stronger effects of the therapeutic touch intervention could have been due to the anxiety-provoking content of the other two interventions, that is, the symbolic meaning of pulse-taking and verbal discussion of the patient's illness (Lynch, Thomas, Mills, Malinow, & Katcher, 1974; Thomas, Lynch, & Mills, 1975; Weiss, 1986).

A second study of the cognitive parameters of emotional arousal was conducted by Longworth (1982). She found that anxiety scores significantly decreased after women received a slow-stroke back massage. In this research, the tactile intervention was standardized nicely with controls for important moderators such as other modes of communication, temperature, and environmental distractors.

Eight studies have been conducted to investigate the physiological parameters of emotional arousal. The first of these studies was done by Randolph (1984) to determine the response to a stressful film when treated by either therapeutic touch or physical touch during the film. Both groups had significant increases in skin conductance level and muscle tension, indicating significant stress responses to the film. No change was seen in either direction for skin temperature. Neither type of touch appeared to have any influence on preventing emotional arousal in the subjects.

Two investigators examined the effects of back massage on anxiety as measured by such indicators as heart rate, blood pressure, muscle tension, galvanic skin response, and skin temperature (Kaufmann, 1964; Longworth, 1982). Although there was not convergence across all indicators in Longworth's (1982) study, the heart rate and blood pressure increases during the intervention would indicate an increase in autonomic nervous system arousal rather than any relaxation or anxiety-reduction effect during the massage. The investigator suggested that results provided evidence of a delayed relaxation effect after the massage, but they might also have indicated increased relaxation once touch that was anxiety-producing had stopped.

Kaufmann (1964) concluded from her results that there were no differences in anxiety after the backrub. She also found substantial individual differences in response to the backrub, with males showing greater variability than women and a somewhat greater increase in relaxation from the backrub. In general, both the Kaufmann (1964) and Longworth (1982) studies were well designed, with attempts to use multiple measures for greater convergent validity and to standardize the intervention.

The four remaining studies on emotional arousal took place with critically ill patients. Lynch, Thomas, et al. (1974) studied the effects of social and clinical interactions on heart rate and rhythm changes of cardiac patients, with particular attention to the effects of touch such as pulse-taking and hand-holding. Lynch, Flaherty, Emrich, Mills, and Katcher (1974) conducted a study in which they observed the monitored heart responses of curarized patients in a shock–trauma unit to nurses' pulse-taking and hand-holding. In both of these studies, a few case examples were described showing variable changes in heart rate in reaction to diverse kinds of touch. However, there was no synthesis of the data across subjects to develop some nomothetic perspective on their meaning. In contrast, these same investigators conducted two further studies that yielded a systematic analysis of common outcomes. Mills, Thomas, Lynch, and Katcher (1976) found that the frequency of cardiac arrhythmias in coronary care patients increased during and after pulse palpation by nurses. With a larger sample, Lynch, Thomas, Paskewitz, Katcher, and Weir (1977) found no change in atrial arrhythmias as a result of pulse palpation and a decrease in ventricular arrhythmias, but only for those patients with greater numbers of arrhythmias at baseline. There were no changes in heart rate during or after pulse palpation evidenced in either study. Gender, age, race, and medication did not appear to influence the outcomes.

In a final study, Knable (1981) measured the effect of nurses holding the hands of critically ill patients on blood pressure, heart rate, and respiratory rate. No systematic changes were observed in any of the physiologic parameters, and a tremendous degree of variability in response was noted across subjects. These data provided evidence that soothing or arousing effects of touch may be dependent on individual differences in perception of touch as comforting or anxiety-producing.

This cluster of studies would indicate that touch was not particularly effective in reducing emotional arousal and, in some cases, may have increased it. Although touch would appear to have some important individual effects on emotional states, observed responses seemed based on various person-related variables that have not been examined well. For example, age may be an important consideration based on the Triplett and Arneson (1979) findings that touch was effective in reducing emotional distress of infants and preschool children.

SYNTHESIS OF RESEARCH FINDINGS

Results of nursing research on touch point to four areas of coherence that may indicate potentially reliable knowledge. The first area is in regard to the effects of touch on developmental responses of infants. This area of research represents the largest concentration of nursing investigations on touch, suggesting the value of intensive study by a number of investigators. Findings would support three propositions. First, skin contact with the mother during the first few minutes after birth is as effective as heated beds in maintaining the newborn's temperature. There appears to be no research from other disciplines to either support or negate this proposition. Second, the use of touch by nurses in caring for neonates has the potential to enhance their behavioral organization by modulating arousal levels and inducing states of quiet relaxation. This proposition has been supported by the clinical observations of investigators from other disciplines (Als & Duffy, 1983; Gorski, Davison, & Brazelton, 1979).

The third proposition is that programs of tactile stimulation do not seem effective in enhancing the physical development of preterm infants. In contrast to the findings of nurse investigators, data from research in other disciplines provide support for the effectiveness of stimulation programs, indicating that handling can have a significant effect on such parameters as weight gain and incidence of apnea (Kattwinkel, Hearman, Fanaroff, Katona, & Klaus, 1975; Rice, 1977; Scarr-Salapatek & Williams, 1973; Solkoff & Matuszak, 1975; Solkoff, Yaffe, Weintraub, & Blase, 1969; White & LaBarba, 1976). In light of these findings, it seems far too early to assume that touch has no effect on preterm physical response, particularly because some of the nurse researchers have depended upon historical control groups whose data were unreliable.

A second area of coherence is related to the effects of touch on attachment. A potential proposition from these studies is that brief physical contact with the infant during the first few hours or even days of life is not by itself a major predictor of the parent's attachment or bonding to the infant. This postulate is in conflict with the work of neonatologists who have suggested that contact during an early sensitive period seems important to attachment (Klaus et al., 1972; Kennell, Trause, & Klaus, 1975). However, some authors suggest that there is no evidence to support the existence of critical periods for attachment (Denenberg, 1984). More careful consideration of potential moderating variables may help to clarify the disparity among these research outcomes.

A proposition from the third area of coherence is that caregivers use instrumental or task-related touch to a much greater extent than expressive or comforting types of touch. In support of this proposition are findings from the Spitz (1945) research with institutionalized infants and the more recent Watson (1975) work with patients in a nursing home.

Coherence in the last area leads to the proposition that use of touch by nurses may improve the patient's affective response to the nurse–patient interaction. This proposition would be supported by the work of two psychologists, Whitcher and Fisher (1979), who found that for female patients touching of the hand by the nurse was associated with a perception that the nurse was interested in their well-being. Other psychologists have shown positive effects of even very brief touch on interpersonal relationships across many non-health-related contexts (Alagna, Whitcher, Fisher, & Wicas, 1979; Cooper & Bowles, 1973; Fisher, Rytting, & Heslin, 1976; Pattison, 1973).

In reviewing research outcomes on touch, the only major area of conflicting findings relates to anxiety. Anxiety has received a substantial amount of attention from nurse investigators interested in touch, second only to research on developmental responses of infants. The controversial questions pertain to whether touch induces anxiety, reduces it, or does not affect it at all. Although some findings provide evidence that touch may produce anxiety, multiple measures across different kinds of tactile contexts show varying effects.

The interest in effects of touch on anxiety are shared with investigators from the discipline of psychology. Similar to outcomes in nursing research, they have shown conflicting findings regarding the effect of touch on anxiety as measured by skin conductance (Geis & Viksne, 1972; Patterson, 1978; Patterson, Jordan, Hogan, & Frerker, 1981), as well as blood pressure, heart rate, and self-report (Whitcher & Fisher, 1979). It seems likely that the meaning of touch changes with each different context, mediating the response to touch at any point in time.

RECOMMENDATIONS FOR FUTURE RESEARCH

As can be seen from the great variety of approaches to touch research, the phenomenon is multifaceted in nature, with an overt association to both the person and the environment. As a result, it is critical that investigators consider the many personal and environmental variables that may influence use of touch as well as responses to it. For example, six of the studies described in this review dealt with age differences, and researchers found differences in either use or perception of touch as a function of age. Similarly, eight of the investigators found gender differences in thresholds for touch, use of touch, or responses to touch. Such individual differences have been evidenced in research of other disciplines as well (Hochreiter, Jewell, Barber, & Browne, 1983; Kenshalo, 1977; Maier & Ernest, 1978; Nguyen, Heslin, & Nguyen, 1975).

In regard to the environment, factors such as the particular social context, the relationship of the individuals involved in touching, and the effects of other modes of communication must be taken into consideration. These and other variables have been identified by some of the investigators as influencing outcomes, yet there has not been systematic examination of these variables across most research. There is clearly a need for an integrated theoretical model in studying touch whereby all investigators would begin to use a multivariate, biopsychosocial, person–environment interaction approach.

In addition, the phenomenon of touch needs to be defined operationally within research. Existing studies regarding properties of touch can be exceptionally useful in this regard. Is the touch being examined instrumental or expressive? Is it technical, comforting, or caregiving? What are its dimensional qualities in terms of action, duration, location, or intensity? Unless investigators carefully define and describe the phenomenon they are studying, comparison across studies will be relatively impossible and the meaning of outcomes will not be understood fully.

Lastly, investigators need to consider carefully the most significant focus for future efforts. Although the existing areas of research emphasis are important, there are other areas of study that must also be addressed. For example, nurse researchers must examine (a) the role of tactile perception and tactile interventions in adaptation to pain, (b) the utility of touch in helping children to cope with illness and to recover effectively, (c) tactile patterns within families that can support or impede healthy development of infants and children, and (d) the specific qualities of touch that must be avoided or encouraged in caring for high-risk, critically ill patients. These areas of research are central to nursing.

The research described in this review covers a spectrum in terms of its methodological rigor: some studies are designed carefully, whereas others barely warrant being labeled as research. In general, methodological limitations prevail. In certain cases, the problems are as simple as a sample that is too small, lack of an appropriately determined control group for an intervention study, or failure to collect pretest or baseline data. Other concerns are of an even more basic nature: invalid criterion measures for validity testing of an instrument or for measurement of a key concept, no clarity regarding the coding or analytic system for observational analysis, lack of independence of observational categories, lack of consideration for the effects of observation on the variables being studied, or issues of social desirability in asking for patient evaluations of one's own behavior or interventions.

In addition, there are some major methodological drawbacks that seem consistently to appear across studies: (a) the development and use of observational measures without any prior validity or reliability testing, (b) the lack of adequate training for observers in the use of observational systems, (c) the lack of standardization for tactile interventions, and (d) inadequate controls for other communication occurring during the touch or for other intervening variables that could influence outcomes. In particular, the person and environment variables discussed earlier must be considered.

If these conceptual and methodological issues are given careful attention, nursing research on touch will progress more rapidly toward a major contribution to science. Regardless, the contributions to date provide a good foundation for future improvements in the quality of scientific endeavors.

REFERENCES

Aguilera, D. C. (1967). Relationship between physical contact and verbal interaction between nurses and patients. *Journal of Psychiatric Nursing, 5*(1), 5–21.

Alagna, F. J., Whitcher, S. J., Fisher, J. D., & Wicas, E. A. (1979). Evaluative reaction to interpersonal touch in a counseling interview. *Journal of Counseling Psychology, 26*, 465–472.

Als, H., & Duffy, F. H. (1983). The behavior of the premature infant. In T. B. Brazelton & B. M. Lester (Eds.), *New approaches to developmental screening of infants* (pp. 153–173). Amsterdam: Elsevier Science Publishing.

Barnett, K. (1972). A survey of the current utilization of touch by health team personnel with hospitalized patients. *International Journal of Nursing Studies, 9*, 195–209.

Blackburn, S. T., & Barnard, K. E. (1985). Analysis of caregiving events relating to preterm infants in the special care unit. In A. W. Gottfried & J. L. Gaiter (Eds.), *Infant stress under intensive care* (pp. 113–129). Baltimore: University Park Press.

Cannon, R. B. (1977). The development of maternal touch during early mother–infant interaction. *Journal of Obstetric, Gynecologic, and Neonatal Nursing, 6*(2), 28–33.

Cashar, L., & Dixson, B. K. (1967). The therapeutic use of touch. *Journal of Psychiatric Nursing, 5*(5), 442–451.

Chamorro, I. L., Davis, M. L., Green, D., & Kramer, M. (1973). Development of an instrument to measure premature infant behavior and caretaker activities: Time-sampling methodology. *Nursing Research, 22*, 300–309.

Cooper, C. L., & Bowles, D. (1973). Physical encounter and self-disclosure. *Psychological Reports, 33*, 451–454.

Copstead, L. C. (1980). Effects of touch on self-appraisal and interaction appraisal for permanently institutionalized older adults. *Journal of Gerontological Nursing, 6*, 747–752.

Curry, M. A. (1982). Maternal attachment behavior and the mother's self-concept: The effect of early skin-to-skin contact. *Nursing Research, 31*, 73–78.

De Augustinis, J., Isani, R. S., & Kumler, F. R. (1969). Ward study: The meaning of touch in interpersonal communication. In S. F. Burd & M. A. Marshall (Eds.), *Some clinical approaches to psychiatric nursing* (pp. 271–306). New York: Macmillan.

Denenberg, V. (1984). Stranger in a strange situation: Commentary by a comparative psychologist. *The Behavioral and Brain Sciences, 7*, 150–152.

DeWever, M. K. (1977). Nursing home patients' perception of nurses' affective touching. *The Journal of Psychology, 96*, 163–171.

Dunbar, J. (1977). Maternal contact behaviors with newborn infants during feedings (Monograph 6). *Maternal–Child Nursing Journal, 6*, 209–295.

Ellis, L., Taylor, J., & Walts, N. (1979). Reach out and touch. *The Journal of Nursing Care, 12*(9), 19–21.

Farrah, S. (1971). The nurse—the patient—and touch. In M. Duffey, E. H. Anderson, B. S. Bergersen, M. Lohr, & M. H. Rose (Eds.), *Current concepts in clinical nursing* (Vol. III) (pp. 247–259). St. Louis: Mosby.

Fisher, J. D., Rytting, M., & Heslin, R. (1976). Hands touching hands: Affective and evaluative effects of an interpersonal touch. *Sociometry, 39*, 416–421.

Gardner, S. (1979). The mother as incubator—after delivery. *Journal of Obstetric, Gynecologic, and Neonatal Nursing, 8*, 174–176.

Geis, F., & Viksne, V. (1972). Touching: Physical contact and level of arousal. *Proceedings of the 80th Annual Convention of the American Psychological Association. Part I, 7*, 179–180.

Gorski, P. A., Davison, M. F., & Brazelton, T. B. (1979). Stages of behavioral organization in the high-risk neonate: Theoretical and clinical considerations. *Seminars in Perinatology, 3*(1), 61–72.

Hasselmeyer, E. G. (1963). Handling and premature infant behavior: An experimental study of the relationship between handling and selected physiological, pathological, and behavioral indices related to body functioning among a group of prematurely born infants who weighed between 1,501 and 2,000 grams at birth and were between the ages of seven and twenty-eight days of life. *Dissertation Abstracts International, 24*, 2874–2875. (University Microfilms No. 64–257)

Heidt, P. (1981). Effect of therapeutic touch on anxiety level of hospitalized patients. *Nursing Research, 30*, 32–37.

Hill, S. T., & Shronk, L. K. (1979). The effect of early parent–infant contact on newborn body temperature. *Journal of Obstetric, Gynecologic, and Neonatal Nursing, 8*, 287–290.

Hochreiter, N., Jewell, M., Barber, L., & Browne, P. (1983). Effect of vibration of tactile sensitivity. *Physical Therapy, 63*, 934–937.

Jay, S. S. (1982). The effects of gentle human touch on mechanically ventilated very-short-gestation infants (Monograph 12). *Maternal–Child Nursing Journal, 11*, 199–256.

Jones, C. (1981). Father to infant attachment: Effects of early contact and characteristics of the infant. *Research in Nursing and Health, 4*, 193–200.

Kattwinkel, J., Hearman, H., Fanaroff, A. A., Katona, P., & Klaus, M. H. (1975). Apnea of prematurity. *Journal of Pediatrics, 86*, 588–592.

Kaufmann, M. A. (1964). Autonomic responses as related to nursing comfort measures. *Nursing Research, 13*, 45–55.

Kennell, J., Trause, M., & Klaus, M. (1975). Evidence for a sensitive period in the human mother. In *CIBA Foundation Symposium 33*. Amsterdam: Elsevier Science Publishing.

Kenshalo, D. (1977). Age changes in touch, vibration, temperature, kinethesis and pain sensitivity. In J. Birren & K. Schaie (Eds.), *Handbook of the psychology of aging* (pp. 562–579). New York: Von Nostrand Reinhold.

Klaus, M., Jerauld, R., Kreger, N., McAlpine, W., Steffa, M., & Kennell, J. H. (1972). Maternal attachment: Importance of the first post-partum days. *The New England Journal of Medicine, 286*, 460–463.

Klaus, M., & Kennell, J. (1976). *Maternal-infant bonding.* St. Louis: Mosby.

Knable, J. (1981). Handholding: One means of transcending barriers of communication. *Heart and Lung, 10*, 1106–1110.

Kramer, M., Chamorro, I., Green, D., & Knudtson, F. (1975). Extra tactile stimulation of the premature infant. *Nursing Research, 24,* 324–334.

Krieger, D. (1975). Therapeutic touch: The imprimatur of nursing. *American Journal of Nursing, 75,* 784–787.

Langland, R. M., & Panicucci, C. L. (1982). Effects of touch on communication with elderly confused clients. *Journal of Gerontological Nursing, 8,* 152–155.

Longworth, J. C. D. (1982). Psychophysiological effects of slow stroke back massage in normotensive females. *Advances in Nursing Science, 4*(4), 44–61.

Lynch, J. J., Flaherty, L., Emrich, C., Mills, M. E., & Katcher, A. H. (1974). Effects of human contact on the heart activity of curarized patients in a shock–trauma unit. *American Heart Journal, 88,* 160–169.

Lynch, J. J., Thomas, S. A., Mills, M. E., Malinow, K., & Katcher, A. H. (1974). The effects of human contact on the cardiac arrhythmia in coronary care patients. *The Journal of Nervous and Mental Disease, 158*(2), 88–99.

Lynch, J. J., Thomas, S. A., Paskewitz, D., Katcher, A. H., & Weir, L. (1977). Human contact and cardiac arrhythmia in a coronary care unit. *Psychosomatic Medicine, 39,* 188–192.

Maier, R., & Ernest, R. (1978). Sex differences in the perception of touching. *Perceptual and Motor Skills, 46*(2), 577–578.

McBride, M. R., & Mistretta, C. M. (1982). Light touch thresholds in diabetic patients. *Diabetes Care, 5,* 311–315.

McCorkle, R. (1974). Effects of touch on seriously ill patients. *Nursing Research, 23,* 125–132.

McCoy, P. (1977). Further proof that touch speaks louder than words. *RN, 40*(11), 43–46.

Mills, M., Thomas, S., Lynch, J., & Katcher, A. (1976). Effect of pulse palpation on cardiac arrhythmia in coronary care patients. *Nursing Research, 25,* 378–382.

Morse, J. M. (1983). An ethnoscientific analysis of comfort: A preliminary investigation. *Nursing Papers: The Canadian Journal of Nursing Research, 15*(1), 6–19.

Nguyen, J., Heslin, R., & Nguyen, M. (1975). The meaning of touch: Sex differences. *Journal of Communication, 25,* 92–103.

Pannabecker, B. J., & Emde, R. N. (1977). Effect of extended contact on father–newborn interaction. In M. Batey (Ed.), *Communicating nursing research: Vol. 10. Optimizing environments for health: Nursing's unique perspective* (pp. 97–114). Boulder, CO: Western Interstate Commission on Higher Education.

Patterson, M. L. (1978). Arousal change and cognitive labeling: Pursuing the mediators of intimacy exchange. *Environmental Psychology and Nonverbal Behavior, 3,* 17–22.

Patterson, M. L., Jordan, A., Hogan, M. B., & Frerker, D. (1981). Effects of nonverbal intimacy on arousal and behavioral adjustment. *Journal of Nonverbal Behavior, 5,* 184–197.

Pattison, J. E. (1973). Effects of touch on self-exploration and the therapeutic relationship. *Journal of Consulting and Clinical Psychology, 40,* 170–175.

Penny, K. S. (1979). Postpartum perceptions of touch received during labor. *Research in Nursing and Health, 2,* 9–16.

Phillips, C. R. N. (1974). Neonatal heat loss in heated cribs vs. mothers' arms. *Journal of Obstetric, Gynecologic, and Neonatal Nursing, 3*(6), 11–15.

Randolph, G. L. (1984). Therapeutic and physical touch: Physiological response to stressful stimuli. *Nursing Research, 33*, 33-36.

Rausch, P. B. (1981). Effects of tactile and kinesthetic stimulation on premature infants. *Journal of Obstetric, Gynecologic, and Neonatal Nursing, 10*, 34-37.

Rice, R. D. (1977). Neurophysiological development in premature infants following stimulation. *Developmental Psychology, 13*, 69-76.

Rubin, R. (1963). Maternal touch. *Nursing Outlook, 11*, 828-831.

Scarr-Salapatek, S., & Williams, M. L. (1973). The effects of early stimulation on low birth weight infants. *Child Development, 44*, 94-104.

Solkoff, N., & Matuszak, D. (1975). Tactile stimulation and behavioral development among low-birthweight infants. *Child Psychiatry and Human Development, 6*(1), 33-37.

Solkoff, N., Yaffe, S., Weintraub, D., & Blase, B. (1969). Effects of handling on the subsequent developments of premature infants. *Developmental Psychology, 1*, 765-768.

Spitz, R. (1945). Hospitalism — An inquiry into the genesis of psychiatric conditions of early childhood. *Psychoanalytic Study of the Child, 1*, 53-74.

Thomas, S. A., Lynch, J. J., & Mills, M. E. (1975). Psychosocial influences on heart rhythm in the coronary care unit. *Heart and Lung, 4*, 746-750.

Thornbury, J. M., & Mistretta, C. M. (1981). Tactile sensitivity as a function of age. *Journal of Gerontology, 36*, 34-39.

Tobiason, S. J. B. (1981). Touching is for everyone. *American Journal of Nursing, 81*, 728-730.

Toney, L. (1982). The effects of holding the newborn at delivery on paternal bonding. *Nursing Research, 32*, 16-19.

Triplett, J. L., & Arneson, S. W. (1979). The use of verbal and tactile comfort to alleviate distress in young hospitalized children. *Research in Nursing and Health, 2*, 17-23.

Tulman, L. J. (1985). Mothers' and unrelated persons' initial handling of newborn infants. *Nursing Research, 34*, 205-210.

Watson, W. (1975). The meanings of touch: Geriatric nursing. *Journal of Communication, 25*(3), 104-112.

Weiss, S. (1984). Parental touch and the child's body image. In C. Brown (Ed.), *The many facets of touch* (pp. 130-138). New York: International Universities Press.

Weiss, S. (1985). *Tactile interaction indicator: Video cassette and handbook.* San Francisco: University of California, San Francisco, School of Nursing, Department of Mental Health, Community and Administrative Nursing.

Weiss, S. (1986). Psychophysiologic effects of caregiver touch on incidence of cardiac arrhythmia. *Heart and Lung, 15*, 495-505.

Weiss, S. (in press). Parental touching: Correlates of body image in children. In T. B. Brazelton & K. Barnard (Eds.), *Touch: The foundation of experience.* New York: International Universities Press.

Whitcher, S. J., & Fischer, J. D. (1979). Multidimensional reaction to therapeutic touch in a hospital setting. *Journal of Personality and Social Psychology, 37*(1), 87-96.

White, J. L., & LaBarba, R. C. (1976). The effects of tactile and kinesthetic stimulation on neonatal development in the premature infant. *Developmental Psychobiology, 9*, 569-577.

Chapter 2

Patient Education

CAROL A. LINDEMAN
SCHOOL OF NURSING
OREGON HEALTH SCIENCES UNIVERSITY

CONTENTS

The intent of the reviewer was to summarize published nursing research on patient education and to draw inferences for a theory of instruction for patient education. In the world of patient care, influencing human learning is a complex process affected by six major categories of variables: (a) characteristics of the patient as learner; (b) characteristics of the nurse as teacher; (c) nurse–patient interaction as instructional strategy; (d) characteristics of the target group; (e) health care setting as learning environment; and (f) content. The first five categories were used as the organizing framework for this review. A subsequent chapter in this series will be focused on studies relating to instructional content in patient education.

A search of the literature to identify studies for review was performed in several ways. Computerized searches using MEDLINE for 1965 through 1986 and the Educational Resources Information Center (ERIC) for 1966 through 1982 were done with the following subtitles: *patient education, comparative studies, clinical trials, evaluation studies*, and *preoperative education*. The *International Nursing Index* and *Cumulative Index to Nursing and Allied Health Literature* were hand-searched for the years 1965 to 1986, and the bibliographies of all retrieved articles were examined for additional studies. Those articles having a nurse as the first author and reporting adequate information about every phase of the research process were included. The data base included 120 research articles: 20 related to the patient as learner; 2 to the nurse as teacher; 92 to instructional strategy and specific patient groups; and 6 to the health care setting.

Each study was analyzed to identify the independent and dependent variables, method for sample selection, size and characteristics of the sample, setting, data-gathering devices and psychometric properties, types of statistical analysis, and conclusions. Based on traditional standards of scientific merit, many of the studies were flawed. Small convenience samples were used in many studies; research instruments were specific to the study, and reliability and validity information was not provided. Frequently the investigator was the patient educator.

Recently the traditional definition of scientific merit has been the subject of extensive and intensive criticism, particularly in relation to the human sciences. Users of research are urged to analyze research critically from their own knowledge base rather than to apply predetermined criteria of merit. The latter approach to a review of research is particularly significant for patient education research given that investigators evaluating the effect of patient education using meta-analytic analysis have raised questions about the relative importance of some aspects of design on research outcomes (Devine & Cook, 1983). The chapter includes descriptive information about most of the studies reviewed. Emphasis is on the contribution to a theory of instruction. The reader will have to apply personal knowledge and judgment when using individual studies cited in the review.

CHARACTERISTICS OF THE PATIENT AS LEARNER

Twenty studies were related to the patient as learner and included exploration of the impact of patient characteristics on learning outcomes. Three investigators explored the impact of psychological variables; five focused on intellectual ability and related phenomena; five used a trait–treatment interaction model; four examined timing of teaching; and three studied family involvement.

Psychological Variables

Lowery and DuCette (1976) explored the relationship between locus of control and control of diabetes over time. They used a cross-sectional sample of 30 newly diagnosed diabetics, 30 diagnosed for 3 years, and 30 diagnosed for 6 years. Subjects completed the Internal–External Control Scale (Rotter, 1966) and a Diabetes and Health Information Test developed for the study. Results showed that subjects with internal locus of control had more diabetic information than those with external locus of control, although this superiority decreased as the length of time from diagnosis increased.

Gierszewski (1983) studied locus of control in relation to weight loss for people in a weight-control program ($N = 46$). Social support was included as a third variable. The findings did not support a significant relationship between locus of control and success in weight reduction. Subjects with high social support scores were not more successful at weight reduction than the others.

Kinney (1977) used a theoretical framework linking situational anxiety and typical response to threat (repressor, sensitizer, neutral) in order to study individual differences and effect of preoperative teaching. Thirty male candidates for cardiac surgery served as subjects. There were no statistically significant differences between the three groups on the measurements of anxiety after preoperative teaching.

Educational Level and
Demographic Characteristics

Mohammed (1964) investigated patients' abilities to understand health information. The intent of the study was to provide a method for quick assessment of a person's reading comprehension and understanding. In this exploratory study the investigator used a random sample of patients attending a diabetic clinic. A total of 300 subjects participated by completing (a) a reading test of five paragraphs and (b) questions on health information constructed at the fourth, sixth, and eighth grade reading levels. The average amount of education was 6.8 school grades completed. Results of the study showed that for this sample education was not a reliable predictor of ability to comprehend written health information. Written materials at the clinic were primarily at the eighth grade reading level; approximately 22% of the clinic population could comprehend this literature.

Using 30 hypertensive male subjects, Smeltzer (1980) explored the relationship between the understanding of medical terminology and several variables such as educational level, race, age, and duration and severity of illness. The findings showed that race, educational level and age could serve as significant predictors of level of understanding of terminology. Duration of diagnosed illness, severity of the disease, and recent hospitalization were not statistical predictors.

Taylor, Skelton, and Czajkowski (1982) compared the reading and comprehension ability of 200 patients from various settings to the readability of 94 patient education brochures. In general, about 30% of the materials exceeded the patients' educational levels; pharmacy material exceeded the educational level of 40 to 45% of the sample.

Whitley (1979) compared the characteristics of 19 couples who attended regular prenatal classes and prepared childbirth classes to 92 couples who attended only the regular prenatal classes. The couples selecting the prepared childbirth classes were better educated, older, of higher socioeconomic status, nulliparas, and planning to breastfeed, compared to the couples selecting only the regular prenatal classes.

Vinal (1982) surveyed a random sample of 201 patients from the postpartum units of four hospitals to determine why some women chose not to attend childbirth education classes. Those who had not attended reported they already knew what they needed to know, had no interest, had scheduling problems, or had physicians who did not recommend attendance. Those who attended classes were younger, had fewer children, were married fewer years, and had more education than those not attending.

Trait-Treatment Interaction

Sime (1976) investigated the relationship of preoperative fear level, extent of information seeking, and amount of information received to recovery from surgery. The sample consisted of 57 females undergoing abdominal surgery. The results showed (a) a linear relationship between level of preoperative fear and recovery, and (b) a significant interaction between level of preoperative fear and amount of preoperative information. High levels of preoperative fear were associated with a longer recovery period, a greater use of analgesics and sedatives, and higher levels of postoperative negative affect. High fear subjects who reported little preoperative information experienced the least favorable recovery period as measured by number of analgesics, number of sedatives, and days to discharge.

Lum et al. (1978) explored the significance of patient characteristics in a study using a process-outcome quality assurance framework. Selected nursing activities, including educational interventions, were analyzed in terms of patient outcomes for 57 oncology subjects. The content and the quality of the explanation of the treatment and care regimen were correlated positively with the patients' self-esteem.

Rottkamp and Donohue-Porter (1982) studied the relationship between preference for instructional approach and needs as measured on the Personality Research Form E (Jackson, 1974). A sample of 46 diabetics was used. Anticipated preferences were not supported fully. The data did support a relationship between preference for structured teaching and need for control.

Adler, Rawlinson, Crabtree, and Hallburg (1983) examined the relationships between teaching strategy, patient characteristics, and knowledge and behavior outcomes. Chronically ill patients with complex medication regimens were the focus of the investigation; 61 renal and 60 cardiac patients served as subjects. Data analysis gave evidence that all three teaching strategies were effective in producing knowledge acquisition and retention. Findings also revealed that renal subjects learned significantly more than cardiac subjects regardless of teaching strategy. The profile of a patient who acquired and retained the most knowledge was a relatively young person who had a good memory, was in the hospital longer than the average time, and perceived him- or herself as resistant to illness.

Mills, Barnes, Rodell, and Terry (1985) conducted an exploratory study using 342 patients with ischemic heart disease to determine the effect of a patient education program on knowledge level. Also studied was the relationship between compliance and sociodemographic variables, intelligence, problem-solving ability, motivation, and knowledge. Results showed a significant increase in knowledge following the patient education program. Of the other variables studied, motivation was correlated most highly with compliance.

Timing of Teaching

Four studies were focused on the timing of patient education; in three of the studies surgical subjects were used, and in one study maternity subjects were used. Christopherson and Pfeiffer (1980) compared anxiety scores of subjects who read an informational booklet 1 to 2 days preoperatively with subjects who read the same booklet 3 to 35 days preoperatively. Subjects who chose not to read the booklet served as a control group. A total of 41 patients served as subjects. Results showed that anxiety scores were significantly lower postoperatively for the subjects reading the booklet 1 to 2 days preoperatively. Subjects reading the booklet showed a significant increase in knowledge scores compared to the control subjects.

Rice and Johnson (1984) evaluated the effects of preadmission self-instructional booklets on levels of performance and time needed to achieve mastery of exercise behaviors. A total of 130 patients was assigned randomly to one of three instructional groups: no preadmission information, specific preadmission instructions, and nonspecific preadmission instructions. Findings indicated that the specific preadmission instruction group performed significantly more of the exercise behaviors than those in the nonspecific group. Required postadmission teaching time did not differ significantly between the specific and nonspecific groups, but both groups required significantly less teaching time than the nonpreadmission instruction group.

Levesque, Grenier, Ke'rouac, and Reidy (1984) compared the effects of a preoperative teaching program given on the evening of surgery to a program given at a preadmission visit about 15 days prior to admission. One hundred twenty five cholecystectomy patients were assigned randomly to one of the teaching groups or a control group. Dependent variables included anxiety, ventilatory function, self-rating pain scale, functional ability, use of analgesics, and length of hospitalization. Findings showed no significant differences for the three groups except that anxiety on the evening of surgery was significantly higher for the control group.

Petrowski (1981) used an experimental approach to assess the effect of timing of teaching postpartum material to 40 maternity patients randomly assigned to one of four groups. The timing of teaching ranged from the last trimester of pregnancy to 4 days postpartum. There were no significant differences in knowledge gain associated with the timing of teaching.

Family Involvement

Three studies were concerned with the involvement of family in the educational experience. Serving as subjects were children, surgical patients, and patients in a critical care unit. Mahaffy (1965) used an experimental approach to determine the impact on the hospitalized child of providing support and information to the mother. A sample of 43 randomly selected children was divided into control and experimental groups. Experimental group children had lower temperatures, pulse rates, and systolic blood pressures; voided sooner; cried and vomited less; incurred fever less frequently after discharge; and recovered sooner than the control group children.

Dziurbejko and Larkin (1978) tested the hypothesis that preoperative teaching that included the family would be more beneficial than preoperative instructions given to the patient alone. A total of 21 female patients served as subjects in this posttest-only control group design. They were assigned randomly to one of three groups: patient alone; patient with family; and control. Significant main effects from teaching were shown on 9 of the 13 dependent variables. The patient with family group differed significantly from the controls on duration of hospital stay and number of injectable narcotics.

Doerr and Jones (1979) examined the effect of family preparation on the anxiety level of the patient. The family preparation consisted of reading an informational booklet before visiting a patient in the critical care unit. A pretest–posttest control group design was used, and 12 subjects were assigned randomly to the experimental or control group. Results showed that family preparation led to lower anxiety scores for the patients.

**Generalizations for
Theory of Instruction**

The data base for the category Characteristics of the Patient as Learner included 20 studies addressing five types of variables. The following generalizations are offered:

1. Psychological factors studied in isolation of other characteristics are not strong predictors of patient teaching outcomes. When an interaction model is used psychological factors appear to interact with teaching strategy to influence patient teaching outcomes.
2. Educational level and demographic characteristics influence the outcomes of patient teaching. Patient education materials tend to be developed at reading levels beyond the reading capabilities of most patients.
3. The timing of teaching does not appear to be related to patient education outcomes. Teaching, not the timing of it, is the stronger variable.
4. Instruction of the family benefits the patient.

CHARACTERISTICS OF THE NURSE AS TEACHER

Two studies were focused on characteristics of the nurse in the role of patient educator. Linde and Janz (1979) studied the impact of educational level of the nurse in an investigation of the effect of a structured, comprehensive teaching program on knowledge and compliance of cardiovascular patients. Twenty-five patients were taught by two cardiovascular clinical nursing specialists prepared at the master's level; 23 were taught by four staff nurses with less than master's preparation. The investigators concluded that although non-master's-prepared staff nurses did influence patient knowledge, the master's-prepared nurses had a much greater impact.

Kishi (1983) investigated the verbal communication patterns of health care providers in relation to client recall. The theoretical rationale for the study was derived from Flanders Interaction Analysis System (Flanders, 1965). The findings did not support Flanders's notion that higher indirect influence by the teacher leads to higher achievement by the learner.

The studies in this category offer promising leads for further research. It would appear that the category Characteristics of the Nurse as Teacher is an important component of a theory of instruction. With only two studies, however, no generalizations can be offered.

NURSE–PATIENT INTERACTION AND TARGET POPULATIONS

In reviewing the articles in this category, it was difficult to separate a primary focus on instructional strategy from a focus on group characteristics. The investigator frequently designed the instructional strategy with a particular patient population in mind. In this section the two categories of variables are combined. The organization of the material is by patient population: maternal–infant, surgical, cardiovascular, chronic illness, psychiatric, and diagnostic procedures. In each section the subcategories of research questions on effectiveness, teaching strategies, and group and individual approaches are discussed.

Maternal–Infant

Ten studies were designed to examine the effectiveness of teaching. In seven of these researchers used nonexperimental approaches. Nunnally and Aguiar (1974) found that women who attended prenatal classes had a more positive attitude toward their labor and delivery experience and higher scores on a knowledge test than women who did not attend prenatal classes. Allen and Ries (1985) reported significant decreases in alcohol consumption and smoking following prenatal education. Fawcett and Burritt (1985) received positive evaluations of an antenatal program of cesarian birth information. Halstead and Fredrickson

(1978) concluded that more than 5 hours of structured prenatal education had a positive impact on maternal–child health. Dickerson and Ouellette (1982) reported a significant gain in knowledge from a program designed for pregnant adolescents. Bull and Lawrence (1984) found that mothers believed the prenatal teaching was useful and recommended more information in the areas of psychosocial changes and infant behavior. Orstead, Arrington, Kamath, Olson, and Kohrs (1985) found that positive weight gain, fewer low-birth-weight infants, and infants weighing 100 grams more at birth were associated with prenatal counseling.

Timm (1979) and Henderson (1983) used experimental approaches to determine the effects of prenatal teaching. Timm reported that subjects receiving prenatal teaching during pregnancy used significantly less medication during labor than women assigned to control groups. Henderson's experimental subjects had significantly higher perineometer readings than the control subjects who had no teaching. Cohen (1980) evaluated the effectiveness of breastfeeding instruction and reported that the experimental group had a significantly lower incidence of supplementation with formula at 6 weeks than the control group, but not beyond that time.

Seven studies were designed to compare the effectiveness of various teaching strategies. Because the teaching strategies in these investigations reflect diverse educational theories, each study is presented separately.

Dalzell (1965) compared three teaching strategies for delivering a prenatal program. Three hundred women were assigned randomly to one of four groups: prenatal group classes, home visit, individual counseling, and control. Women in the three teaching groups did significantly better on the knowledge test than did the control group. The home visit and individual counseling groups did significantly better than the prenatal class group.

Packard and Van Ess (1969) used an experimental design to compare informal teaching with role-delineated teaching. A control group having no teaching was included. One hundred and two postpartum patients alternately were assigned to one of the three groups. The dependent variable was change in food selection behavior. Both teaching methods resulted in significant changes from preteaching behavior.

Lowe (1970) compared the effectiveness of typical prenatal education in the clinic setting with an experimental program that supplemented the clinic program with home instruction by public health nurses. The sample consisted of 56 black primigravidae randomly assigned to either the control or experimental groups. No significant differences were found between the two groups on compliance with the medical regimen.

Downs and Fernbach (1973) reported an experimental study designed to assess the effect of a prenatal leaflet series on knowledge and subsequent behavior. A Solomon Four Group Design was used with a starting sample of 286 subjects drawn from the Maternity and Infant Care Family Planning Projects. No differences in information level were found, nor were knowledge and behavior related.

With respect to success at breastfeeding, Hall (1978) described the outcomes of three educational approaches: regular care, a slide tape presentation, and a slide tape presentation plus nurse support. Six weeks after discharge, 80% of the mothers experiencing the slide tape plus nurse support approach still were breastfeeding, compared to 50% of mothers in the other two groups.

Manderino and Bzdek (1984) conducted an experiment to evaluate the effects of modeling and information in the context of a labor preparation analogue. Sixty nulliparous female college students were assigned randomly to one of four treatment conditions: videotaped modeling, videotaped information, combination, control video. Following the treatment, subjects were exposed to a pain stimulator. Subjects in the combined modeling and information group reported significantly lower pain ratings than those in the other groups.

Dooher (1980) compared marital adjustment and feeling of crisis in the postpartum period of 10 couples who had attended Lamaze classes with similar measures on 10 couples who had not. Couples who attended Lamaze classes had lower marital adjustment scores than the other couples, and the males reported greater stress.

McNeil and Holland (1972) compared the effectiveness of group teaching with individual teaching in the home on mothers of newborn infants. Knowledge of infant care was the dependent variable. The sample consisted of 107 mothers; a static group design was used. Findings showed that mothers who attended the group classes scored significantly higher than the in-home individual group.

Surgical

The effectiveness of preoperative teaching has been the focus of a series of studies. In five of the studies researchers reported significant effects, and in two researchers reported no significant main effect. Healy (1968) reported an exploratory study in which patients who had received structured teaching were discharged earlier, spent less time on narcotics, and had fewer complications than patients who had regular care. Lindeman and Van Aernam (1971) found significantly increased postoperative ventilatory function and reduced length of hospital stay for experimental subjects. In a replication of that study, King and Tarsitano (1982) supported the conclusion regarding significant improvement in ability to cough and deep-breathe postoperatively. They found no difference in length of hospital stay. Marshall, Penckofer, and Llewellyn (1986) found significantly higher self-care compliance scores for subjects receiving structured teaching. A significant reduction in anxiety following instruction was reported by Shimko (1981). Carrieri (1975) and Midgley and Osterhage (1973) did not find evidence of a significant main effect for preoperative teaching.

Three studies on effectiveness of preoperative teaching are reported separately. In two studies the preoperative teaching content had a unique focus, and in the third a unique design was used.

Krueger et al. (1979) conducted an exploratory study of the relationships between sexual counseling during hospitalization and postoperative adjustment of hysterectomy patients after hospital discharge. Only 80 of the sample of 108 premenopausal women returned the postdischarge questionnaire. In general, subjects reported that discussion was more helpful than written information. Only 12 identified the nurse as the source of the most valuable information. No significant correlations were found between knowledge scores and the person identified by the respondents as giving them the most valuable information or as the person with whom they felt most comfortable in discussing questions about sexuality.

Lindeman and Stetzer (1973) used an experimental design to evaluate the effects of preoperative visits by operating room nurses on effectiveness, efficiency, and safety of nursing care; anxiety; emergence from anesthesia; postoperative analgesics; postoperative physiological problems; and length of hospital stay. Preoperative visits were designed to prepare the patient for the surgical experience by providing information and reassurance. The sample consisted of 176 surgical patients randomly assigned to either the visit or no-visit group. Findings supported the preoperative visit as an effective means of improving the safety and effectiveness of care in the operating room. There were no significant effects on anxiety level or recovery.

Hinshaw, Gerber, Atwood, and Allen (1983) used a quasi-experimental, causal modeling approach to test the impact of a perioperative teaching program on patient outcomes including coping, anxiety, pain, recovery, and satisfaction. A sample of 88 patients participated, with 54 receiving the teaching and 34 not. Data analysis led to the conclusion that perioperative teaching affected patient outcomes indirectly through increased nurse attention to patient safety and individualization of care in the operating room.

The seven studies on teaching strategies reflect a diverse range of educational approaches. Cross and Parsons (1971) compared two alternate teaching strategies using a pre–post control group design. The subjects were patients hospitalized for orthopedic surgery and randomly assigned to one of three groups: diet teaching, diet teaching and goal-setting, and no teaching (control). Menu selection cards were used to collect data over a 3-day period. Postteaching mean scores showed a significant difference between the experimental and control groups and supported the hypothesis that health teaching by nurses is an effective stimulus for behavior change.

Fortin and Kirouac (1976) evaluated the effects of a preoperative teaching program given 15 to 20 days preoperatively to 65 patients randomly assigned to experimental or control groups. Dependent variables included physical functional capacity, length of hospitalization, and length of delay before normal activities were resumed. Data were collected at 2, 10, and 33 days postoperatively. Subjects receiving the structured preoperative teaching had significantly higher levels of physical functioning at all time periods.

Felton, Huss, Payne, and Srsic (1976) studied the outcomes of three nursing approaches to the preoperative preparation of the surgical patient on frequency of postoperative complications, ventilatory function, manifest anxiety level, and patients' perceptions of psychological well-being. Sixty-two patients having major surgery under general anesthesia were distributed into three groups: routine instruction, therapeutic communication, and experimental. Data were collected through self reports, pre- and postoperative scores on the Personal Orientation Inventory (Knapp, 1976) and the Multiple Affect Adjective List (Zuckerman & Lubin, 1965), and medical records. The findings supported two hypotheses: (a) patients having the experimental preoperative teaching had a significant decrease in pre- to postoperative level of anxiety, and (b) patients having experimental teaching had higher postoperative psychological well-being.

Goodwin (1979) investigated the use of programmed instruction to enhance self-care following pulmonary surgery. The 26 subjects were assigned randomly to an experimental or control group. Results indicated that those in the experimental group significantly increased their knowledge, performed more recommended activities, and coughed less than control subjects.

Ferguson (1979) evaluated the timing of teaching and the method of teaching in a four-group experimental study. Eighty-two children scheduled for tonsillectomy were randomly assigned to one of four groups: regular care, regular care and a peer-modeling film, preadmission home visit, or preadmission home visit and the peer-modeling film. The dependent variables included both psychological measures and behavioral ratings. The preadmission visit resulted in less maternal anxiety during and after the hospitalization and greater satisfaction. The peer-modeling film was associated with less anxiety among the children and less undesirable behavior posthospitalization.

Parrinello (1983) surveyed 28 patients hospitalized for vascular surgery to determine the effectiveness of a preoperative teaching booklet. The booklet was rated as very helpful by 85% of the patients. Its helpfulness was increased when discussed with a member of the health care team.

Wong and Wong (1985) evaluated the effectiveness of an individualized learning activity package to teach hip replacement patients to perform postoperative exercises. The 98 subjects were assigned randomly to an experimental or control group. Dependent variables included compliance, satisfaction, and complications. Experimental subjects showed a significantly higher degree of compliance and were more satisfied than the others.

Four studies were designed to evaluate the effectiveness of group and individual patient education for surgical patients. Mezzanotte (1970) concluded that group teaching was effective and that patients liked the group environment because they learned from others. Lindeman's (1972) experimental study gave evidence that group teaching was as effective as individual teaching and was more efficient. In a descriptive study Phillips (1977) revealed that those not attending the class had more unanswered questions and that the class benefited those attending. Adom and Wright's (1982) survey of patients' and nurses' perceptions of individual and group teaching modalities showed patients and nurses holding different preferences. Only one-third of the patients preferred individual teaching, whereas nurses indicated a greater preference for that modality.

Cardiovascular

In 10 studies researchers examined the effectiveness of patient education for cardiovascular patients. Two were surveys of patients' perceptions; three used a single-group design; and five used a control group.

Open-heart surgical patients reported problems with respiration and physical condition in the immediate postoperative period as the most difficult according to Miller and Shada (1978). Allendorf and Keegan (1975) concluded from their survey of patients under treatment for coronary artery disease that (a) patients were poorly informed and (b) teaching by both the nurse and doctor resulted in greater knowledge. Deberry, Jefferies, and Light (1975), Owens, McCann, and Hutelmyer (1978), and Tanner and Noury (1981) all used a single group design and reported significant gains in knowledge for subjects participating in a teaching program.

The five studies in which investigators used control groups also gave support to the effectiveness of patient education. Finesilver (1978) reported that experimental subjects had significantly lower distress and were more satisfied with the information received than control subjects. Hill and Madison (1980) concluded that experimental subjects had a significantly greater mean weight loss than control subjects. Owens and Hutelmyer's (1982) findings showed that experimental subjects were better able to cope than control subjects. Ventura et al. (1984) found significant differences in frequency, distance, and length of walks for experimental subjects choosing to increase their exercise. This finding was not supported with subjects choosing to alter foot care or smoking. The study by Scalzi, Burke, and Greenland (1980) was the only one in which there were no significant differences between experimental and control groups.

Two studies were concerned with adherence among hypertensives. Swain and Steckel (1981) compared routine clinic care, patient education, and contingency contracting as strategies for influencing adherence among hypertensives. The sample consisted of 115 patients randomly selected and randomly assigned to one of the three groups. The findings showed contingency contracting to be an effective intervention strategy for improving knowledge and adherence and for decreasing diastolic blood pressure.

Kerr (1985) compared an educational strategy, a self-monitoring approach, and a combination of these for promoting adherence to treatment in 116 subjects from three occupational sites. They were randomly assigned to one of the treatment groups or the control group. There were no significant differences on adherence scores, knowledge, or blood pressure.

Four articles included evaluation of structured or formal teaching. Billie (1977) compared the effectiveness of structured and unstructured teaching on knowledge of disease and compliance of 24 myocardial infarction patients from two hospitals. Knowledge was measured at discharge and compliance at one month. No significant differences were found between groups, and the correlation between knowledge and compliance was not significant.

Toth (1980) compared the effects of structured and unstructured pretransfer teaching on the anxiety level of 20 myocardial infarction patients being transferred from the coronary care unit. Ten received unstructured teaching from the unit nurses, and the other 10 received that instruction plus structured teaching. Subjects who received the structured teaching were significantly less anxious on the day and at the time of transfer than the others as measured by systolic blood pressure and heart rate.

Milazzo (1980) investigated the effects of formal and informal teaching on knowledge level of 25 coronary patients randomly assigned to one of three groups: informal teaching with a pre- and posttest, formal teaching with a pre- and posttest, or formal teaching with a posttest only. There were no significant differences between the two groups receiving formal teaching. Subjects receiving formal teaching scored significantly higher on the posttest than those receiving informal teaching.

Sivarajan et al. (1983) investigated the effects of exercise combined with a teaching–counseling program in facilitating changes in behavior relevant to risk factors of smoking, diet, and weight for myocardial infarction patients. A total of 258 subjects from seven hospitals were assigned randomly to one of the three treatment groups. At 6 months posthospital discharge there were no significant differences between the groups.

Four studies included examination of instructional strategies making use of audiovisual materials and printed matter. Rankin (1979) compared programmed instruction with routine teaching practices using knowledge acquisition and retention as the dependent variable. Nineteen subjects recovering from myocardial infarctions served as subjects. Subjects receiving the programmed instruction scored significantly higher initially and retained that knowledge after 3 weeks compared to the others.

Barbarowicz, Nelson, DeBusk, and Haskell (1980) compared routine teaching with a slide–sound module and booklet program. Dependent variables included knowledge, anxiety, and health-enhancing behaviors. A total of 230 patients from three hospitals served as subjects and were assigned randomly to either group. Findings gave evidence that both groups experienced significant increases in knowledge scores, that the experimental group scores were significantly higher than those of the control group, and that the finding held for knowledge retention at 3 months.

Gregor (1981) compared the effects of a self-instructional booklet designed to teach basic facts about myocardial infarction, unstable angina, and treatment with routine instruction. A total of 100 patients from two hospitals were assigned randomly to the control or experimental group. The dependent variable was knowledge acquisition and retention. Those completing the self-instructional booklet had significantly higher posttest and retention scores.

Lamb (1984) evaluated the effectiveness of a teaching manual about cardiac catheterization for use by patients. A total of 30 patients scheduled for elective cardiac catheterization served as subjects. They were pretested, given the booklet, and then given the posttest. Findings supported a significant increase in mean scores from pretest to posttest.

Two studies were focused on comparisons of group and individual instruction. Nath and Rinehart (1979) compared group and individual instruction on relaxation therapy for patients with essential hypertension. Findings showed that group and individual instruction were equally effective. Falkiewicz (1980) compared knowledge scores of cardiac patients attending group classes in one hospital with comparable patients not receiving group instruction in two other hospitals. Test scores of the subjects receiving group instruction increased significantly and were significantly higher than test scores of the other subjects.

Chronic Illness

There were seven studies in which researchers evaluated the effectiveness of patient education for patients with chronic illness. Two studies were exploratory; one investigator used a single-group design; and four made use of a control group.

Watkins, Williams, Martin, Hogan, and Anderson (1967) conducted an exploratory study to determine the relationships among what diabetics know, what they do, and their state of control. Results showed that (a) a large number were making errors in their care; (b) the longer individuals had the disease the more errors were made; (c) those who knew more managed better; (d) there was no relationship between management and control; and (e) those in poorer control knew more about the disease.

Hoffart (1982) reported a descriptive study of decision making for renal transplant patients. Skills and facts were used more frequently than rules to aid decision making. Perry (1981) used a single group design with rehabilitation patients and reported a significant increase in knowledge and skills associated with a four-phase educational program.

Hecht (1974), Johnson (1982), and Spelman (1984) all reported significant positive effects from educational programs for experimental subjects. Hecht studied medication compliance of tuberculosis patients. Johnson analyzed anxiety, perceptions of meaningfulness in life, and knowledge of cancer patients. Spelman evaluated adherence to an exercise regimen by low back pain patients. In contrast, Tagliacozzo, Luskin, Lashof, and Ima (1974) reported no significant effects from an educational intervention on attitudes and behaviors of black clinic patients.

Thirteen studies were focused on teaching strategies. Brock (1978) conducted an exploratory study with eight subjects to assess the effectiveness of a learning activity package for diabetes mellitus. Newly diagnosed diabetics receiving the experimental treatment scored higher on all dependent variables except administering insulin and urine testing than the previously diagnosed control group.

Kim and Grier (1981) explored the effects of pacing of medical instruction on the learning of elderly clients. A sample of 45 subjects was assigned to a control group or a normal-paced or a slow-paced group. The slow-paced group scored significantly higher on knowledge gain scores and lower on mean number of response errors than the others.

Dodd (1983) used a pretest–posttest, four-group design to evaluate side-effect management techniques singly and in combination with information on drugs for cancer patients. A sample of 48 patients was assigned randomly to one of the four groups. A self-care questionnaire was administered to collect data. Those patients who learned side-effect management techniques performed significantly more self-care behaviors and initiated them sooner than the others.

Garvey and Kramer (1983) compared the effects of a structured self-paced educational program to the effects of a previous method of one-on-one teaching by a nurse. The instruction was designed to help 32 cancer patients self-administer chemotherapy with a portable infusion pump. Results showed that the self-paced program decreased teaching time by 50%, eliminated the need for outpatient teaching, reduced the number of nighttime phone calls for help, and resulted in higher patient satisfaction.

Deimling et al. (1984) tested the hypothesis that chronic hemodialysis patients who received additional teaching about phosphorus control and participated in their care by using an algorithm and contingency contracting would show better phosphorus control than either patients who received routine care or patients who received the additional phosphorus information but did not use the algorithm. A total of 37 patients was divided randomly into a control and two experimental groups. None of the groups had significant improvements in serum phosphorus levels over the study period.

Watchous, Thurston, and Carter (1980) reported a pilot study with 10 volunteer dialysis patients to determine the effect of programmed instruction on knowledge regarding renal failure. There was a significant gain in knowledge from pre- to posttest.

Heston and Lazar (1980) evaluated the effectiveness of a learning device, a book and game, in increasing knowledge of diabetic children aged 7 to 12 years. Six children served as the control group, and 31 as the experimental group. Children in the experimental group had a significant increase in mean knowledge scores.

Edlund (1981) evaluated the effectiveness of an ostomy care guide designed to improve documentation of care and to increase the self-care abilities of the patient. Patients using the guide reported more opportunities for return demonstration, more awareness that a step-by-step process was being used, and fewer problems following discharge.

Minton (1983) used a quasi-experimental design to compare the relative effectiveness of lecture and videotape for teaching bowel and bladder management to 14 patients with traumatic spinal cord injuries divided into two groups. Subjects in both groups had significant gains in knowledge scores. There were no significant differences between the groups.

Young and Brooks (1986) used 16 multiple sclerosis patients randomly assigned to an experimental and control group to determine the effectiveness of a teaching manual concerning medication. Both groups were given instruction by a physician and a nurse, and the experimental subjects also received a patient information manual. The experimental group had significantly higher posttest scores than the others.

Ankenbrandt and Tanner (1971) investigated the effects of role-delineated nutrition teaching compared to usual nutrition teaching on the food selection behavior of geriatric patients. A total of 85 patients over the age of 55 were assigned randomly to one of five treatment groups and compared on food selection of hospital menus. There was no evidence of significant changes in food selection behavior in any group; neither formal nor informal teaching nor the use or lack of visual aids influenced learning.

Israel and Mood (1982) evaluated the effect of a set of three media presentations made for the purpose of reducing stress during radiation therapy for the treatment of cancer. The presentations provided information about treatment, side effects, and possible emotional reactions. Findings from 36 subjects randomly assigned to experimental or control groups showed that the experimental group had significantly higher gains in knowledge in all areas.

Nield (1971) examined the effects of health teaching on the anxiety level of 20 patients with chronic lung disease, randomly assigned to one of three treatment groups: group teaching, individual teaching, or no teaching. Results showed no significant differences for the three groups.

Psychiatric–Mental Health

In five studies psychiatric patients were used as subjects in research on medications and teaching strategies. Witt (1981) studied 33 psychiatric patients to assess the effects of locus of control, health values, and patient education method on medication compliance determined by pill count. The patient education methods were nondirective to harmonize with the needs of an internally oriented patient and directive to harmonize with the needs of an externally oriented patient. Medication compliance was not influenced by teaching method or locus of control.

Battle, Halliburton, and Wallston (1982) evaluated the effects of two teaching programs on ability to handle self-medication before discharge and on compliance 1 year after discharge. Sixty hospitalized psychiatric patients on oral phenothiazines were divided into three groups: lecture and discussion on self-medication; group sessions once a week for 2 weeks; and control. There were no significant differences between groups.

Osguthorpe, Roper, and Saunders (1983) investigated the effectiveness of three teaching methods on medication knowledge. The three methods were a drug information sheet, videotaped nurse explanation, and a combination of the two. A total of 202 psychiatric patients from general psychiatric wards served as subjects. Results showed no significant differences across teaching methods using pretest–posttest change scores.

Whiteside, Harris, and Whiteside (1983) studied the effects of a structured educational program that included written reinforcements. A pre–post control group design was used. The subjects were 28 psychiatric patients attending a cardiology clinic. Medication knowledge was the dependent variable. The experimental group subjects showed significant improvement in knowledge from pretest to posttest.

C. Hart, Craig-Williams, and Gladwell (1985) compared a traditional informal teaching method with a systematic, group approach that included using a consumer medication education form. A pre–post control group design was used. A total of 28 psychiatric patients were matched and assigned randomly to either the experimental or control group. Whereas all subjects learned something, those in the experimental group demonstrated significant learning.

Diagnostic Procedures

In four studies researchers explored the effectiveness of patient education with patients undergoing diagnostic procedures in either inpatient or ambulatory care settings. In one study the researchers surveyed patient and nurse perceptions, and three studies included a control group design.

Schuster and Jones (1982) explored possible differences in nurse and patient opinions about patient education for the barium enema. Nurses believed the patient should have more information than patients believed necessary. Nurses also believed that they should give more information than they actually do in practice.

Findings from studies by Barnett (1978), Latta and Wiesmeier (1981), and Lumsden and Hyner (1985) all showed positive effects from patient education. Barnett evaluated the effect of informing patients having a barium meal and those having a barium enema before and during the procedure. Informed subjects having a barium enema reported significantly less anxiety. Latta and Wiesmeier's experimental subjects showed significantly increased positive attitudes at the time of a gynecological examination. Lumsden and Hyner's experimental subjects had a significant reduction in the recurrence of urinary tract infections.

Clark and Bayley (1972) compared three teaching methods for patients on long-term anticoagulant therapy. A total of 45 subjects were assigned randomly to one of three groups: programmed instruction, printed information sheet, or no specific format. Subjects receiving the programmed instruction had significantly higher knowledge scores than subjects in the other groups.

Choi-Lao (1976) compared the influence of group and individual instruction on self-medication. Dependent variables were knowledge and medication errors. The subjects were nine patients at two hospitals who were taking antibiotics. Subjects receiving group instruction demonstrated more knowledge and were more compliant than the others.

Generalizations for Theory of Instruction

The following generalizations are based on the review of the 92 articles focused on instructional strategy and group characteristics:

1. Patient education does influence learning. The greatest impact is on knowledge and skills. Patients tend to retain and transfer the knowledge acquired. More complex outcomes such as compliance are the product of variables over and above exposure to patient education.
2. Most teaching strategies, for example, booklet, programmed instruction, modeling, and lecture–discussion, are effective. The finding that most strategies are effective may be an artifact of the research design or simply may underscore the strength of patient education as an intervention.
3. Group teaching is as effective as individual teaching, may lead to benefits apart from knowledge gained, and may be preferred by patients.
4. All patient groups represented responded to patient education.

HEALTH CARE SETTING AS LEARNING ENVIRONMENT

Organizational Structure

Two studies dealt with the organizational structure of nursing service and its impact on patient education. Girouard (1978) explored the impact of the clinical nurse specialist on preoperative teaching. A pretest–posttest–control–group design was used. A total of 36 nurses and 80 patients served as subjects. Dependent variables included patient and nurse satisfaction, frequency of teaching, and documentation of teaching. The investigator functioned as a clinical specialist on the experimental unit for 4 weeks. Data collected from the kardex and patient interviews showed a significant increase in preoperative teaching on the experimental unit. Nurses on the experimental unit did not have more positive feelings, nor did they claim that they did more teaching. Documentation did not differ.

Barton and Wirth (1985) explored the effects of primary nursing on patient education. A total of 22 renal transplant recipients comprised the subjects in this posttest-only static-group design to compare education under routine nursing care with education under primary nursing. Discharge preparedness and knowledge of self-care were the dependent variables. There were no significant differences between the groups.

Quality Assurance

Hageman and Ventura (1981) used a quality assurance framework to evaluate the effects of a medication routine. Imbedded in the study design were questions regarding the effectiveness of patient education programs and the use of a particular instrument. Findings showed that (a) the patient outcome instrument was a reliable criterion for measuring the effects of the teaching regimen and (b) the teaching regimen had a positive effect on patients by increasing knowledge of medication in two of the five areas measured.

Evaluation

Weiler (1968) surveyed postsurgical patients regarding preoperative preparation on a sample of 100 patients who had open-heart surgery. Data were collected approximately 1 week after surgery. According to patients the most important areas for preoperative teaching were deep breathing, coughing, pain, oxygen and chest tubes, and information describing the intensive care unit.

Pender (1974) reported on interviews with 138 patients regarding the health information received during hospitalization. Most information was given by physicians and consisted of diagnosis, treatment type, and treatment procedure. Patients reported a need for more information about self-care, possible complications of the present illness, and prevention of future illness.

L. Hart and Frantz (1977) surveyed hospitals to determine the characteristics of patient education programs for subjects having open-heart surgery and the effects of teaching strategies and timing on patient compliance. Questionnaires were sent to 512 hospitals and 402 responded; open-heart surgery was performed in 358 hospitals. Only 66% of the hospitals in which open-heart surgery was performed offered a patient education program. Only 45% of the hospitals with a program used a planned teaching sequence. Most frequently the nurse was the instructor for the areas of drugs, activity, and support services and was second most frequently involved in instruction on diet and complications. Most hospitals used an individual approach supplemented by pamphlets, pictures, and diagrams. Most frequently noted as supportive of a teaching program was a knowledgeable staff who thought teaching was important. Inadequate staffing and time were the major impediments.

**Generalizations for
Theory of Instruction**

Using the six studies addressing three variables as the basis for drawing generalizations, the following statements are offered:

1. The organizational structure of the hospital is less important than the value the staff and administration attach to patient teaching.
2. Patients view patient education as important.
3. The quality assurance system can be used to assess the effectiveness of patient education programs.

SUMMARY

The 120 studies included in this review were grouped in relation to five categories of variables basic to a theory of instruction in patient education. Findings in the studies related to the characteristics of the patient as learner support the following variables as significant for a theory of instruction: demographic characteristics including age, race, duration and type of illness, educational level, and family preparedness. Selected psychological variables are significant as they interact with teaching approaches.

Given only two studies in which the characteristics of the nurse as teacher were the main variables, no inferences for a theory of instruction could be drawn. However, the findings from those studies combined with results from studies in which characteristics of the nurse were secondary variables support the importance of this category of variables. The educational preparation, motivation, values, and job description of the nurse implementing patient teaching appear to be significant variables for a theory of instruction.

Investigators explored a wide range of teaching strategies in the studies of patient teaching. The setting for teaching, group and individual teaching, and a variety of instructional strategies all prove promising at the operational level. The instructional strategies were too diverse to allow analysis at a level of abstraction beyond the operational.

Findings in this review also support characteristics of the health care setting as an important category of variables for a theory of instruction. The organizational structure, a quality assurance framework, and valuing patient teaching appear to be significant variables.

Patient education research provides a rich data source for future developments in theory, practice, and research. The effectiveness of patient education as a nursing intervention is clearly established. Furthermore, positive learning outcomes are associated with a broad range of teaching strategies, content areas, and patient populations. Systematic explorations of the characteristics of the patient as learner, the nurse as teacher, and the health care setting as a learning environment are still necessary for developing a theory of instruction for patient education. Future researchers should attend to phenomena unique to patient education rather than to duplicating general educational research. Instead of the investigator-driven research approach that characterizes research to date, replication should be encouraged. Future research should be designed to link theory and research and thereby contribute to the further development of a theory of instruction in patient education.

REFERENCES

Adler, P., Rawlinson, M., Crabtree, K., & Hallburg, J. (1983). Effectiveness of teaching methods for renal patients. *American Association of Nephrology Nurses and Technicians Journal, 10,* 9–16.

Adom, D., & Wright, A. (1982). Dissonance in nurse and patient evaluations of the effectiveness of a patient-teaching program. *Nursing Outlook, 30*, 132–136.

Allen, C., & Ries, C. (1985). Smoking, alcohol and dietary practices during pregnancy: Comparison before and after prenatal education. *Journal of the American Dietetic Association, 85*, 605–606.

Allendorf, E., & Keegan, H. (1975). Teaching patients about nitroglycerin. *American Journal of Nursing, 75*, 1168–1170.

Ankenbrandt, M., & Tanner, L. (1971). Role-delineated and informal nurse-teaching and food selection behavior of geriatric patients. *Nursing Research, 20*, 61–63.

Barbarowicz, P., Nelson, M., DeBusk, R., & Haskell, W. (1980). A comparison of in-hospital education approaches for coronary bypass patients. *Heart & Lung, 9*, 127–133.

Barnett, J. (1978). Patients' emotional responses to barium x-rays. *Journal of Advanced Nursing, 3*, 37–46.

Barton, C., & Wirth, P. (1985). Evaluating the education of renal transplant patients after primary nursing. *American Association of Nurse Anesthetists Journal, 12*, 357–359.

Battle, E., Halliburton, A., & Walston, K. (1982). Self-medication among psychiatric patients and adherence after discharge. *Journal of Psychosocial Nursing and Mental Health Services, 20*(5), 21–28.

Billie, D. (1977). A study of patients' knowledge in relation to teaching format and compliance. *Supervisor Nurse, 8*(3), 55–57, 60–62.

Brock, A. (1978). A study to determine the effectiveness of a learning activity package for the adult with diabetes mellitus. *Journal of Advanced Nursing, 3*, 265–275.

Bull, M., & Lawrence, D. (1984). A pilot study: Postpartum mothers' perception of the information received in the hospital and its usefulness during the first weeks at home. *Journal of Community Health Nursing, 1*, 111–124.

Carrieri, V. (1975). Effect of an experimental teaching program on post-operative ventilatory capacity. In M. V. Batey (Ed.), *Communicating nursing research* (Vol. 7) (pp. 121–141). Boulder, CO: Western Interstate Commission for Higher Education.

Choi-Lao, A. (1976). A preliminary study designed to explore the difference in effectiveness of group and individual teaching in self-medication. *Nursing Papers, 8*, 22–29.

Christopherson, B., & Pfeiffer, C. (1980). Varying the timing of information to alter preoperative anxiety and postoperative recovery in cardiac surgery patients. *Heart & Lung, 9*, 854–861.

Clark, C., & Bayley, E. (1972). Evaluation of the use of programmed instruction for patients maintained on warfarin therapy. *American Journal of Public Health, 62*, 1135–1139.

Cohen, S. (1980). Postpartum teaching and the subsequent use of milk supplements. *Birth and the Family Journal, 7*, 163–167.

Cross, J., & Parsons, C. (1971). Nurse-teaching and goal-directed nurse-teaching to motivate change in food selection behavior of hospitalized patients. *Nursing Research, 20*, 454–458.

Dalzell, I. (1965). Evaluation of prenatal teaching program. *Nursing Research, 14*, 160–163.

Deberry, P., Jefferies, L., & Light, M. (1975). Teaching cardiac patients to manage medications. *American Journal of Nursing, 75*, 2191-2193.

Deimling, A., Denny, M., Harrison, M., Kerr, B., Mayfield, M., Pelle-Shearer, M., Seaby, N., & Townsend, S. (1984). Effect of an algorithm and patient information on serum phosphorous levels. *American Association of Nephrology Nurses and Technicians Journal, 2*, 35-38, 50.

Devine, E.C., & Cook, T.D. (1983). A meta-analytic analysis of effects of psychoeducational interventions on length of postsurgical hospital stay. *Nursing Research, 32*, 267-274.

Dickerson, P., & Ouellette, M. (1982). Prenatal education for adolescents in a delinquent youth facility. *Journal of Obstetric, Gynecologic, and Neonatal Nursing, 11*, 39-44.

Dodd, M. (1983). Self-care for side effects in cancer chemotherapy: An assessment of nursing interventions — part II. *Cancer Nursing, 6*, 63-67.

Doerr, C., & Jones, J. (1979). Effect of family preparation on the state anxiety level of the CCU patient. *Nursing Research, 28*, 315-316.

Dooher, M. (1980). Lamaze method of childbirth. *Nursing Research, 29*, 220-224.

Downs, F., & Fernbach, V. (1973). Experimental evaluation of prenatal leaflet series. *Nursing Research, 22*, 498-506.

Dziurbejko, M., & Larkin, J. (1978). Including the family in preoperative teaching. *American Journal of Nursing, 78*, 1892-1894.

Edlund, B. (1981). Determining the effectiveness of an ostomy care guide in facilitating comprehensive patient care. *Oncology Nursing Forum, 8*(3), 43-46.

Falkiewicz, J. (1980). Are group classes helpful in teaching cardiac patients? *American Journal of Nursing, 80*, 444.

Fawcett, J., & Burritt, J. (1985). An exploratory study of antenatal preparation for cesarean birth. *Journal of Obstetric, Gynecologic, and Neonatal Nursing, 14*, 224-230.

Felton, G., Huss, K., Payne, E., & Srsic, K. (1976). Preoperative nursing intervention with the patient for surgery: Outcomes of three alternative approaches. *International Journal of Nursing Studies, 13*, 83-96.

Ferguson, B. (1979). Preparing young children for hospitalization: A comparison of two methods. *Pediatrics, 64*, 656-664.

Finesilver, C. (1978). Preparation of adult patients for cardiac catheterization and coronary cineangiography. *International Journal of Nursing Studies, 15*, 211-221.

Flanders, N. A. (1965). Teacher influence, pupil attitudes, and achievement (U.S. Office of Education Cooperative Research Monograph No. 12). Washington, DC: U.S. Government Printing Office.

Fortin, G., & Kirouac, S. (1976). A randomized controlled trial of preoperative patient education. *International Journal of Nursing Studies, 13*, 11-24.

Garvey, E., & Kramer, R. (1983). Improving cancer patients' adjustment to infusion chemotherapy: Evaluation of a patient education program. *Cancer Nursing, 6*, 373-378.

Gierszewski, S. (1983). The relationship of weight loss, locus of control, and social support. *Nursing Research, 32*, 43-47.

Girouard, S. (1978). The role of the clinical specialist as change agent: An experiment in preoperative teaching. *International Journal of Nursing Studies, 15*, 57-65.

Goodwin, J. (1979). Programmed instruction of self-care following pulmonary surgery. *International Journal of Nursing Studies, 16*, 29–40.

Gregor, F. (1981). Teaching the patient with ischemic heart disease: A systematic approach to instructional design. *Patient Counseling and Health Education, 3*, 57–61.

Hageman, P., & Ventura, M. (1981). Utilizing patient outcome criteria to measure the effects of a medication teaching regimen. *Western Journal of Nursing Research, 3*, 25–33.

Hall, J. (1978). Influencing breast feeding success. *Journal of Obstetric, Gynecologic, and Neonatal Nursing, 7*(6), 28–32.

Halstead, J., & Fredrickson, T. (1978). Evaluation of a prepared childbirth program. *Journal of Obstetric, Gynecologic, and Neonatal Nursing, 7*(3), 39–42.

Hart, C., Craig-Williams, N., & Gladwell, C. (1985). A deliberative and group approach to inpatient consumer medication education. *Journal of the New York State Nurses Association, 16*(1), 33–42.

Hart, L., & Frantz, R. (1977). Characteristics of post-operative patient-education programs for open-heart surgery patients in the U.S. *Heart & Lung, 6*, 137–142.

Healy, K. (1968). Does preoperative instruction make a difference? *American Journal of Nursing, 68*, 62–67.

Hecht, A. (1974). Improving medication compliance by teaching outpatients. *Nursing Forum, 13*(2), 112–119.

Henderson, J. (1983). Effects of prenatal teaching program on postpartum regeneration of the pubococcygeal muscle. *Journal of Obstetric, Gynecologic, and Neonatal Nursing, 12*, 403–408.

Heston, J., & Lazar, S. (1980). Evaluating a learning device for juvenile diabetic children. *Diabetes Care, 3*, 668–671.

Hill, D., & Madison, R. (1980). A health education program for weight reduction in a hypertension clinic. *Public Health Reports, 95*, 271–275.

Hinshaw, A., Gerber, R., Atwood, J., & Allen, J. (1983). The use of predictive modeling to test nursing practice outcomes. *Nursing Research, 32*, 35–42.

Hoffart, N. (1982). Self-care decision making by renal transplant recipients. *American Association of Nephrology Nurses and Technicians Journal, 9*(6), 43–47.

Israel, M., & Mood, D. (1982). Three media presentations for patients receiving radiation therapy. *Cancer Nursing, 5*, 57–63.

Jackson, D. N. (1974). *Personality research form manual.* Goshen, NY: Research Psychologists Press.

Johnson, J. (1982). The effects of a patient education course on persons with a chronic illness. *Cancer Nursing, 5*, 117–123.

Kerr, J. (1985). Adherence and self-care. *Heart & Lung, 14*, 24–31.

Kim, K., & Grier, M. (1981). Pacing effects of medication instruction for the elderly. *Journal of Gerontology, 7*, 464–468.

King, I., & Tarsitano, B. (1982). The effect of structured and unstructured preoperative teaching: A replication. *Nursing Research, 31*, 324–329.

Kinney, M. R. (1977). Effects of preoperative teaching upon patients with differing modes of response to threatening stimuli. *International Journal of Nursing Studies, 14*, 49–59.

Kishi, K. (1983). Communication patterns of health teaching and information recall. *Nursing Research, 32*, 230–235.

Knapp, R. R. (1976). *Handbook for the Personal Orientation Inventory.* San Diego, CA: Educational and Industrial Testing Service.

Krueger, J., Hassell, J., Goggins, D., Ishimatsu, T., Pablico, M., & Tuttle, E. (1979). Relationship between nurse counseling and sexual adjustment after hysterectomy. *Nursing Research, 28,* 145-150.

Lamb, L. (1984). Patient understanding of a teaching manual on cardiac catheterization. *Heart & Lung, 13,* 267-271.

Latta, W., & Wiesmeier, E. (1981). Effects of an educational gynecological exam on women's attitudes. *Journal of Obstetric, Gynecologic, and Neonatal Nursing, 10,* 242-245.

Levesque, L., Grenier, R., Ke'rouac, S., & Reidy, M. (1984). Evaluation of a presurgical group program given at two different times. *Research in Nursing and Health, 7,* 227-236.

Linde, B., & Janz, N. (1979). Effect of teaching program on knowledge and compliance of cardiac patients. *Nursing Research, 28,* 282-286.

Lindeman, C. (1972). Nursing intervention with the presurgical patient. *Nursing Research, 21,* 196-209.

Lindeman, C., & Stetzer, R. (1973). Effect of preoperative visits by operating room nurses. *Nursing Research, 22,* 4-16.

Lindeman, C., & Van Aernam, B. (1971). Nursing intervention with the presurgical patient – the effects of structured and unstructured preoperative teaching. *Nursing Research, 20,* 319-332.

Lowe, M. (1970). Effectiveness of teaching as measured by compliance with medical recommendations. *Nursing Research, 19,* 59-63.

Lowery, B., & DuCette, J. (1976). Disease-related learning and disease control in diabetics as a function of locus of control. *Nursing Research, 25,* 358-362.

Lum, J., Chase, J., Cole, S., Johnson, A., Johnson, J., & Link, M. (1978). Nursing care of oncology patients receiving chemotherapy. *Nursing Research, 27,* 340-346.

Lumsden, L., & Hyner, G. (1985). Effects of an educational intervention on the rate of recurrent urinary tract infections in selected female outpatients. *Women & Health, 10*(1), 79-86.

Mahaffy, P. (1965). The effects of hospitalization on children admitted for tonsillectomy and adenoidectomy. *Nursing Research, 14,* 12-19.

Manderino, M., & Bzdek, V. (1984). Effects of modeling and information on reactions to pain: A childbirth-preparation analogue. *Nursing Research, 33,* 9-14.

Marshall, J., Penckofer, S., & Llewellyn, J. (1986). Structured postoperative teaching and knowledge and compliance of patients who had coronary artery bypass surgery. *Heart & Lung, 15,* 76-82.

McNeil, H., & Holland, S. (1972). A comparative study of public health nurse teaching in groups and in home visits. *American Journal of Public Health, 62,* 1629-1636.

Mezzanotte, E. (1970). Group instruction in preparation for surgery. *American Journal of Nursing, 70,* 89-91.

Midgley, J., & Osterhage, R. (1973). Effect of nursing instruction and length of hospitalization on postoperative complications in cholecystectomy patients. *Nursing Research, 22,* 69-72.

Milazzo, V. (1980). A study of the difference in health knowledge gained through formal and informal teaching. *Heart & Lung, 9,* 1079-1082.

58 RESEARCH ON NURSING PRACTICE

Miller, Sister P., & Shada, E. (1978). Preoperative information and recovery of open-heart surgery patients. *Heart & Lung, 7*, 486–493.

Mills, G., Barnes, R., Rodell, D., & Terry, L. (1985). An evaluation of an inpatient cardiac patient/family education program. *Heart & Lung, 14*, 400–406.

Minton, P. (1983). Video tape instruction: An effective way to learn. *Rehabilitation Nursing, 8*(3), 15–17.

Mohammed, M. (1964). Patients' understanding of written health information. *Nursing Research, 13*, 100–108.

Nath, C., & Rinehart, J. (1979). Effects of individual and group relaxation therapy on blood pressure in essential hypertensives. *Research in Nursing and Health, 2*, 119–126.

Nield, M. A. (1971). The effect of health teaching on the anxiety level of patients with chronic obstructive lung disease. *Nursing Research, 20*, 537–541.

Nunnally, D., & Aguiar, M. (1974). Patients' evaluation of their prenatal and delivery care. *Nursing Research, 23*, 469–474.

Orstead, C., Arrington, D., Kamath, S., Olson, R., & Kohrs, M. (1985). Efficacy of prenatal counseling: Weight gain, infant birth weight and cost-effectiveness. *Journal of the American Dietetic Association, 85*, 40–45.

Osguthorpe, N., Roper, J., & Saunders, J. (1983). The effect of teaching on medication knowledge. *Western Journal of Nursing Research, 5*, 205–215.

Owens, J., & Hutelmyer, C. (1982). The effect of preoperative intervention on delirium in cardiac surgical patients. *Nursing Research, 31*, 60–62.

Owens, J., McCann, C., & Hutelmyer, C. (1978). Cardiac rehabilitation: A patient education program. *Nursing Research, 27*, 148–150.

Packard, R., & Van Ess, H. (1969). A comparison of informal and role-delineated patient-teaching situations. *Nursing Research, 18*, 443–446.

Parrinello, K. (1983). Patients' evaluation of a teaching booklet for arterial bypass surgery. *Patient Counseling and Health Education, 5*, 183–188.

Pender, N. (1974). Patient identification of health information received during hospitalization. *Nursing Research, 23*, 262–267.

Perry, J. (1981). Effectiveness of teaching in the rehabilitation of patients with chronic bronchitis and emphysema. *Nursing Research, 30*, 219–222.

Petrowski, D. (1981). Effectiveness of prenatal and postnatal instruction in postpartum care. *Journal of Obstetric, Gynecologic, and Neonatal Nursing, 10*, 386–389.

Phillips, C. (1977). The hysterectomy patient in the obstetrics service: A presurgery class helps to meet her needs. *Journal of Obstetric, Gynecologic, and Neonatal Nursing, 6*(1), 45–49.

Rankin, M. (1979). Programmed instruction as a patient teaching tool: A study of myocardial infarction patients receiving warfarin. *Heart & Lung, 8*, 511–516.

Rice, V., & Johnson, J. (1984). Preadmission self-instruction booklets, postadmission exercise performance, and teaching time. *Nursing Research, 33*, 147–151.

Rotter, J. B. (1966). Generalized expectancies for internal versus external control of reinforcements. *Psychology Monographs, 80*(1, Whole No. 609), 1–28.

Rottkamp, B., & Donohue-Porter, P. (1982). The role of patient needs and preferences for instructional approaches in self-management of diabetes. *Patient Counseling and Health Education, 4*, 137–145.

Scalzi, C., Burke, L., & Greenland, S. (1980). Evaluation of an inpatient educational program for coronary patients and families. *Heart & Lung, 9*, 846–853.

Schuster, P., & Jones, S. (1982). Preparing the patient for a barium enema: A comparison of nursing and patient opinions. *Journal of Advanced Nursing, 7*, 523–527.

Shimko, C. (1981). The effect of preoperative instruction on state anxiety. *Journal of Neurosurgical Nursing, 13*, 318–322.

Sime, A. M. (1976). Relationship of preoperative fear, type of coping, and information received about surgery to recovery from surgery. *Journal of Personality and Social Psychology, 34*, 716–724.

Sivarajan, E., Newton, K., Almes, M., Kempf, T., Mansfield, L., & Bruce, R. (1983). Limited effects of outpatient teaching and counseling after myocardial infarction: A controlled study. *Heart & Lung, 12*, 65–73.

Smeltzer, C. (1980). Hypertensive patients' understanding of terminology. *Heart & Lung, 9*, 498–502.

Spelman, M. (1984). Back pain: How health education affects patient compliance with treatment. *Occupational Health Nursing, 30*, 649–651.

Swain, M. A., & Steckel, S. (1981). Influencing adherence among hypertensives. *Research in Nursing and Health, 4*, 213–222.

Tagliacozzo, D., Luskin, D., Lashof, J., & Ima, K. (1974). Nurse intervention and patient behavior. *American Journal of Public Health, 64*, 596–603.

Tanner, G., & Noury, D. (1981). The effect of instruction on control of blood pressure in individuals with essential hypertension. *Journal of Advanced Nursing, 6*, 99–106.

Taylor, A., Skelton, J., & Czajkowski, R. (1982). Do patients understand patient-education brochures? *Nursing & Health Care, 3*, 305–310.

Timm, M. (1979). Prenatal education evaluation. *Nursing Research, 28*, 338–341.

Toth, J. (1980). Effect of structured preparation for transfer on patient anxiety on leaving coronary unit. *Nursing Research, 29*, 28–34.

Ventura, M., Young, D., Feldman, M., Pastore, P., Pikula, S., & Yates, M. (1984). Effectiveness of health promotion interventions . . . peripheral vascular disease. *Nursing Research, 33*, 162–167.

Vinal, D. (1982). Childbirth education programs: A study of women participants and non-participants. *Birth, 9*, 183–185.

Watchous, S., Thurston, H., & Carter, M. (1980). The nurse educator and the adult dialysis patient. *Nursing Forum, 19*(1), 68–84.

Watkins, J., Williams, T., Martin, D., Hogan, M., & Anderson, E. (1967). A study of diabetic patients at home. *American Journal of Public Health, 57*, 452–457.

Weiler, Sister M. C. (1968). Postoperative patients evaluate preoperative instruction. *American Journal of Nursing, 68*, 1465–1467.

Whiteside, S., Harris, A., & Whiteside, H. D. (1983). Patient education: Effectiveness of medication programs for psychiatric patients. *Journal of Psychosocial Nursing and Mental Health Services, 21*(10), 16–21.

Whitley, N. (1979). A comparison of prepared childbirth couples and conventional prenatal class couples. *Journal of Obstetric, Gynecologic, and Neonatal Nursing, 8*, 109–111.

Witt, R. (1981). Medication compliance among discharged psychiatric patients. *Issues in Mental Health Nursing, 3*, 305–317.

Wong, J., & Wong, S. (1985). A randomized controlled trial of a new approach to preoperative teaching and patient compliance. *International Journal of Nursing Studies, 22*, 105–115.

Young, F., & Brooks, B. (1986). Patient teaching manuals improve retention of treatment information—a controlled clinical trial in multiple sclerosis. *Journal of Neuroscience Nursing, 18*(1), 26–28.

Zuckerman, M., & Lubin, B. (1965). *Manual for the Multiple Affect Adjective Check List*. San Diego, CA: Educational and Industrial Testing Service.

Chapter 3

The Physical Environment and Patient Care

MARGARET A. WILLIAMS
SCHOOL OF NURSING
UNIVERSITY OF WISCONSIN–MADISON

CONTENTS

In this chapter research linking physical environmental factors and patient care is reviewed. The physical environment cannot constitute a total environment for care; social factors and, in institutions, organizational factors also are highly important. The intent, however, is to review research in which dimensions of the physical environment are an explicit focus or are identified elements in an environment for care.

The goal of the review is to stimulate research. The physical environment is of substantial importance in nursing practice, and concern with it has a distinguished early history in the profession. However, there is limited empirical research by nurses.

The physical environment consists of the natural and built environments. The topics under those headings that are particularly relevant to patient care and that form the major part of this review are hospital and unit design, space, sound, light, color, temperature, and weather. Research on the use of certain elements or their artificial equivalents for prescribed therapy, such as controlled auditory stimulation, phototherapy, or heat treatment, is not included; the focus is on setting.

The criterion for selection of studies was that they be data based. Manual searches were the best means of locating studies; computerized retrieval systems were helpful but not efficient because terminology was diverse. Journals searched from their initial publication date through 1985 were *Advances in Nursing Science, Heart and Lung, International Journal of Nursing Studies, Journal of Advanced Nursing, Nursing Science* (Volumes 1–3), *Nursing Research*, and *Research in Nursing and Health. Dissertation Abstracts International* was searched from the years 1974 to 1985. *Communicating Nursing Research* was searched for the years 1968 through 1977, during which period the complete reports of research were available rather than abstracts.

The literature from which relevant research could be drawn is voluminous because the topical areas are all part of the broad field of environment and behavior. The interrelatedness of human behavior with the natural and built environments interests persons in a variety of fields. Various investigators pose both basic and practical questions about that relationship. In this review, selected landmark studies or ones that are especially relevant to nursing practice are cited whatever the profession or discipline of the authors. For a wider view of the field, illustrative reviews, books, or chapters include (a) an early analysis of the concepts of privacy, crowding, territory, and personal space by Altman (1975); (b) reviews of research in environmental psychology (Russell & Ward, 1982; Stokols, 1978), environmental sociology (Dunlap, 1979), and human spatial behavior (Baldassare, 1978); and (c) works related to environment and health (Baum & Singer, 1982), environmental stress (Evans, 1982), therapeutic environments (Canter & Canter, 1979), and social ecology (Moos, 1976, 1979).

PERSPECTIVES ON ENVIRONMENT
AND PATIENT CARE

Persons concerned with physical environments for patient care use perspectives principally from environment and health or from environmental psychology. The notion that both physical and social environments influence health and disease is central to the environment and health field. In that field two orientations to cause of disease are: (a) a disease-specific orientation in which specific diseases can be linked to specific agents; and (b) a holistic–ecological orientation in which a variety of stressors and pollutants endured over time have an impact upon the individual (Moos, 1979). Researchers in the field address both of those causes as well as the factors that affect host resistance. The latter (factors that affect host resistance) are less studied and understood (Lindheim & Syme, 1983).

The relatively new area of environmental psychology is considered by some persons to be a branch of psychology and by others to be an interdisciplinary study of environment and behavior (Russell & Ward, 1982). Theory building has progressed slowly due to the breadth of the field, although a number of theoretical approaches have been suggested, particularly by those interested in aging and the environment (Lawton, Windley, & Byerts, 1982). Several focused research domains, however, have evolved, including spatial cognition, proxemics, stress, and ecological psychology (Stokols, 1978). A simple stimulus-response model has been used in many studies of the psychological effects of environmental variables. More recently, the effects of mediating variables such as perceived control on behavior and the reciprocal relationship of people with their milieu have received increased attention (Russell & Ward, 1982; Stokols, 1978). An optimization theme is common; that is, individuals and groups attempt to create environments that are maximally supportive of their goals and activities (Stokols, 1978).

Environmental impact is of particular importance in the care of certain vulnerable populations. Persons who are ill, mentally handicapped, or frail are limited in the amount of control they can exert over their environment. Therefore, the impact of the environment becomes greater for them than for those who can voluntarily enter, leave, or control their environments. This concept, termed the *environmental docility hypothesis*, has been used particularly by Lawton (1974) and other gerontologists.

The desire to optimize environments to achieve health and well-being goals has led directly to attempts to create *therapeutic environments.* Interpretation of what constitutes a therapeutic environment has varied. Some define therapeutic environment as a location in which therapy occurs, and others define environment as the major therapeutic agent (Canter & Canter, 1979). An intermediate meaning of the term therapeutic environment is that both the physical design of the setting and the social environment are oriented toward enhancing therapeutic goals and activities. Closely allied to this concept is that of the *prosthetic environment,* in which prostheses are provided to compensate for deficits in physical and social skills (Lindsley, 1964).

Other models of environments for care include normalization, custodial, enhancement, medical, and individual growth models (Canter & Canter, 1979). In any model, as noted, both the physical and social environments are important. In institutions, organizational factors also contribute to the treatment climate. Moos (1974) has been a proponent of the view that social environments have identifiable and measurable dimensions. Although the scales Moos and his colleagues constructed have been criticized on the basis of the paradigm employed and confusion about the unit of analysis (Richards, 1978), they nevertheless are a step forward in an attempt to measure an important facet of the treatment environment.

In this review, discussion of research on dimensions of the physical environment is followed by examples of studies in which the focus is on either examination of specific types of environments in relation to support of care goals or attempts to create such environments. The examples are illustrative only, since a comprehensive review is beyond the scope of this chapter.

TRENDS IN NURSING'S CONCERN WITH ENVIRONMENT

Nightingale was an environmentalist *non pareil.* Her two best-known works, *Notes on Nursing* (1859) and *Notes on Hospitals* (1859), blend perspectives from both environment and health and environmental psychology. The former publication is a cogent discussion on the importance to the health of patients of adequate ventilation, warmth, control of noise, light, cleanliness, variety in the sick room, a social environment free of "chattering hopes and advices," and an environment characterized by orderliness and good management. *Notes on Hospitals* contains explicit instructions on how to design wards that foster recuperation of patients by provision of safe, sanitary, light, airy, and pleasant surroundings as well as instructions about where to locate hospitals and provide for clean water and drainage. Nightingale's prescriptions are buttressed by detailed statistics and her own field observations. Although *Notes on Nursing* is better known within the nursing profession, *Notes on Hospitals* was an enormous influence on hospital architecture throughout the world (Thompson & Goldin, 1975).

Early nursing leaders in the United States such as Goodrich (1903/1973) addressed hospital construction and environment and nurses' responsibility for participating in the planning of hospitals. However, advances in infection control, heating, and construction methods gradually made hospitals less hazardous to health; delegation of housekeeping and maintenance tasks to nonnursing personnel also contributed to making environmental concerns less salient in hospital nursing.

Following World War II there was great interest in establishing therapeutic communities in psychiatric hospitals; "nontraditional environments" also became characteristic of many rehabilitation hospitals. With the exception of some pediatric and maternity services, however, environmental changes were limited in acute care hospitals. Brown, a social anthropologist, used data from field observations made by "walking" hospitals throughout the United States as the basis for suggestions regarding potential therapeutic uses of the physical and social environment of the general hospital. Widely read and acclaimed within nursing, her monograph on those potential therapeutic uses was the first of a three-part series, *Newer Dimensions of Patient Care* (1961).

Rogers (1970) introduced a widely disseminated conceptual model in nursing about the relationship of human beings to their physical environment. One of the principles within her model was that the individual and the environment are continuously exchanging matter and energy with each other. The emphasis on environment, although broadly stated and lacking in operational definitions, was the impetus for a number of studies by Rogers' students on the effects of factors such as light and sound.

Currently, concern with the environment is most evident in nursing literature on care of the elderly. Environments for labor and delivery and neonatal and adult intensive care also are receiving attention because of concern for probable effects on both patients and personnel. Some of that literature is a source of potential hypotheses for investigation, but systematic, data-based studies are few.

RESEARCH ON DIMENSIONS OF THE PHYSICAL ENVIRONMENT

Hospital and Unit Design

Characteristics of the literature on hospital design and human behavior were summarized by Reizenstein (1982). The literature was scattered widely, creating problems of utilization, and more came from the United Kingdom than from the United States. It contained more empirical work on nonacute-care hospitals, especially psychiatric ones, than on acute-care hospitals. The articles were divided equally between empirical and nonempirical studies and were of varying quality, many anecdotal. Empirical studies included a variety of dependent variables, but potentially important ones still remain unexamined. Reizenstein also concluded that those who make design decisions in health facilities tend not to use the research that exists.

A series of studies in Great Britain sponsored by the Nuffield Provincial Hospitals Trust (1955) was the first systematic approach to the problem of hospital design since Nightingale's *Notes on Hospitals* (Stones, cited by Kenny & Canter, 1979). The intent was to produce a ward design that would maximize nursing efficiency and patient-centered care. Although the patient was the person for whom design was to be maximized, the work involved primarily job analyses, ergonomic studies of nursing procedures, and analyses of nurses' movements in the wards. Patients' views were solicited minimally (Kenny & Canter, 1979).

Nursing staff behaviors or outcomes that hospital and, more particularly, unit design reasonably can affect include ease and frequency of interaction with patients and families, travel time, staffing requirements, infection control practices, satisfaction with ability to carry out treatment, surveillance, communication processes, and general satisfaction with the work setting. Literature on ward design and nurse staffing was reviewed by Seelye (1982), who found the majority of evaluation studies to be concentrated on nurses' time, particularly in travel, and on user opinion of wards. Seelye concluded that two main aspects of unit design related to effective and efficient nursing care: short travel distances and features that facilitate maximum contact between nurses and patients. Maximizing contact and visibility may, however, cause distractions when there are no off-scene places for activities such as report-giving (Gagneaux & Shaver, 1977).

Patient behaviors or outcomes that could be affected by design of the nursing unit have been more ambiguous than nurse-related behaviors; orientation, anxiety, interaction with others, feelings of privacy and security, and general satisfaction with setting may be included. The issue of privacy has been addressed primarily by surveys in which patients were asked preferences about single, double, or multibed rooms. Thompson and Goldin (1975) concluded that the issue would always remain an open question. An attempt by Wood (1977) to determine whether there were differences in sensory disturbances between patients randomly assigned to single and two-bed rooms revealed more disturbances among the patients in single units. Reduced sensory stimulation and social isolation were considered probable causes.

One extensive unit redesign study has been reported. Kraegel, Mousseau, Goldsmith, and Arora (1974) reported on the nurse-led restructuring of the entire care delivery system on a medical–surgical nursing unit. Of particular interest were the processes involved and rationale for changes made in the system once the focus shifted from a design to promote nurse utilization to one based on meeting patient needs. Architectural changes were an important but not the sole part of the redesign. Evaluation postimplementation included certain cost and quality factors compared to a control unit. Physical conversion costs, primarily for installation of professional supply cabinets in patients' rooms and a new communication system, were incurred on the demonstration unit. However, personnel costs did not increase, savings were realized in the materials supply system, and substantial indirect cost savings were estimated to occur through reallocation of tasks, personnel, and responsibility. Nurses direct care time with patients was doubled. Quality of care and patient satisfaction increased on the demonstration unit, but personnel satisfaction did not increase significantly.

In the literature on psychiatry, positive changes have been cited in patient behavior after certain unit design changes were made (e.g., Holahan & Saegert, 1973; Whitehead, Polsky, Crookshank, & Fik,

1984). Many of the concepts for redesign are drawn from Osmond's seminal work (1957). To date, there is little evidence that the physical design of general medicine and surgical nursing units is the sole variable related to patients' emotional comfort or their satisfaction with nursing care. Campbell (1984) examined patients' self-reported levels of anxiety and satisfaction with nursing care in physical designs that provided variable proximity between nurses and patients through nuclear (radial, triangular, and cluster) and linear (rectangular) unit designs. Hypotheses that predicted more satisfaction with care and less anxiety in the nuclear designs were not supported.

Some evidence exists that nurses, at least in intensive care units, find circular or semicircular designs more desirable than rectangular or other designs (Macdonald, Schentag, Ackerman, & Walsh, 1981). Whether that perception translates into differences in patient care is not known. It has been suggested, however, that the physical design of the work environment also can be an influence on the nature of interpersonal interactions between supervisor and subordinate and, consequently, the extent to which they agree about performance-related matters (Ferris & Rowland, 1985).

The Spatial Environment

The spatial setting of human behavior has interested persons in a number of disciplines, and various subareas of study have evolved. Baldassare (1978), a sociologist, identified three subareas: interpersonal distancing, small-group ecology, and crowding. Stokols (1978), a psychologist, used Hall's term (1966), proxemics, as the overall study of human spatial behavior with four phenomena encompassed: privacy, personal space, territoriality, and crowding.

Literature in the field as a whole is enormous but few nurse investigators are represented. Kerr (1982) used nonnursing research of the 1960s and early 1970s on space use in hospitals to pose questions for future study. As with much of that literature, however, the probable effects of mediating variables were discussed minimally. In an observational study of staff use of space on four hospital units, Kerr (1985) concluded that the relationship between space use and staff role was defined by the hospital social organization. Spatial norms were evident in the relative lack of unwarranted intrusion of one category of staff into space assigned to another category.

Allekian (1973) administered questionnaires to hospitalized patients to assess whether intrusions of territory and personal space were anxiety-producing. Territorial intrusions were found to be anxiety-producing, but personal space intrusions were not. Reliability and validity of the instrument were not reported. Using two projective tests, Gioiella (1978) found that the preferred personal space of a group of elderly women increased as their self-esteem decreased. Louis (1981) assessed the personal space boundary of persons in retirement apartments. Both elderly men and women approached the stimulus-individual (a nurse) less closely than they allowed themselves to be approached. This finding contradicted results with younger subjects but may have been a result of the role identity of the stimulus-individual. Males', but not females', perceived personal space was related significantly and inversely to body temperature and perception of time duration (Collett, 1974). Johnson (1979), using Allekian's questionnaire, found that 68% of one nursing home's residents had high anxiety about territorial intrusion. Intrusion by other patients produced higher anxiety than intrusion by staff. Females were significantly more anxious about intrusion than males. The congruency of questionnaire responses with actual behavioral responses to intrusions under a variety of conditions has not been tested.

Using a figure placement test, Geden and Begeman (1981) reported that hospitalized patients' personal space preferences differed between hospital and home settings and by role of the other person (nurse, doctor, family member, or stranger). Preferred distances were smaller in the hospital than in the home. In both settings the family member figure was placed closest to the self figure, but the space preference for the doctor was not significantly different from that placement. Questions were raised about the "knownness" of nurses to the patient compared to that of the physician.

Case studies might furnish important clues to persons' use of space in different health-related situations. Only one case report was found, however, in which a depressed patient's changes in spatial behavior over time were recorded by the nurse therapist (Murphy, 1981).

Sound

Studies of the aural environment in health care settings have generally taken the form of (a) measuring sound levels in various areas and then projecting the potential physiologic effects based on laboratory research, or (b) obtaining data about effects such as heart rate change, sleep disturbance, or annoyance under different sound conditions. Populations considered to be particularly vulnerable to adverse effects of continual loud sound are infants, especially premature infants in incubators; seriously ill patients in high-technology-intensive care areas; persons with heightened cardiovascular or psychological reactivity to unwanted sound; and persons taking ototoxic drugs. In occupational health nursing a major concern in certain industries is loss of hearing with continued exposure to excessive sound.

Studies in which levels of sound were measured in various hospital areas and discussed in terms of possible adverse effects on patients were reported by Falk and Woods (1973), Woods and Falk (1974), Ogilvie (1980), Topf (1983a), and Keefe (1984). In the first two reports, levels of sound in infant incubators, a recovery room, and an acute-care unit were judged to be potentially capable of interfering with sleep and of damaging hearing in patients receiving aminoglycosidic antibiotics. Topf found average sound levels in patient rooms on a surgical nursing unit to exceed recommended levels. Ogilvie also found excessive nocturnal sound levels on two surgical nursing units in an English hospital, and in addition this researcher found the levels to be related to unit design. Sound levels in a normal newborn nursery exceeded those in nearby postpartum rooming-in rooms (Keefe, 1984).

Hilton (1985) augmented her study of sound levels in six acute-care units of three hospitals in Canada with interviews of selected patients. Generally, strong annoyance was not expressed until sound levels were above roughly normal conversational level. Haslam (1970) found that patients were more disturbed by conversation from other patients, staff, and visitors than by sound from mechanical sources.

Hypothesizing that high sound levels could intensify the discomfort of postoperative patients, Minckley (1968) investigated the amount of pain medication given in a recovery room during periods of high and low sound levels. The hypothesis that more pain medication would be given during periods of high sound levels was supported, although the actual number of patients given medications was relatively few (40 out of 644) during the observation period. This study has not been replicated. Storlie (1976) attempted to associate heart rate change with sound levels among patients in coronary care units. During times of high sound level on the unit, the majority of subjects' average heart rates increased significantly over readings taken at low sound intensities. Substantial conceptual and methodological problems have been identified (Donaldson, 1977; Lewis, 1972) in both Marshall's exploratory (1972) attempt to link heart rate responses of patients in a coronary care unit with selected sounds and Putt's attempt (1977) to determine effects of noise on fatigue in healthy adults.

The effect of sound on sleep of adults has been assessed by self-report (Davies & Peters, 1983; Keefe, 1984) and by continuous polygraph recording combined with observation of sleep-disturbing factors (Hilton, 1976). In the Hilton study, sounds created by staff were most frequently the disturbing factor. Results of studies of sound effects on sleep are notoriously difficult to evaluate, however, because age, sex, meaningfulness of the sound, stage of sleep, and pattern and intensity of sound can all be modifying factors (Lukas, 1975).

The most theoretical study to date was done by Topf (1983b). A model, modified from Moos (1979), of the effects of aversive physical characteristics of the environment on health was specified (Topf, 1984), and hypotheses and variables for study were drawn from the model. The latter included personal variables, namely locus of control, socioeconomic status, and seriousness of illness; control over noise; and reactivity to noise as factors influencing postoperative recovery. The experimental condition, instruction for control over noise, did not account for significant amounts of variance in patients' reported disturbance due to noise or in their recovery outcomes. Contrary to hypotheses, subjects in the control group with internal locus of control experienced less disturbance due to noise than subjects with external locus of control. In the experimental group, internal and external locus of control subjects did not differ in the degree to which they exercised actual control over noise. In contrast to several prior studies, social desirability was accounted for in responses, and instruments were employed that had established reliability and validity. The investigator pointed out the several limitations of the study, but, nevertheless, it was a promising move toward a multidimensional conceptualization of noise and its possible effect on patient outcomes.

Suggestions for reduction of sound levels in patient care areas were made consistently by investigators. Reports of actual institution of such measures with follow-up evaluation were lacking, however. Limited data reported from the one follow-up study (Hurst, 1966) suggested that the phenomenon of adaptation to high sound levels among staff would be a continuing problem in making such programs successful.

Light

A large literature exists on the biological effects of natural light on animals and humans. Such effects relate to hormonal and metabolic balance, entrainment of biological rhythms, and skin and eye effects. Some of this knowledge has been translated into therapeutic use through employment of the artificial equivalent, phototherapy, for the treatment of neonatal jaundice and dermatologic and other disorders. Less research attention has been paid to effects of the artificial luminous environment in which much of the care of patients takes place. Clinical articles about newborn nurseries and neonatal and adult intensive care units consistently have contained conjectures about possible effects of continuous lighting on sleep, biological rhythms, and, in adults, psychological reactance. There is evidence now of the association of continuous bright nursery illumination with the incidence of retinopathy in premature infants (Glass et al., 1985).

Knowledge of age-related changes in the human eye has alerted persons to problems of glare, distinguishing between colors, and boundary recognition among older persons. Increased knowledge about ultraviolet irradiation and Vitamin D synthesis in relation to calcium metabolism and bone fragility in the aged also has created interest in the metabolic effects of long-term artificial light conditions on aged or immobilized persons who spend their time indoors (Dattani, Exton-Smith, & Stephen, 1984; Neer et al., 1971).

Shoobs (1973) treated light as a potential developmental stimulus. Day–night lighting was alternated as an experimental condition for low-birth-weight infants to determine whether this would effect differences in developmental behavior compared to infants kept in the usual continuous light of the nursery. No differences were found.

Other nurse investigators who have examined presumed effects of light have framed their studies within Rogers' conceptualization (1970) that human beings and their environments are comprised of electrical and magnetic energy fields, with change in the patterning of energy waves of either giving rise to simultaneous change in the other. Studies based on that conceptualization have included investigation of differing wavelengths of light on heart rate (Cortes, 1976), visual selective-attention behavior in hyperactive and nonhyperactive children (Joyce, 1982), the experience of pain (McDonald, 1981), and judgment about loudness of sound (Singel, 1980). Malinski (1980) hypothesized that the more hyperactive a child, the more preference there would be for hues associated with short wavelength light and the more ability to identify numbers illuminated with that wavelength. Results of these studies have shown no support, or equivocal support, for stated hypotheses. Although the theoretical underpinnings of the studies are of interest, the difficulties of attempting to study these phenomena as bivariate relationships also were demonstrated.

Color

Color is known to have biological cue functions in certain organisms, to elicit certain psychophysiologic reactions in humans, and to have aesthetic and symbolic meaning (Schaie, 1966). Color discrimination also is known to be affected by advancing age (Gilbert, 1957). However, probably because there is no evidence that certain hues actually affect health, the use of color in patient care areas has been left largely to administrators' or decorators' preferences. Birren (1979) stated that certain principles should guide use of color in hospitals, but studies of patient behavior under different color conditions are lacking.

During the 1960s color in nurses' uniforms was a cause of debate, and a number of rather poorly designed studies appeared that purported to show evidence for or against the wearing of colored versus white uniforms. At present the clinical literature in gerontological nursing contains discussions of the potential positive results of using color for stimulus, identification, and orienting purposes. Evaluation studies of such use have not been done.

The Thermal Environment

Concern with the thermal environment in patient care usually takes the form of questions about patient comfort in different ambient temperatures, or the physiologic effects of variant temperatures on vulnerable populations. Populations considered vulnerable to adverse effects of temperature extremes include patients under anesthesia; patients with spinal cord injuries; infants, especially those of low birth weight; persons with cardiac conditions or burns; and the elderly. In the medical literature, temperature and humidity are noted to affect specific processes such as wound healing (Pollack, 1979).

Neal and Nauen (1968) studied the ability of low-birth-weight infants to maintain their body temperature when transferred from incubators to regular cribs in a nursery. The results were difficult to interpret, but over half of the infants achieved normal axillary temperatures within 24 hours after the transfer. This study was the only empirical nursing research found on the thermal environment. A model of adaptation to the thermal environment, however, was presented by Erickson (1982).

Weather

Numerous atmospheric stimuli are believed to have physiologic and psychologic effects on human beings. Human biometeorology commands limited attention and funding in this country, however. The lack of attention may be due partially to skepticism about inferring cause and effect in this field. Inquiry suffers, too, because of frequent identification of the topic with folklore.

Weather is experienced as a combination of thermal and light stimuli, air pressure, air movement, and humidity; of all the atmospheric stimuli, weather is acknowledged most frequently as an influence on health. Certain disorders such as asthma, bronchitis, and rheumatic diseases are reported to change in symptomatology in accord with weather changes. Climatotherapy is prescribed frequently for persons with weather-sensitive disorders, but evaluation of effect tends to be anecdotal.

Mood and behavior changes also have been linked with changes in season, altitude, barometric pressure, humidity, temperature, air turbulence, and climate (Moos, 1976). Tromp noted particularly the physiologic effects of weather (1963, 1971) and strongly advocated greater scientific development of human biometeorology (1971). Changes in therapeutic properties of drugs under different environmental conditions may be of special relevance (Rosen, 1978–1979; Tromp, 1963).

In the nursing literature, Flynn's study (1965) was an attempt to examine the diurnal relationship of blood pressure readings in healthy young women to atmospheric pressure, ambient temperatures, and relative humidity. The findings were negative or equivocal with respect to those relationships. In retrospect, the study demonstrated the gain that access to climate-controlled chambers rather than natural conditions would have provided.

Attempts have been made to link phases of the moon with number of births and with psychologic effects. Indices such as number of suicides, homicides, and psychiatric hospital admissions have been used as presumed evidence of the latter effect. Campbell and Beets (1978), however, concluded after a review of such studies that the few positive findings were undoubtedly Type I error. Bonk (1979) also found that the number of untoward events that occurred in one hospital over 4 years bore no relationship to lunar phases.

TOWARD THERAPEUTIC ENVIRONMENTS

The physical environment serves two important, related functions in therapeutic environments: a symbolic role and a role in facilitating therapeutic processes (Canter & Canter, 1979). Difficulties in structuring the physical environment to serve those functions occurs when the therapeutic goals are ambiguous or when one setting must serve many users and functions.

The report by Kraegel and others (1974) exemplified the value of setting explicit goals for optimizing a total environment. With that exception, planned, comprehensive efforts spearheaded by nurses to create and evaluate therapeutic environments for patient populations were not found in the literature. Large-scale efforts, of course, involve facility administrators, architects, and planners, as well as the several groups who will use the facility. Furthermore, government and private funding for demonstration units has been minimal.

A few examples illustrate avenues nurses have taken in investigating the effect of existing or experimentally created environments relative to limited therapeutic goals. In an early study, Ringholtz and Morris (1961) examined the possible differential extent to which multiparous and primiparous mothers in a new rooming-in setting experienced satisfaction, anxiety, and rest. They found little difference between the two groups on these variables but concluded that an important influencing factor was the enthusiasm and positive attitude of the staff toward rooming-in. Keefe (1984) found that mothers' sleep did not vary significantly in a rooming-in setting compared to non-rooming-in. Differences occurred, however, in the sleep–wake patterns of infants in the rooming-in group compared to those in the nursery environment.

The goal of reducing further the "unnatural" fragmentation of the family that occurs during childbirth in traditional hospital settings resulted in the concept of alternative birthing environments, a natural extension of rooming-in. The goal also was to reduce the possibility of cross-infections. Whether such environments have long-term effects on family and sibling relationships has not been investigated. Griffing (1983) found no differences in prenatal and postnatal complications, anxiety, or stress in mothers delivering in a traditional labor and delivery setting and in a hospital-based alternate birthing center. Littlefield and Adams (1987) found that women in an alternative birthing center had higher satisfaction with and a greater sense of participation in the birth experience than those who delivered in a conventional labor and delivery setting. Self-selection effects and staff preferences and enthusiasm are always possibilities, however, whenever choice of setting is voluntary and when the setting is "new."

An excellent example of how information on environment can be examined relative to a future goal of care was Ryden's study (1985) of environmental supports for autonomy in nursing home residents. Three aspects of the environment — physical, social, and organizational — had certain characteristics that were unsupportive of self-determination. Several of those characteristics were judged to be potentially amenable to change.

Some investigators have attempted to create orienting environments for older patients. Williams, Campbell, Raynor, Mlynarczyk, and Ward (1985) demonstrated that it was possible to reduce the extent of older patients' postoperative confusion after hip fracture repair by a combination of environmental changes and interpersonal approaches. The difficulty, though, of ascribing relative effectiveness to the individual methods employed was acknowedged. Nagley (1984) also used interventions that included environmental manipulations in her study of confusion in older patients. The control and experimental groups were on different units and had differing diagnoses, which may have introduced factors contributing to the finding of no outcome difference.

Provisions of an orienting environment is an assumed central feature of the reality orientation programs carried out in many nursing homes. However, two reviewers (Burton, 1982; Campos, 1984) of the equivocal, and even negative, results to date have suggested that a reason for those results may be that the total environmental context actually is given limited attention.

Provision of a more positive environment for patients also has been facilitated through formative evaluation by users. This approach was used in a study by Hoffman, Donckers, and Hauser (1978) in which physical and social environmental stressors identified by patients in a coronary care unit were the basis for in-service classes on suggested interventions. Postintervention results from a comparable group of patients showed that the interventions had reduced overall stress levels. Comparisons of the physical and social environments of 24 hospital units and the effects of introduced changes were reported by Porter and Watson (1985). Whether differences in environmental ratings could be related to patient care outcomes was not examined, however.

SUMMARY AND RESEARCH DIRECTIONS

It is evident from this review that the physical environment for patient care has commanded limited attention from nurse researchers. A number of reasons can be advanced for that, but an overarching reason, perhaps, is that the physical environment has been incorporated minimally into the mainstream of behavioral science (Lawton, 1982). Much of the nursing literature on patient care is drawn explicitly from the behavioral sciences. These sciences are characterized by defining environmental influences as social, that is, those from family, peers, work supervisors, group processes, norms, and the like (Lawton, 1982). The physical environment, unlike the social environment, then becomes an explicit focus in nursing only when concepts from the field of environment and health are under consideration. In the field of environment and health the physical environment is linked primarily with stress and disease. The net result is that conscious use of the physical environment in enhancing therapeutic goals and activities in patient care is not emphasized.

The studies reviewed here share several characteristics in addition to being few in number. Consistent with much of the literature in both environment and health and environmental psychology, a limited number of variables were included in study designs. In addition, there was a striking gap between most of the studies, which were largely atheoretical, and those that were based on Rogers' (1970) abstract conceptual framework. The general lack of significant findings using that framework was apparent, and for the most part the reports have remained in dissertation form. It is clear that grand theories about environment and person relations leave much to be desired in guiding empirical study. Development of conceptual frameworks with more empirical referents is needed, as is attention to the role of mediating variables in persons' response to dimensions of the environment.

Beyond the foregoing observations, it is difficult to draw conclusions based on the few studies that appeared in each of the seven topical areas. The purpose of this chapter, however, is to stimulate research. The following suggestions are offered in that sense.

To begin, the need is not simply for more research. A large amount of information already exists that is not yet incorporated into patient care. For example, one hardly needs more "proof" that changing seating arrangements in institutions will change patterns of interaction among those who use the area, or that excess noise will keep some patients awake at night, although such studies may sensitize persons to the problem. Nor does one need further documentation that more travel time is needed to reach patients in a single or double corridor unit plan with service areas clustered at one end than is needed when service areas are centrally located.

At the same time, other types of solid descriptive studies are needed. For example, most of the existing information that is used in the design or redesign of facilities was obtained from well persons. Little is known about changes in perceptions of the environment when one is physically ill or mentally or emotionally impaired. There is a need to "get into the patient's world," a process that requires skilled and sensitive observation and interaction over time. Use of projective techniques and other qualitative research methods might be incorporated usefully.

The clinical literature in geriatric nursing increasingly contains references to the need to modify environments for the elderly. Adoption of many of those ideas is long overdue, but comparative studies need to be done relative to the effectiveness of certain modifications. Older persons, in effect, are in danger of prescription as a homogeneous group. Many of the environmental modifications urged for nursing homes and retirement residences also should be considered for incorporation in acute-care hospitals, with the same proviso that comparative evaluations be made.

At the other end of the age continuum are newborns, another group highly vulnerable to their environment. The environmental docility hypothesis nowhere is epitomized better than in the case of neonates, who can exert no control over their environment and, hence, are highly open to its effects. Concerns about effects of institutional light and noise are particularly relevant here. Longitudinal studies of individuals who have spent prolonged periods in intensive care units are indicated relative to a variety of possible physical and social-environmental effects.

Studies especially are needed that evolve from the question, "What therapeutic goal or functional process needs to be supported?" The creation of an environment that will support that goal or function then can proceed. Both the physical and social environment may need modification, and insofar as possible the research design should incorporate evaluation of both the extent of goal achievement and the processes served by the environmental manipulations. The difficulties involved in the latter are several, however. Changes in the physical environment generally are measurable, but changes in the social environment are measured with difficulty. Existing assessment tools need to be scrutinized carefully for their appropriateness to the situation, and, undoubtably, new tools are needed.

Study is needed relative to how environments can be structured to allow patients more control. Often this is interpreted as meaning providing more input into decision making about treatment. That is important, but in many instances increased control of one's immediate physical environment also can be implemented. Allied questions for study concern the conditions under which persons want or do not want increased control over their environment.

Finally, demonstration units are needed. Environmental changes to facilitate processes for care often are extensive, and their implementation in existing settings may be prohibitively difficult. Such demonstration units should incorporate means of varying the social and organizational environment as well as the physical environment.

REFERENCES

Allekian, C. I. (1973). Intrusions of territory and personal space. *Nursing Research, 22,* 236–241.

Altman, I. (1975). *The environment and social behavior.* Monterey, CA: Brooks/Cole.

Baldassare, M. (1978). Human spatial behavior. *Annual Review of Sociology, 4,* 29–56.

Baum, A., & Singer, J. E. (Eds.). (1982). *Advances in environmental psychology: Vol. 4. Environment and health.* Hillsdale, NJ: Erlbaum.

Birren, F. (1979). Human response to color and light. *Hospitals, 53*(14), 93–96.

Bonk, J. R. (1979). Don't pass the buck: The full moon is not responsible for an increase in the occurrence of untoward events in a hospital setting. *Journal of Psychiatric Nursing and Mental Health Services, 17*(5), 33–36.

Brown, E. L. (1961). *Newer dimensions of patient care, Part 1, The use of the physical and social environment of the general hospital for therapeutic purposes.* New York: Russell Sage Foundation.

Burton, M. (1982). Reality orientation for the elderly: A critique. *Journal of Advanced Nursing, 7,* 427–433.

Campbell, D. E., & Beets, J. L. (1978). Lunacy and the moon. *Psychological Bulletin, 85,* 1123–1129.

Campbell, J. L. (1984). Anxiety and satisfaction of patients in four hospital designs. *Dissertation Abstracts International, 46,* 112-B. (University Microfilms No. 8504987)

Campos, R. G. (1984). Does reality orientation work? *Journal of Gerontological Nursing, 10,* 53–64.

Canter, D., & Canter, S. (Eds.). (1979). *Designing for therapeutic environments: A review of research.* Chichester, England: Wiley.

Collett, B. A. (1974). Variation in body temperature, perceived duration and perceived personal space. *International Journal of Nursing Studies, 11,* 47–60.

Cortes, R. A. (1976). An investigation of the relationship between lightwaves and cardiac rate. *Dissertation Abstracts International, 37,* 696-B. (University Microfilms No. 76-19,018)

Dattani, J. T., Exton-Smith, A. N., & Stephen, J. M. L. (1984). Vitamin D status of the elderly in relation to age and exposure to sunlight. *Human Nutrition: Clinical Nutrition, 38C,* 131–137.

Davies, A. D. M., & Peters, M. (1983). Stresses of hospitalization in the elderly: Nurses' and patients' perceptions. *Journal of Advanced Nursing, 8,* 99–105.

Donaldson, S. K. (1977). Critique of "Effects of noise on fatigue in healthy middle-aged adults." In M. Batey (Ed.), *Communicating nursing research: Vol. 8. Nursing research priorities: Choice or change* (pp. 35–40). Boulder, CO: Western Interstate Commission for Higher Education.

Dunlap, R. E. (1979). Environmental sociology. *Annual Review of Sociology, 5,* 243–273.

Erickson, R. (1982). A model of adaptation to the thermal environment. *Advances in Nursing Science, 4*(4), 1–12.

Evans, G. W. (Ed.). (1982). *Environmental stress.* Cambridge, England: Cambridge University Press.

Falk, S. A., & Woods, N. F. (1973). Hospital noise—levels and potential health hazards. *New England Journal of Medicine, 289,* 774–781.

Ferris, G. R., & Rowland, K. M. (1985). Physical design implications for the performance evaluation process. *Nursing Administration Quarterly, 9*(3), 55–63.

Flynn, E. D. (1965). Diurnal relationships between ambient meteorological phenomena and blood pressure in women. *Nursing Science, 3,* 392–413.

Gagneaux, V., & Shaver, D. V. (1977). Distractions at nurses' stations during intershift report. *Nursing Research, 26,* 42–46.

Geden, E. A., & Begeman, A. V. (1981). Personal space preferences of hospitalized adults. *Research in Nursing and Health, 4,* 237–241.

Gilbert, J. G. (1957). Age changes in color matching. *Gerontologist, 12,* 210–215.

Gioiella, E. C. (1978). The relationship between slowness of response, state anxiety, social isolation and self-esteem, and preferred personal space in the elderly. *Journal of Gerontological Nursing, 4,* 40–43.

Glass, P., Avery, G. B., Subramanian, K. N. S., Keys, M. P., Sostek, A. M., & Friendly, D. S. (1985). Effect of bright light in the hospital nursery on the incidence of retinopathy of prematurity. *New England Journal of Medicine, 313*, 401–404.

Goodrich, A. W. (1973). Some common points of weakness in hospital construction. In A. W. Goodrich, *The social and ethical significance of nursing: A series of addresses* (pp. 97–104). New Haven: Yale University School of Nursing. (Original work published in 1903)

Griffing, D. R. (1983). The effects of birthing environment upon maternal stress and anxiety during labor and delivery. *Dissertation Abstracts International, 44*, 1781-B–1782-B. (University Microfilms No. 8324438)

Hall, E. T. (1966). *The hidden dimension*. New York: Doubleday.

Haslam, P. (1970). Noise in hospitals: Its effect on the patient. *Nursing Clinics of North America, 5*, 715–724.

Hilton, B. A. (1976). Quantity and quality of patients' sleep and sleep-disturbing factors in a respiratory intensive care unit. *Journal of Advanced Nursing, 1*, 453–468.

Hilton, B. A. (1985). Noise in acute patient care areas. *Research in Nursing and Health, 8*, 283–291.

Hoffman, M., Donckers, S., & Hauser, M. (1978). The effect of nursing intervention on stress factors perceived by patients in a coronary care unit. *Heart and Lung, 7*, 804–809.

Holahan, C. J., & Saegert, S. (1973). Behavioral and attitudinal effects of large-scale variation in the physical environment of psychiatric wards. *Journal of Abnormal Psychology, 82*, 454–462.

Hurst, T. W. (1966). Is noise important in hospitals? *International Journal of Nursing Studies, 3*, 125–135.

Johnson, F. L. P. (1979). Response to territorial intrusion by nursing home residents. *Advances in Nursing Science, 1*(4), 21–34.

Joyce, B. S. (1982). An investigation of the effects of different wavelengths of visible light on visual selective attention behavior in hyperactive and nonhyperactive children. *Dissertation Abstracts International, 43*, 3536-B. (University Microfilms No. 8307681)

Keefe, M. R. (1984). The effect of the hospital environment on newborn state behavior and maternal sleep. *Dissertation Abstracts International, 45*, 1429-B. (University Microfilms No. 8418015)

Kenny, C., & Canter, D. (1979). Evaluating acute general hospitals. In D. Canter & S. Canter (Eds.), *Designing for therapeutic environments: A review of research* (pp. 309–332). Chichester, England: Wiley.

Kerr, J. A. C. (1982). An overview of theory and research related to space use in hospitals. *Western Journal of Nursing Research, 4*, 395–405.

Kerr, J. A. C. (1985). Space use, privacy, and territoriality. *Western Journal of Nursing Research, 7*, 199–219.

Kraegel, J., Mousseau, V., Goldsmith, C., & Arora, R. (1974). *Patient care systems*. Philadelphia: Lippincott.

Lawton, M. P. (1974). The human being and the institutional building. In J. Lang, C. Burnette, W. Moleski, & D. Vachon (Eds.), *Designing for human behavior: Architecture and the behavioral sciences* (pp. 60–71). Stroudsberg, PA: Dowden, Hutchinson & Ross.

Lawton, M. P. (1982). Competence, environmental press, and the adaptation of older people. In M. P. Lawton, P. G. Windley, & T. O. Byerts (Eds.), *Aging and the environment: Theoretical approaches* (pp. 33–59). New York: Springer Publishing Co.

Lawton, M. P., Windley, P. G., & Byerts, T. O. (1982). *Aging and the environment: Theoretical approaches.* New York: Springer Publishing Co.

Lewis, L. (1972). Critique of "Patient reaction to sound in an intensive coronary care unit." In M. Batey (Ed.), *Communicating Nursing Research: Vol. 5. The many sources of nursing knowledge* (pp. 93–97). Boulder, CO: Western Interstate Commission for Higher Education.

Lindheim, R., & Syme, S. L. (1983). Environments, people, and health. *Annual Review of Public Health, 4,* 335–359.

Lindsley, O. R. (1964). Geriatric behavioral prosthetics. In R. Kastenbaum (Ed.), *New thoughts on old age* (pp. 41–60). New York: Springer Publishing Co.

Littlefield, V. M., & Adams, B. N. (1987). Patient participation in alternative perinatal care: Impact on satisfaction and health locus of control. *Research in Nursing & Health, 10,* 139–148.

Louis, M. (1981). Personal space boundary needs of elderly persons: An empirical study. *Journal of Gerontological Nursing, 7,* 395–400.

Lukas, J. S. (1975). Noise and sleep: A literature review and a proposed criterion for assessing effect. *Journal of the Acoustical Society of America, 58,* 1232–1242.

Macdonald, M. R., Schentag, J. J., Ackerman, W. B., & Walsh, M. A. (1981). ICU nurses rate their work places. *Hospitals, 55*(2), 115–116, 118.

Malinski, V. M. (1980). The relationship between hyperactivity in children and perception of short wavelength light: An investigation into the conceptual system proposed by Dr. Martha E. Rogers. *Dissertation Abstracts International, 41,* 4459-B. (University Microfilms No. 8110669)

Marshall, L. A. (1972). Patient reaction to sound in an intensive coronary care unit. In M. V. Batey (Ed.), *Communicating Nursing Research: Vol. 5. The many sources of nursing knowledge* (pp. 81–92). Boulder, CO: Western Interstate Commission for Higher Education.

McDonald, S. F. (1981). A study of the relationship between visible lightwaves and the experience of pain. *Dissertation Abstracts International, 42,* 569-B. (University Microfilms No. 8117084)

Minckley, B. B. (1968). A study of noise and its relationship to patient discomfort in the recovery room. *Nursing Research, 17,* 247–250.

Moos, R. H. (1974). *Evaluating treatment environments.* New York: Wiley.

Moos, R. H. (1976). *The human context: Environmental determinants of behavior.* New York: Wiley.

Moos, R. H. (1979). Social-ecological perspectives on health. In G. C. Stone, F. Cohen, & N. E. Adler (Eds.), *Health psychology: A handbook* (pp. 523–547). San Francisco: Jossey-Bass.

Murphy, K. E. (1981). Use of territoriality in psychotherapy. *Journal of Psychiatric Nursing and Mental Health Services, 19*(3), 13–16.

Nagley, S. J. (1984). Prevention of confusion in hospitalized elderly persons. *Dissertation Abstracts International, 46,* 1732-B–1733-B. (University Microfilms No. 8420848)

Neal, M. V., & Nauen, C. M. (1968). Ability of premature infant to maintain his own body temperature. *Nursing Research, 17,* 396–402.

Neer, R. M., Davis, T. R. A., Walcott, A., Koski, S., Schepis, P., Taylor, I.,

Thorington, L., & Wurtman, R. J. (1971). Stimulation by artificial lighting of calcium absorption in elderly human subjects. *Nature, 229,* 255–257.

Nightingale, F. (1859). *Notes on nursing.* London: Harrison & Sons.

Nightingale, F. (1859). *Notes on hospitals* (2nd ed.). London: Longmans, Green and Co.

Nuffield Provincial Hospitals Trust. (1955). *Studies in the function and design of hospitals.* London: Oxford University Press.

Ogilvie, A. J. (1980). Sources and levels of noise on the ward at night. *Nursing Times, 76,* 1363–1366.

Osmond, H. (1957). Function as the basis of psychiatric ward design. *Mental Hospitals, 8,* 23–29.

Pollack, S. V. (1979). Wound healing: A review. II. Environmental factors affecting wound healing. *Journal of Dermatology, Surgery, and Oncology, 5,* 477–481.

Porter, R., & Watson, P. (1985). Environment: The healing difference. *Nursing Management, 16*(6), 19–24.

Putt, A. M. (1977). Effects of noise on fatigue in healthy middle-aged adults. In M. V. Batey (Ed.), *Communicating Nursing Research: Vol. 8. Nursing research priorities: Choice or chance* (pp. 24–34). Boulder, CO: Western Interstate Commission for Higher Education.

Reizenstein, J. E. (1982). Hospital design and human behavior: A review of the recent literature. In A. Baum & J. E. Singer (Eds.), *Advances in environmental psychology: Vol. 4. Environment and health* (pp. 137–169). Hillsdale, NJ: Erlbaum.

Richards, J. M., Jr. (1978). Review of the Social Climate Scales. In O. Buros (Ed.), *Eighth mental measurements yearbook* (pp. 1085–1087). Highland Park, NJ: Gryphon.

Ringholtz, S., & Morris, M. (1961). A test of some assumptions about rooming-in. *Nursing Research, 10,* 196–199.

Rogers, M. (1970). *An introduction to the theoretical basis of nursing.* Philadelphia: Davis.

Rosen, S. (1978–1979). Weathering: How the atmosphere conditions health. *Medical Dimensions, 7*(9), 21–33.

Russell, J. A., & Ward, L. M. (1982). Environmental psychology. *Annual Review of Psychology, 33,* 651–688.

Ryden, M. B. (1985). Environmental support for autonomy in the institutionalized elderly. *Research in Nursing and Health, 8,* 363–371.

Schaie, K. W. (1966). On the relation of color and personality. *Journal of Projective Techniques and Personality Assessment, 30,* 512–524.

Seelye, A. (1982). Hospital ward layout and nurse staffing. *Journal of Advanced Nursing, 7,* 195–201.

Shoobs, D. S. (1973). The relationship between exposure to light and neonatal developmental behavior in the infant of low birth weight. *Dissertation Abstracts International, 34,* 2740-B. (University Microfilms No. 73-30,126)

Singel, J. F. (1980). A study of white light, blue light, and red light and the judgment of loudness. *Dissertation Abstracts International, 41,* 2123-B. (University Microfilms No. 8027488)

Stokols, D. (1978). Environmental psychology. *Annual Review of Psychology, 29,* 253–295.

Storlie, F. J. (1976). Does urban noise represent a hazard to health? *Dissertation*

Abstracts International, 38, 148-B-149-B. (University Microfilms No. 77-14,260)

Thompson, J., & Goldin, G. (1975). *The hospital: A social and architectural history.* New Haven: Yale University Press.

Topf, M. (1983a). Noise pollution in the hospital. *New England Journal of Medicine, 309,* 53-54.

Topf, M. (1983b). Physiological and psychological effects of hospital noise upon postoperative patients. *Dissertation Abstracts International, 38,* 148-B-149-B. (University Microfilms No. 8309650)

Topf, M. (1984). A framework for research on aversive physical aspects of the environment. *Research in Nursing and Health, 7,* 35-42.

Tromp, S. W. (1963). *Medical biometeorology.* Amsterdam: Elsevier Publishing.

Tromp, S. W. (1971). Future scientific developments in human biometeorology. *Annals of the New York Academy of Sciences, 184,* 43-61.

Whitehead, C. C., Polsky, R. H., Crookshank, C., & Fik, E. (1984). Objective and subjective evaluation of psychiatric ward redesign. *American Journal of Psychiatry, 141,* 639-644.

Williams, M. A., Campbell, E. B., Raynor, W. J., Mlynarczyk, S. M., & Ward, S. E. (1985). Reducing acute confusional states in elderly patients with hip fracture. *Research in Nursing and Health, 8,* 329-337.

Wood, M. (1977). Clinical sensory deprivation: A comparative study of patients in single care and two-bed rooms. *Journal of Nursing Administration, 7,* 28-32.

Woods, N. F., & Falk, S. A. (1974). Noise stimuli in the acute care area. *Nursing Research, 23,* 144-150.

Chapter 4

Social Support

JANE S. NORBECK
SCHOOL OF NURSING
UNIVERSITY OF CALIFORNIA, SAN FRANCISCO

CONTENTS

Nurses have played an important role from the beginning in the interdisciplinary field of social support research. As the field changes from its current predominant emphasis on methodological and descriptive research to emphasis on applied research, the contributions of nurses might expand because of the natural access that nurses have to people undergoing life transitions, crises, and illnesses.

This chapter contains a review of the studies conducted by nurse investigators in a variety of areas of social support. The work done by this group is similar to that conducted by colleagues in other disci-

Appreciation is expressed to Lou Ellen Barnes for assistance in locating articles for this review and to the anonymous reviewers for their insightful criticism and helpful suggestions in revising this manuscript.

plines. A complete understanding of the state of knowledge in any subarea of social support research requires consideration of research results from all sources. The objectives of this chapter were to organize, describe, and analyze the research conducted about social support by nurses and to suggest avenues for future research to optimize the contribution that nurses can make to this field.

INTERDISCIPLINARY PROGRESS IN SOCIAL SUPPORT RESEARCH

Interest in the concept of social support began in the mid-1970s with the publication of review articles by Caplan (1974), Cassel (1976), and Cobb (1976). These authors described the deleterious effects of social isolation or low social integration on health outcomes. A classic among the studies that predated the use of the term *social support* was the study of pregnancy complications by the nurse investigator Nuckolls, which was published with Cassel and Kaplan (Nuckolls, Cassel, & Kaplan) in 1972.

With the use of the term social support and several complementary definitions, a rapid surge of research activity unfolded in the fields of anthropology, behavioral medicine, epidemiology, nursing, psychiatry, psychology, and sociology. To date, several hundred research articles have been published in a wide variety of journals as well as numerous conceptual and literature review articles and several books devoted exclusively to the concept. Within nursing both national (cf. R. A. O'Brien, 1985) and international (cf. Norbeck, 1986) research conferences on social support were held in 1985, and a research roundtable was held in 1982 that resulted in a book on social support in relation to vulnerable infants (Barnard, Brandt, Raff, & Carroll, 1984).

The basic conceptual model underpinning social support research is shown in Figure 4.1. This model is oversimplified, but it is useful to depict the essential relationships proposed in most research in this field. The model shows that stress is related to health outcomes (arrow d) and that social support buffers the effect of stress on health (arrow b). Social support also has direct effects on stress (arrow a) and on health outcomes (arrow c). These relationships have been supported in many correlational studies, but many authors have noted that

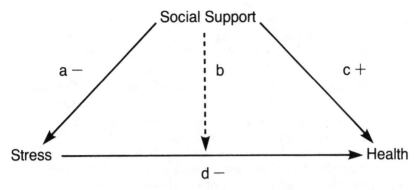

Figure 4.1. Simplified conceptual model of stress, social support, and health.

the relationships in the social support model are likely to be bidirectional and that longitudinal studies are needed to unravel the actual cause and effect relationships that exist. In addition, other variables not in the model also may contribute to health outcomes.

Just as agreement has not been reached as to the exact components that should be included in the definition of social support, optimal measurement of social support has not been attained as yet. There are, however, at least 10 published instruments with acceptable levels of reliability and validity (Norbeck, 1985a). These first-generation instruments will be supplanted in time by instruments based on sound conceptual definitions and advanced formats. In the meantime it is now possible to compare findings from study to study because many researchers have moved beyond the use of idiosyncratic, unvalidated measures.

SELECTION OF STUDIES FOR REVIEW

Nurse-authored studies on social support from 1972 to 1985 were located through the (a) *Cumulative Index of Nursing and Allied Health Literature, Index Medicus,* and *Social Sciences Citation Index*; (b) hand searches of current contents for the following nursing journals: *Advances in Nursing Science, International Journal of Nursing Studies, Journal of Advanced Nursing, Nursing Research,*

Research in Nursing and Health, Western Journal of Nursing Research, and many clinical nursing journals; (c) hand searches of current contents of the interdisciplinary journals that frequently publish social support articles: *American Journal of Community Psychology, Journal of Behavioral Medicine, Journal of Community Psychology, Journal of Health and Social Behavior,* and *Social Science and Medicine*; (d) hand searches of bibliography entries of recently published articles; and (e) correspondence with authors active in the field. The search was limited to sources published or in press in readily available journals and books rather than proceedings or abstracts. References concerning the related construct of social network were not included unless social support also was addressed.

Among the nurse-authored publications, 67 were research articles that represented 53 studies. Correlational designs were used in 62% of the studies, and sampling by convenience in 85%. In the 40 studies in which social support was measured directly as a variable, only 28% of the investigators used instruments with established reliability and validity. Fifty-five percent of the studies were designed using measures with no reported reliability or validity, except for occasional mention of content validity. The remaining 18% of the studies were designed using instruments in which only reliability was known, and this was usually limited to internal consistency reliability.

CONTRIBUTIONS OF NURSE RESEARCHERS TO THE FIELD

The studies were organized for review into three categories: (a) instrument development; (b) descriptive studies in the areas of life transitions, role performance, health behavior, and crisis or illness behavior; and (c) intervention studies.

Instrument Development

In 1981 two research teams reported on general social support instruments that now have well-established reliability and validity. The Personal Resources Questionnaire (PRQ) developed by Brandt and Weinert (1981) was based on Weiss' (1974) five categories of relational functions. The PRQ measured number of social support resources, satisfaction with assistance received, and perceived social support. Continued work with the instrument has resulted in careful revisions and additional testing of psychometric properties with various populations (Weinert, in press; Weinert & Brandt, 1987). Overall, the authors have provided evidence for content validity, internal consistency reliability, test–retest reliability, predictive validity, and freedom from social desirability response bias.

The Norbeck Social Support Questionnaire (NSSQ) (Norbeck, Lindsey, & Carrieri, 1981, 1983) was based on the definition of social support proposed by Kahn (1979). The format of this instrument was one in which respondents listed their social support network members and then rated these individuals on a series of questions related to functional properties of social support and to structural network properties. The two reports presented a basis for content validity and data to support internal consistency reliability, test–retest reliability, concurrent validity, predictive validity, construct validity, freedom from social desirability response bias, and normative data from employed adults.

Preliminary work has been reported for two special-purpose instruments. Ellison (1983) described an instrument to measure parental support to school-aged children and presented data on internal consistency reliability and normative data from parents and children. Although the overall internal consistency of the instrument was acceptable, further work is needed to improve the internal consistency of the subscales and to establish other types of reliability and validity. Tilden and Galyen (1987) reported work on an instrument, Cost and Reciprocity of Social Support, based on social exchange and equity theories. Internal consistency reliability was acceptable for the instrument as a whole and for all but the conflict subscale. The conceptual underpinning of this instrument was derived from dimensions of social network interaction that need attention in the social support literature. Because the full instrument has not been used in conjunction with the other variables in the stress and social support model of health, it will be important to determine empirically if information on cost, conflict, and reciprocity increases the predictive power over instruments that only measure positive aspects of social support.

Through empirical results from factor analysis, two nurse researchers have challenged the frequently stated notion that social support is a multidimensional construct. Brown (1986a) developed a 45-item instrument based on House's (1981) four categories for use with expectant mothers and fathers. Through several methods of analysis, data from 626 respondents revealed only one dominant factor that explained 48% of the variance in partner support and 61% in support from others. In a similar fashion, Ide (1983) analyzed the data from 85 elderly clients on a measure that produced a single score for each of nine dimensions of social network support. All but the dimension of density loaded on a single factor that explained 70% of the variance. Because density did not have health-protective effects in a larger study, Ide recommended deleting it from the measure. The results from these studies provided evidence that social support may not have been a multidimensional construct. Neither investigator used an instrument with fully developed reliability and validity, so further work is needed to clarify the issue of dimensionality. However, an important assumption has been challenged by both Brown and Ide.

Descriptive Studies

Research with clinical populations encountered in nursing practice has been a major contribution of nurse investigators to the social support field. Studies of this type have been categorized into four areas: (a) life transitions, (b) role performance, (c) health behavior, and (d) crisis or illness behavior.

Life Transitions.   Of the life transitions of interest to nursing, social support has been studied with pregnancy and aging. The results of seven studies affirmed that social support was important in relation to complications of pregnancy (Norbeck & Tilden, 1983; Nuckolls et al., 1972), psychological or physical health of expectant parents (Brown, 1986b; Tilden, 1983, 1984), and adaptation to parenthood (Cranley, 1984; Cronenwett, 1984, 1985a, 1985b; Mercer, Hackley, & Bostrom, 1983, 1984). All were correlational studies; four were designed using prospective or longitudinal measures, and three with concurrent measures. These studies were designed using unvalidated social support instruments and convenience sampling. All of the studies had middle-class subjects, with the exception of a teenage subsample in one study (Mercer et al., 1983, 1984); thus, the results have limited generalizability to most groups of high-risk pregnant women.

The results of the prospective correlational study by Nuckolls et al. (1972) showed that among high-stress pregnant women, those with high psychosocial assets had a complication rate of 33% compared to 91% for women with low psychosocial assets, a threefold increase.

This study predated the social support era, and the variable of psychosocial assets was a confounding of social support with emotional states and attitudes toward pregnancy. Thus, replication of this important study was needed.

Norbeck and Tilden (1983) designed a prospective correlational study of pregnancy complications to examine the effects of life stress, social support, and emotional disequilibrium as separately measured variables in a medically normal population of middle-class women. In the full sample of 117 women, only life stress was predictive of overall complications, and emotional disequilibrium of infant complications. In the subsample of 81 women for whom data on life stress during the second half of the pregnancy was available, the interaction of stress during pregnancy and tangible social support accounted for 6% of the variance in both gestation and labor and delivery complications and 9% in infant complications. Although the size of the social support buffering effects was smaller than Nuckolls et al. (1972) found, the findings from this study showed that the relationships remained even when preexisting medical risk factors were controlled and psychosocial variables were measured as separate constructs. In an expanded sample ($n = 141$) from this population, Tilden (1983, 1984) reported on the relationships among life stress, social support, and emotional disequilibrium and the relationship of partner status to eight subscale scores for these variables. The amount of variance in emotional disequilibrium explained by life stress was 30%, and by social support only 3%. In the 1984 report, three of the seven hypotheses regarding differences between single and partnered women were reported to be supported: single women had higher stress, higher state anxiety, and lower tangible social support than partnered women; however, only the difference in tangible support would be significant if the study alpha level were controlled (Reid, 1983).

Mercer et al. (1983, 1984) studied 294 primiparous women of three age groups in a longitudinal correlational study of perception of childbirth and maternal role attainment. Over 25 psychosocial and obstetric variables were measured with interview questions. Perception of childbirth was found to be most highly related to emotional support from the mate and early interaction with the infant (Mercer et al., 1983). In the 1984 report, the relationship of social support to the maternal role attainment of the 66 teenage mothers was presented. This age group presented both response rate (48%) and attrition problems (40% lost) to the investigators over the year-long study. At early postpartum, both informational support and the presence of the mate in labor and delivery were related to maternal role attainment. At 1 month, many social support and other variables were related significantly to maternal role attainment; however, at 4, 8, and 12 months only isolated social support variables were related to maternal role attainment and in an inconsistent manner.

Cranley (1984) studied the construct of fetal attachment in relation to social support and dyadic adjustment with 30 pregnant women and 326 expectant couples. Fetal attachment had low but significant correlations with social support from family and friends and with dyadic adjustment, and high correlations with social support from physicians.

Cronenwett (1984, 1985a, 1985b) reported on a longitudinal correlational study of 58 middle-class couples who were expecting their first child. The subjects were tested before delivery and at three time periods postpartum. The response rate of about 45% was low; however, the dropout rate of 14% was not high. The 1984 report showed that size of network was the most consistent network property related to social support. Men and women had very similar network characteristics. In the 1985b report the investigator gave evidence that over time new parents reshaped the composition of their networks by replacing certain network members with people who were also parents. In the 1985a article Cronenwett reported that emotional and instrumental support were related to adaptation to parenthood, but informational and appraisal support were not. The network properties of size, percent kin, and density also were related to adaptation to parenthood, but differently for fathers and mothers.

In a correlational study, Brown (1986b) studied the influence of social support and stress on health with 313 expectant couples. For expectant fathers, partner support explained most of the variance in their health, whereas for mothers, stress explained more of the variance in their health than did support variables. The overall pattern of results gave evidence that for men the spouse was the primary source of support; in contrast, women benefited from both partner support and support from other people, at least during pregnancy.

In the area of aging, social support was studied in relation to home care (Lindsey & Hughes, 1981), institutionalization (Brock & O'Sullivan, 1985), and physical and psychological health (Fuller & Larson, 1980; Laschinger, 1984; Pohl & Fuller, 1980). All four of these studies were designed using random sampling methods; however, unvalidated measures of social support were used in three studies. One study was descriptive, another ex post facto, and two correlational.

Lindsey and Hughes (1981) described the functions or activities that the support person provided to 112 elderly persons who had participated in a Geriatric Evaluation Service. In this descriptive study the investigators showed that the family provided most of the care to the elderly subject, with little use of community resources.

Brock and O'Sullivan (1985) used an ex post facto design to determine the variables that distinguished elderly persons who were newly institutionalized from those who were residing and functioning in the community. In comparisons between 47 community residents and 40 nursing home residents, social support network measured by the Pattison Social Network Inventory (Pattison, Defrancisco, Wood, Frazier, & Crowder, 1975) accounted for 25% of the variance in group membership after the effects of age had been controlled. No other demographic or health status variables were related significantly to group membership; thus lack of social support resources was the crucial variable in predicting institutionalization.

A correlational study of 110 elderly residents who recently had experienced relocation to a residential unit for the aged (Fuller & Larson, 1980; Pohl & Fuller, 1980) had mixed results. Social interaction and emotional support were related to morale, but emotional support was not related significantly, either as main or buffering effect, to physical health outcomes. Similarly, in a correlational study Laschinger (1984) did not find that social support was related to functional health among 25 elderly persons living in their homes; however, for men social support was related significantly to psychological well-being. The findings of these two studies were consistent in showing association with psychological, but not physical, health outcomes of the elderly.

Role Performance. Six of the 10 studies in this section were concerned with family roles (Brandt, 1984a, 1984b; Fuller & Karlson, 1981; Hentinen, 1983; Lynam, 1985; Norbeck & Sheiner, 1982; Woods, 1980, 1985) and four with worker roles (Cronin-Stubbs & Brophy, 1985; Cronin-Stubbs & Rooks, 1985; Hilbert & Allen, 1985; Hillestad, 1984; Norbeck, 1985b), all primarily with female subjects. These studies were descriptive or correlational, with one correlational study designed using prospective measures. Random sampling was used in four studies and convenience sampling in the rest. In only 4 of the 10 studies was social support measured with instruments with well-established reliability and validity.

In the correlational studies by Woods (1980, 1985) women's roles were examined to determine the effects of role proliferation on mental health and on illness episodes. The 1985 report of 140 married women with 1 to 3 roles (spouse, parent, employee) gave evidence that the number of roles the women performed was not related to their mental health but that those with traditional sex-role norms, little task-sharing support from a spouse, and little support from a confidant had poorer outcomes. The findings reported in 1980 from a subsample of 96 women who completed a family health diary for 3 weeks showed that only two variables, support for the primary role from significant others and number of children, were related to illness episodes.

Three studies of parenting under adverse or unusual conditions have been reported. In a correlational study that used the PRQ to measure social support, Brandt studied 91 mothers with a developmentally delayed child to learn the relationship between social support and negative life events (1984a) and to study the relationships between stress, social support, and restrictive maternal discipline (1984b). Significant associations were found between social support measures and negative life events; however, social support was related to restrictive discipline only for the high stress group, and not when income was controlled. Lynam (1985) presented qualitative descriptive reports of sources of support for 12 immigrant women with young children. These women moved along a pathway from exclusive use of kin for support to other people from their own culture, and finally to members of the larger society. This movement appeared to be motivated by their needs as parents in helping their children adapt and fit into the new culture. Norbeck and Sheiner (1982) studied social support sources in relation to the functioning of 30 low-income, single parents and their preschool children. The results of this correlational study provided support for the hypothesis that not having contact with a close friend was associated with parenting problems, and the mother not being close to a family member was related to child problems.

The roles of family caregiver for the elderly or of wife of an ill spouse have been examined in two studies. In a correlational study, Fuller and Karlson (1981) examined physical, psychological, and social well-being of 44 adult sons or daughters who were named as the primary source of help to their aging parents. Although family cohesiveness was related to psychological well-being, the predicted relationships among other types of social support, personal autonomy, and physical well-being were not significant. Hentinen's (1983) descriptive study of 59 wives of myocardial infarction patients 8 weeks after the infarct was focused on the wives' needs for and sources of support. More than 50% did not receive the information they needed for home care. In descending order, support was provided by relatives, neighbors, registered nurses, and physicians; 17% of the wives did not receive support from anyone. These findings point to the needs of wives for information and support during and after the husband's infarct.

Work-related roles were examined in relation to social support in four studies. Two of these concerned staff nursing, one nursing education, and one nursing administration.

The findings of a correlational study of burnout in four clinical areas with 296 nurses (Cronin-Stubbs & Brophy, 1985; Cronin-Stubbs & Rooks, 1985) showed 35 to 39% of the variance in burnout accounted for by study variables. The strongest predictors of burnout were negative life changes, lack of positive life changes, intensity of occupational stress, and social support characteristics. In another correlational study of job stress using the NSSQ, Norbeck (1985b) found that specific types and sources of social support were 2 to 3 times more predictive of psychological distress than global social support scores for 164 female critical care nurses.

Lack of significant effects of social support on educational outcome measures was reported by Hilbert and Allen (1985). In a correlational study of 125 upper division nursing students, social support, measured by the Inventory of Socially Supportive Behaviors (ISSB) (Barrera, Sandler, & Ramsay, 1981), was not related either to grade point average or nursing licensure examination scores, nor was there a significant interaction effect of social support and test anxiety on these educational outcomes. These results were difficult to interpret because this measure of enacted social support typically has produced either nonsignificant findings or significant relationships in the opposite direction than predicted in the model in Figure 4.1 (Barrera, 1981; Barrera & Balls, 1983; Barrera et al., 1981). Subsequently, Barrera (1986) distinguished among the concepts of social embeddedness, perceived support, and enacted support and proposed six alternative models to account for both positive and negative relationships between social support and stress or distress.

In a report of a pilot study and a correlational study of 80 nursing administrators, Hillestad (1984) noted that 47% reported being professionally lonely. Professional loneliness was associated with supportive relationships, personal loneliness, age, and years in service. This report lacked essential details to evaluate the research methodology or findings.

Health Behavior.   This section contains a review of four studies of compliance with the treatment regimen (Hilbert, 1985; Klinger, 1984; M. E. O'Brien, 1980; Schlenk & Hart, 1984) and three studies of health practices (Gierszewski, 1983; Hubbard, Muhlenkamp, & Brown, 1984; Stephens, 1985) that had mixed results. In one of the compliance studies (Hilbert, 1985) and two of the health practice studies (Gierszewski, 1983; Stephens, 1985) investigators failed to provide evidence for the effect of social support on these behaviors. Although problematic measurement of social support in each of these studies could have accounted for the lack of significant findings, it is also possible that social support is not conceptually valid as a predictor of compliance or health behaviors. Of these seven studies, one was descriptive, and three of the six correlational studies were designed using prospective or panel measures. All made use of convenience samples, and only two incorporated a social support instrument with both reliability and validity established.

Klinger (1984) interviewed 60 postmyocardial infarction patients in a descriptive study to identify areas related to health perception and compliance. Through content analysis the investigator showed that the single most helpful factor cited by patients was support of other people. Lack of significant effects was reported by Hilbert (1985) in a correlational study on the effects of spouse support and compliance with 60 convalescing male patients who ranged from 3 months to 17 years post-myocardial infarction. The use of enacted support as the measure may not have been a conceptually appropriate measure for this problem. Additionally, the 17-year range from the acute illness to the point of data collection may have contributed to the results.

Using a structured interview in a correlational study, M. E. O'Brien (1980) studied compliance of 126 hemodialysis patients and found that both primary group and staff support were related to compliance. Three years later staff support was much more important than primary group support; however, only half of the original sample was still alive or available to participate in the second testing, so the shift in effective sources of support may have been influenced by sample attrition effects.

Compliance with the diabetes regimen was the focus of the correlational study of 30 diabetic adults by Schlenk and Hart (1984). Health locus of control, health value, and perceived social support were independent variables. Social support explained 37% and health locus of control 13% of the variance in compliance. The social support measure was a situation-specific measure based on the chronic illness literature and specific elements of diabetic care. The high effect size points to the value in exploring situation-specific measures of social support.

Promoting a healthy lifestyle through positive health practices was examined in a correlational study by Hubbard, Muhlenkamp, and Brown (1984). Using the PRQ and a validated, investigator-developed Lifestyle Questionnaire, social support accounted for 14% and 34% of the variance in health practices in two samples, 97 upper-middle-class elderly persons from a senior citizens' center and 133 upper-middle-class participants at a health fair. Whether these findings would be applicable to less educated or affluent groups should be studied.

Gierszewski (1983) reported lack of significant findings for the effects of social support and locus of control on weight loss in a prospective correlational study of 46 participants in a company weight-control program. An unexpected finding for individuals with internal locus of control was that higher social support negatively affected weight loss. The lack of support for the study variables was not definitive because of the potential for sampling bias with only a 20% response rate and the use of an unvalidated social support measure. Conversely, the findings may have resulted from a genuine interaction between locus of control and social support, which, if substantiated, could contribute to refined conceptual modeling of the effects of social support and certain health behaviors.

Stephens (1985) studied social support and alcohol consumption in a correlational study of 311 lower-class prenatal patients. None of the social support measures was related to alcohol consumption during pregnancy. Alcohol consumption before pregnancy was related to social support in specific ways that might have been missed if general support and pregnancy support had been combined in the analysis. However, this finding was not conceptually valid because the effect was retrospective: support reported during the 4th month of pregnancy was associated with alcohol consumption prior to the pregnancy.

Crisis or Illness Behavior. Fourteen studies were focused on various crises (Ahmadi, 1985; Burgess & Holmstrom, 1978; Nikolaisen & Williams, 1980), illnesses (Dimond, 1979; Lindsey, Ahmed, & Dodd, 1985; Lindsey, Dodd, & Chen, 1985; Northouse, 1981; Piltz-Kirkby & Fox, 1982; Turner, 1979; Webb & Wilson-Barnett, 1983a; Woods & Earp, 1978), or other symptoms (Elmore, 1984; Jordan & Meckler, 1982; Magilvy, 1985). Three of these studies were descriptive; ten were correlational, and one was ex post facto. All were designed using convenience samples. Eight of the social support measures used in these studies had no evidence to support reliability or validity; two had reliability only, and only four had both reliability and validity established. The correlational studies of adaptation to illness or crises were noteworthy in controlling health status or other clinically relevant variables.

The experience of being hospitalized was studied by Ahmadi (1985) with 100 hospitalized adult patients in a correlational study. She found low but significant correlations between satisfaction with hospitalization and family or friend social support. The relationship between hospital stress and social support from other patients was positive rather than negative, implying that higher levels of hospital stress elicited social support from other patients.

The crisis of rape was studied in a longitudinal correlational study of 92 adult victims by Burgess and Holmstrom (1978). Among the many variables studied in a univariate fashion, lack of social support predicted delayed recovery: 53% of those without social support had not recovered from the rape at the 4 to 6-year follow-up, compared to 20% of those with social support. The crisis of sudden infant death was examined in a descriptive study by Nikolaisen and Williams (1980) with 54 parents. Fathers and married parents had significantly higher perceptions of helpful support than did mothers or single parents, but single status was confounded with lower socioeconomic status. Public health nurses and other parents who had experienced sudden infant death were viewed as helpful by more than 85% of the subjects. Mates also were viewed as supportive, but relatives, although usually supportive, also could be named as making matters worse.

In the area of chronic or life-threatening illness, cancer, hemodialysis, and schizophrenia have been studied. Two descriptive studies (Lindsey, Ahmed, & Dodd, 1985; Lindsey, Dodd, & Chen, 1985) were conducted to provide data on perceived social support of 40 Egyptian and 40 Taiwanese cancer patients. These studies were designed using the NSSQ as a standardized measure of social support; however, the instrument was modified significantly for the Taiwanese study. The descriptive data presented for these two groups will be useful for comparisons with other cultural groups when data from groups comparable in demographic and illness status are available. Care must be taken to avoid drawing cross-cultural conclusions from comparisons that differ not only with respect to culture but also in employment and marital status, education, age, or along extremes of the health–illness continuum. Differences in social support might be due to these extraneous variables rather than culture.

Two studies were conducted to examine emotional outcomes of cancer surgery. In a correlational study of 49 women, Woods and Earp (1978) studied the effects of mastectomy on depression 4 years after surgery. Social support was not related directly to depression, but it buffered the relationship between number of surgical complications and depression. The experience of hysterectomy in the first 4 months after surgery was studied by Webb and Wilson-Barnett (1983a, 1983b) in relation to depression and self-concept with 102 women in a correlational study. The complete pattern of results from this panel study was unclear in the reports; however, it appeared that partner support was more highly predictive of recovery than friend support, even though friend support was more readily available.

Northouse (1981) conducted a correlational study of fear of cancer recurrence with 30 women who were 1 to 4 years postmastectomy and in remission. Significant correlations were found between fear of recurrence and the number of people with whom the women could discuss their fears and the number who understood their health. This study was designed to control for age, marital status, extent of disease, type of treatment, time since surgery, and time since last treatment.

In a correlational study of 36 patients receiving hemodialysis on a renal unit Dimond (1979) found, after controlling for medical status, that family cohesiveness, family expressiveness, and spouse support were related to morale. In addition, family cohesiveness was related also to changes in social functioning. Piltz-Kirkby and Fox (1982) also studied hemodialysis, but with an ex post facto design, to compare patients receiving dialysis in the center or at home. Clients on home dialysis reported a higher level on 14 of 30 support indices than in-center patients; however, only 4 of these differences would be significant if the study alpha level were controlled (Reid, 1983).

Chronically ill schizophrenics have been a challenging group to study, and Turner (1979) was the first to study patients directly, rather than using family informants. In a correlational study, Turner interviewed 103 schizophrenics and classified 25% as disabled according to indices of troublesome behavior and social functioning. To control for extraneous variables, comparisons were made between the disabled and nondisabled groups. No differences were found in age, sex, race, duration or number of hospitalization experiences, amounts or categories of outpatient care, or intake of medication. The disabled group had lower social support scores, more lived with parents, fewer had extrahousehold contacts or friends, fewer could name a helping person, more denied having a confidant, and fewer had helping persons or confidants outside the home. Thus, social support indicators were the main distinguishing characteristics between the two groups.

Three correlational studies were conducted to address isolated symptoms: hearing loss, dysmenorrhea, and depression. Magilvy (1985) studied 66 hearing-impaired older women to examine the major influences on quality of life. Social support, as measured by the NSSQ, social hearing handicap, and perceived health together accounted for 34% of the variance in quality of life. Jordan and Meckler (1982) studied 156 female undergraduate nursing students and found that both life change scores and dysmenorrhea were higher for the low-support group than the high-support group. When multiple regression was used, more of the variance in menstrual distress was accounted for by life events (12%) than by social support (4%). Elmore (1984) divided 72 patients in a nursing stress management clinical program into clinically depressed and nondepressed groups based on their scores on a standardized measure and examined social network size and satisfaction with social support, measured by the Social Support Questionnaire (Sarason, Levine, Basham, & Sarason, 1983), for the two groups. In separate analyses for each group, only social support satisfaction was related to depression in individuals in the clinically depressed group; only life events were related to depression in individuals comprising the nondepressed group. The nondepressed group had higher social support satisfaction scores, but not higher network size scores, than the clinically depressed group.

Intervention Studies

Inclusion criteria for studies in this section were difficult to establish because some nurse authors now use the term social support to include interventions that formerly were described as group therapy, supportive nursing care, or other nursing interventions, such as patient teaching. For purposes of this review, only two types of social support interventions were included: (a) interventions designed to extend or enhance the functioning of the informal social support system, and (b) supportive interventions provided by professionals for individuals or groups who have been identified as lacking adequate social support resources.

Enhancing the Informal Support System.   Three studies were conducted to examine the functions or effectiveness of support groups (Cronenwett, 1980; Gray-Toft & Anderson, 1983; Lipson, 1981, 1982) and one to examine the effect of involving a key network member in a patient rehabilitation program (Dracup, 1985; Dracup et al., 1984). One of these studies was descriptive, one was a field case study, and two were quasi-experimental. All made use of convenience samples. Social support was described or manipulated, but not measured.

Cronenwett (1980) used questionnaire data from 66 participants to describe the characteristics of women who used postpartum support groups and to describe the types of discussions and other factors that contributed to the groups' effectiveness. Only 10% of new mothers who were invited to participate joined support groups, and these women were older, better educated, and more affluent than those who did not participate. This finding raised the question of whether this sociodemographic group was the only one that could benefit from support groups or whether these women had greater needs for support for the role of motherhood.

Lipson (1981, 1982) used a case study approach to examine support groups for women who had experienced cesarian births. The participants were primarily well-educated, middle- to upper-middle-class, married women. Participant observation and interviews were used to identify functions of the groups and problems the women discussed as they worked through their negative and unresolved feelings following cesarian delivery.

In a quasi-experimental study, Gray-Toft and Anderson (1983) developed a 9-week staff support program to assist 17 nurses in a hospice unit to cope with situations involving role conflict and ambiguity. The program resulted in a reduction in the frequency of reported stress, an increase in satisfaction with coworkers, and a reduction in turnover among hospice nurses. Although the multiple-group time-series design with staggered treatment provided control for many sources of threat to internal validity, it was unclear how much the intervention was focused on increasing coworker support or on increasing other coping skills.

In addition to support groups, another intervention to increase support from the informal social support system is to engage key network members in an intervention designed to enhance the support they can provide. The effects of spouse participation in a cardiac rehabilitation program for 58 cardiac patients was evaluated in a quasi-experimental three-group time series study (Dracup, 1985; Dracup et al., 1984). Whether compliance measures or psychological measures were used, the results showed that the two counseling intervention groups were more effective than the no-group control, but the patient-only group was equivalent or better than the spouse-participation group. In retrospect the authors noted that the two counseling groups did not appear to receive comparable interventions. Qualitative differences in group process in the patient-only group compared with the spouse-participation group might have accounted for the findings. Thus, a definitive test of the effects of spouse participation would require an intervention in which spouses receive the cardiac-rehabilitation group counseling intervention in separate groups from the patients. This design would ensure that both patient and spouse groups would experience the type of group process that in the patient-only group seemed to encourage competition and promote compliance.

Surrogate Support.   The term *surrogate support* refers to the provision of support by a professional that is designed to replace the support that is inadequate or unavailable from the patient's support network. This support might be temporary, as during a crisis, or it might be provided on an ongoing basis for socially marginal individuals.

Barnard, Snyder, and Spietz (1984) identified a population of 60 new mothers defined at high social risk because of low income, low education, living alone or with a partner who was unsupportive, inadequate support system of reliable friends and family, or multiproblem family living in a disorganized environment. In addition, these families were also dealing with biologically high-risk infants. A 3-month individualized nursing intervention program was described.

Through process evaluation based on Brammer's (1973) model of the helping process, the authors found that the intervention was ideally suited to 27 mothers who had multiple problems and needed additional support. In contrast, the intervention was not very useful for 27 mothers whose needs for additional support were not great, and the intervention was not very effective for 6 mothers who were stressed so completely that they were unable to form a helping relationship in this short time period. Thus, in this action research patterns were revealed that suggest which high-risk mothers might benefit most from short-term support augmentation.

CONCLUSIONS AND
DIRECTIONS FOR FUTURE RESEARCH

The most important contributions by nurse investigators to the wider social support field have been made through research with populations encountered in clinical practice. These contributions were strengthened further by the careful control in many of these studies of clinically relevant extraneous variables, such as health status or number of prior hospitalizations. The findings presented here will be useful to investigators both in theory development and in efforts to move the field closer to clinical application.

The findings reported in the majority of studies reviewed supported the traditional social support model. The few examples of nonsignificant findings could be accounted for by characteristics of the social support measure, sampling, or other methodological limitations; however, these findings also should stimulate reexamination of the applicability of this model for certain areas, such as health behaviors.

As is true in the broader social support field, nurse investigators of social support need to attend to important measurement and design issues. Considering that the studies reviewed here were conducted in the early years of this field, it is not surprising that unvalidated social support measures were used in the majority of studies. With the existence of several validated general social support instruments, the use of exploratory measures is now appropriate only when new concepts or approaches are studied, such as the use of situation-specific measures.

The correlational studies reviewed here have contributed to establishing the importance of social support in health-related research. Except for testing new models, the value of additional studies using correlational designs should be questioned at this time. The relationships in the traditional social support model have been supported in hundreds of studies, but correlational designs with single concurrent measures of variables are limited in establishing causality. Such designs do not permit statistical control for baseline levels of the symptoms under study.

The value of initial descriptive studies lies in how the findings can be used to design effective assessment and intervention. Now that the effects of social support have been demonstrated in numerous studies and with a great variety of population groups, it is time to shift research agendas. A question that researchers have begun to explore is: What are the key ingredients or features of social support that are protective for a particular population or for people coping with a particular disease or life stressor? Studies designed to examine specific types or sources of support have potential to contribute to this question. Another approach to understanding how social support works for specific groups or individuals is to examine personality or coping patterns, such as in the differential effects or availability of social support for persons with internal rather than external locus of control (Sandler & Lakey, 1982; Thomas & Hooper, 1983). Qualitative research also can be used to understand how social support functions for specific groups or situations.

Another step toward clinical application is the development and validation of clinical assessment measures that are briefer than existing research instruments to identify individuals who are at risk because of a combination of high stress and low social support. The assumption that increasing social support rather than reducing stressful conditions is the best alternative has been questioned only recently (Rook & Dooley, 1985).

Conceptual work is needed to distinguish the various conditions underlying inadequate social support in order to match interventions with the appropriate need. The implicit rationale of self-help or support groups as a social support intervention for certain populations often has come from a synthesis of group dynamics theory and the literature on stigma. The theoretical basis for other forms of social support interventions suggested in the nursing literature usually is not developed clearly.

Controlled intervention trials are needed to test theoretically based social support interventions. The usual difficulties and challenges presented by this form of research are compounded by the likelihood of a strong measurement effect on the control group. Study participants often comment on the insight they gained into their own social isolation after completing a social support questionnaire. If such insight stimulates these subjects to improve their social support resources on their own, the effect of an intervention for the experimental group might be difficult to demonstrate. This is one situation in which the effort required by a Solomon Four-group design would be justified.

Social support is a field of inquiry very central to the goals of nursing. Nursing was one of the first of the human service professions to integrate the physical, psychological, and social needs of patients. Although the term social support has been used in nursing only recently, for decades nurses have been assessing informally the support available to their patients and finding creative ways to supplement inadequate support. Responding to the challenge of conducting clinically relevant research in the social support field also will contribute to an essential part of nursing practice.

REFERENCES

Ahmadi, K. S. (1985). The experience of being hospitalized: Stress, social support and satisfaction. *International Journal of Nursing Studies, 22*, 137–148.

Barnard, K. E., Brandt, P. A., Raff, B. S., & Carroll, P. (Eds.). (1984). *Social support and families of vulnerable infants*. White Plains, NY: March of Dimes Birth Defects Foundation.

Barnard, K. E., Snyder, C., & Spietz, A. (1984). Supportive measures for high-risk infants and families. In K. E. Barnard, P. A. Brandt, B. S. Raff, & P. Carroll (Eds.), *Social support and families of vulnerable infants* (pp. 291–315). White Plains, NY: March of Dimes Birth Defects Foundation.

Barrera, M., Jr. (1981). Social support in the adjustment of pregnant adolescents: Assessment issues. In B. H. Gottlieb (Ed.), *Social networks and social support* (pp. 69–96). Beverly Hills, CA: Sage Publications.

Barrera, M., Jr. (1986). Distinctions between social support concepts, measures, and models. *American Journal of Community Psychology, 14*, 413–445.

Barrera, M., Jr., & Balls, P. (1983). Assessing social support as a preventive resource: An illustrative study. *Prevention in Human Services, 2*(4), 59–74.

Barrera, M., Jr., Sandler, I. N., & Ramsay, T. B. (1981). Preliminary development of a scale of social support: Studies on college students. *American Journal of Community Psychology, 9*, 435–447.

Brammer, L. M. (1973). *The helping relationship process and skills*. Englewood Cliffs, NJ: Prentice-Hall.

Brandt, P. A. (1984a). Social support and negative life events of mothers with developmentally delayed children. In K. E. Barnard, P. A. Brandt, B. S. Raff, & P. Carroll (Eds.), *Social support and families of vulnerable infants* (pp. 205–223). White Plains, NY: March of Dimes Birth Defects Foundation.

Brandt, P. A. (1984b). Stress-buffering effects of social support on maternal discipline. *Nursing Research, 33*, 229–234.

Brandt, P. A., & Weinert, C. (1981). The PRQ—A social support measure. *Nursing Research, 30*, 277–280.

Brock, A. M., & O'Sullivan, P. (1985). A study to determine what variables predict institutionalization of elderly people. *Journal of Advanced Nursing, 10*, 533–537.

Brown, M. A. (1986a). Social support during pregnancy: A unidimensional or multidimensional construct? *Nursing Research, 35*, 4–9.

Brown, M. A. (1986b). Social support, stress, and health: A comparison of expectant mothers and fathers. *Nursing Research, 35*, 72–76.

Burgess, A. W., & Holmstrom, L. L. (1978). Recovery from rape and prior life stress. *Research in Nursing and Health, 1*, 165–174.

Caplan, G. (1974). Support systems. In G. Caplan (Ed.), *Support systems and community mental health: Lectures on concept development* (pp. 1–40). New York: Behavioral Publications.

Cassel, J. (1976). The contribution of the social environment to host resistance. *American Journal of Epidemiology, 104*, 107–123.

Cobb, S. (1976). Social support as a moderator of life stress. *Psychosomatic Medicine, 38*, 300–314.

Cranley, M. C. (1984). Social support as a factor in the development of parents' attachment to their unborn. In K. E. Barnard, P. A. Brandt, B. S. Raff, & P. Carroll (Eds.), *Social support and families of vulnerable infants* (pp. 99–109). White Plains, NY: March of Dimes Birth Defects Foundation.

Cronenwett, L. R. (1980). Elements and outcomes of a postpartum support group program. *Research in Nursing and Health, 3*, 33–41.

Cronenwett, L. R. (1984). Social networks and social support of primigravida mothers and fathers. In K. E. Barnard, P. A. Brandt, B. S. Raff, & P. Carroll (Eds.), *Social support and families of vulnerable infants* (pp. 167–186). White Plains, NY: March of Dimes Birth Defects Foundation.

Cronenwett, L. R. (1985a). Network structure, social support, and psychological outcomes of pregnancy. *Nursing Research, 34*, 93–99.

Cronenwett, L. R. (1985b). Parental network structure and perceived support after birth of first child. *Nursing Research, 34*, 347–352.

Cronin-Stubbs, D., & Brophy, E. B. (1985). Burnout: Can social support save the psych nurse? *Journal of Psychosocial Nursing 23*(7), 9–13.

Cronin-Stubbs, D., & Rooks, C. A. (1985). The stress, social support, and burnout of critical care nurses: The results of research. *Heart & Lung, 14*, 31–39.

Dimond, M. (1979). Social support and adaptation to chronic illness: The case of maintenance hemodialysis. *Research in Nursing and Health, 2*, 101–108.

Dracup, D. (1985). A controlled trial of couples group counseling in cardiac rehabilitation. *Journal of Cardiopulmonary Rehabilitation, 5*, 436–442.

Dracup, K., Meleis, A. I., Clark, S., Clyburn, A., Sheilds, L., & Staley, M. (1984). Group counseling in cardiac rehabilitation: Effect on patient compliance. *Patient Education and Counseling, 6*, 169–177.

Ellison, E. S. (1983). Parental support and school-aged children. *Western Journal of Nursing Research, 5*, 145–153.

Elmore, S. K. (1984). The moderating effect of social support upon depression. *Western Journal of Nursing Research, 6*, 17–22.

Fuller, S. S., & Karlson, S. M. (1981). Social support, personal autonomy, and the well-being of family-member caregivers. In I. G. Mauksch (Ed.), *Primary care: A contemporary nursing perspective* (pp. 91–110). New York: Grune & Stratton.

Fuller, S. S., & Larson, S. B. (1980). Life events, emotional support, and health of older people. *Research in Nursing and Health, 3*, 81–89.

Gierszewski, S. A. (1983). The relationship of weight loss, locus of control, and social support. *Nursing Research, 32*, 43–47.

Gray-Toft, P., & Anderson, J. G. (1983). A hospital staff support program: Design and evaluation. *International Journal of Nursing Studies, 20*, 137–147.

Hentinen, M. (1983). Need for instruction and support of the wives of patients with myocardial infarction. *Journal of Advanced Nursing, 8*, 519–524.

Hilbert, G. A. (1985). Spouse support and myocardial infarction patient compliance. *Nursing Research, 34*, 217–220.

Hilbert, G. A., & Allen, L. R. (1985). The effect of social support on educational outcomes. *Journal of Nursing Education, 24*, 48–52.

Hillestad, E. A. (1984). Is it lonely at the top? *Nursing Administration, 8*(3), 1–13.

House, J. S. (1981). *Work stress and social support*. Menlo Park, CA: Addison-Wesley.

Hubbard, P., Muhlenkamp, A. F., & Brown, N. (1984). The relationship between social support and self-care practices. *Nursing Research, 33*, 266–270.

Ide, B. A. (1983). Social network support among low-income elderly: A two-factor model? *Western Journal of Nursing Research, 5*, 235–244.

Jordan, J., & Meckler, J. R. (1982). The relationship between life change events, social supports and dysmenorrhea. *Research in Nursing and Health, 5*, 73–79.

Kahn, R. L. (1979). Aging and social support. In M. W. Riley (Ed.), *Aging from birth to death: Interdisciplinary perspectives* (pp. 77–91). Boulder, CO: Westview Press.

Klinger, M. (1984). Compliance and the post-MI patient. *The Canadian Nurse, 81*(7), 32–38.

Laschinger, S. J. (1984). The relationship of social support to health in elderly people. *Western Journal of Nursing Research, 6*, 341–350.

Lindsey, A. M., Ahmed, N., & Dodd, M. J. (1985). Social support: Network and quality as perceived by Egyptian cancer patients. *Cancer Nursing, 8*, 37–42.

Lindsey, A. M., Dodd, M. J., & Chen, S. (1985). Social support network on Taiwanese cancer patients. *International Journal of Nursing Studies, 22*, 149–164.

Lindsey, A. M., & Hughes, E. M. (1981). Social support and alternatives to institutionalization for the at-risk elderly. *Journal of the American Geriatrics Society, 29*, 308–315.

Lipson, J. G. (1981). Cesarean support groups: Mutual help and education. *Women & Health, 6*(3/4), 27–39.

Lipson, J. G. (1982). Effects of a support group on the emotional impact of cesarean childbirth. *Prevention in Human Services, 1*(3), 17–29.

Lynam, M. J. (1985). Support networks developed by immigrant women. *Social Science and Medicine, 21*, 327–333.

Magilvy, J. K. (1985). Quality of life of hearing-impaired older women. *Nursing Research, 34*, 140–144.

Mercer, R. T., Hackley, K. C., & Bostrom, A. G. (1983). Relationship of psycho-social and perinatal variables to perception of childbirth. *Nursing Research, 32*, 202–207.

Mercer, R. T., Hackley, K. C., & Bostrom, A. (1984). Social support of teenage mothers. In K. E. Barnard, P. A. Brandt, B. S. Raff, & P. Carroll (Eds.), *Social support and families of vulnerable infants* (pp. 245–272). White Plains, NY: March of Dimes Birth Defects Foundation.

Nikolaisen, S. M., & Williams, R. A. (1980). Parents' view of support following the loss of their infant to sudden infant death syndrome. *Western Journal of Nursing Research, 2*, 593–601.

Norbeck, J. S. (1985a). Measurement of social support: Recent strategies and continuing issues. In R. A. O'Brien (Ed.), *Proceedings of the Symposium on Social Support and Health: New Directions for Theory Development and Research* (pp. 73–106). Rochester, NY: University of Rochester School of Nursing.

Norbeck, J. S. (1985b). Types and sources of social support for managing job stress in critical care nursing. *Nursing Research, 34*, 225–230.

Norbeck, J. S. (Ed.). (1986). *First International Nursing Research Conference on Social Support: Proceedings.* San Francisco, CA: University of California at San Francisco School of Nursing.

Norbeck, J. S., Lindsey, A. M., & Carrieri, V. L. (1981). The development of an instrument to measure social support. *Nursing Research, 30*, 264–269.

Norbeck, J. S., Lindsey, A. M., & Carrieri, V. L. (1983). Further development of the Norbeck Social Support Questionnaire: Normative data and validity testing. *Nursing Research, 32*, 4–9.

Norbeck, J. S., & Sheiner, M. (1982). Sources of social support related to single parent functioning. *Research in Nursing and Health, 5*, 3–12.

Norbeck, J. S., & Tilden, V. P. (1983). Life stress, social support, and emotional disequilibrium in complications of pregnancy: A prospective, multivariate study. *Journal of Health and Social Behavior, 24*, 30–46.

Northouse, L. L. (1981). Mastectomy patients and the fear of cancer recurrence. *Cancer Nursing, 4*, 213–220.

Nuckolls, K. B., Cassel, J., & Kaplan, B. H. (1972). Psychosocial assets, life crisis, and the prognosis of pregnancy. *American Journal of Epidemiology, 95*, 431–441.

O'Brien, M. E. (1980). Hemodialysis regimen compliance and social environment: A panel analysis. *Nursing Research, 29*, 250–255.

O'Brien, R. A. (Ed.). (1985). *Proceedings of the Symposium on Social Support and Health: New Directions for Theory Development and Research.* Rochester, NY: University of Rochester School of Nursing.

Pattison, E. M., Defrancisco, D., Wood, P., Frazier, H., & Crowder, J. (1975). A psychosocial kinship model for family therapy. *American Journal of Psychiatry, 132*, 1246–1251.

Piltz-Kirkby, M., & Fox, M. A. (1982). Support systems as a factor in hemodialysis. *Nephrology Nurse, 4*(5), 19–26.

Pohl, J. M., & Fuller, S. S. (1980). Perceived choice, social interaction, and dimensions of morale of residents in a home for the aged. *Research in Nursing and Health, 3*, 147–157.

Reid, B. J. (1983). Potential sources of Type I error and possible solutions to avoid a "galloping" alpha rate. *Nursing Research, 32*, 190–191.

Rook, K. S., & Dooley, D. (1985). Applying social support research: Theoretical problems and future directions. *Journal of Social Issues, 41*, 5–28.

Sandler, I. N., & Lakey, B. (1982). Locus of control as a stress moderator: The role of control perceptions and social support. *American Journal of Community Psychology, 10*, 65–79.

Sarason, I. G., Levine, H. M., Basham, R. B., & Sarason, B. R. (1983). Assessing social support: The Social Support Questionnaire. *Journal of Personality and Social Psychology, 44*, 127–139.

Schlenk, E. A., & Hart, L. K. (1984). Relationship between health locus of control, health value, and social support and compliance of persons with diabetes mellitus. *Diabetes Care, 7*, 655–574.

Stephens, C. J. (1985). Identifying social support components in prenatal populations: A multivariate analysis on alcohol consumption. *Health Care for Women International, 6*, 285–294.

Thomas, P. D., & Hooper, E. M. (1983). Healthy elderly: Social bonds and locus of control. *Research in Nursing and Health, 6*, 11–16.

Tilden, V. P. (1983). The relation of life stress and social support to emotional disequilibrium during pregnancy. *Research in Nursing and Health, 6,* 167–174.

Tilden, V. P. (1984). The relation of selected psychosocial variables to single status of adult women during pregnancy. *Nursing Research, 33,* 102–106.

Tilden, V. P., & Galyen, R. D. (1987). Cost and conflict: The darker side of social support. *Western Journal of Nursing Research, 9,* 9–18.

Turner, S. L. (1979). Disability among schizophrenics in a rural community: Services and social support. *Research in Nursing and Health, 2,* 151–161.

Webb, C., & Wilson-Barnett, J. (1983a). Hysterectomy: A study in coping with recovery. *Journal of Advanced Nursing, 8,* 311–319.

Webb, C., & Wilson-Barnett, J. (1983b). Self-concept, social support and hysterectomy. *International Journal of Nursing Studies, 20,* 97–107.

Weinert, C. (in press). Revision and further development of a social support measure: The Personal Resource Questionnaire. In C. F. Waltz & O. L. Strickland (Eds.), *Measurement of clinical and educational nursing outcomes.* New York: Springer Publishing Co.

Weinert, C., & Brandt, P. A. (1987). Measuring social support with the PRQ. *Western Journal of Nursing Research, 9,* 589–602.

Weiss, R. S. (1974). The provisions of social relationships. In Z. Rubin (Ed.), *Doing unto others* (pp. 17–26). Englewood Cliffs, NJ: Prentice Hall.

Woods, N. F. (1980). Women's roles and illness episodes: A prospective study. *Research in Nursing and Health, 3,* 137–145.

Woods, N. F. (1985). Employment, family roles, and mental ill health in young married women. *Nursing Research, 34,* 4–10.

Woods, N. F., & Earp, J. A. L. (1978). Women with cured breast cancer: A study of mastectomy patients in North Carolina. *Nursing Research, 27,* 279–285.

Chapter 5

Relaxation

MARIAH SNYDER
SCHOOL OF NURSING
UNIVERSITY OF MINNESOTA

CONTENTS

Relaxation interventions have been used extensively during the past 25 years for reducing anxiety, treating symptoms associated with specific health problems, and promoting increased well-being. Numerous interventions are categorized as relaxation therapies: progressive muscle relaxation, passive muscle relaxation, autogenic therapy, imagery, self-hypnosis, breathing techniques, and yoga (Davis, McKay, & Eshelman, 1980; Rice, Caldwell, Butler, & Robinson, 1986; Smith, 1985; Woolfolk & Lehrer, 1984).

Several factors have contributed to the increased use of relaxation interventions. In the 1960s investigators discovered that functions under the control of the autonomic nervous system such as heart rate, blood pressure, and breathing could be altered by intentional actions or thoughts. Researchers demonstrated that functions previously thought to be regulated automatically by the autonomic nervous system could be brought under volitional control through reinforcement of these functions. During this same time period techniques that were part of Eastern cultures were introduced into the West.

The majority of the research on relaxation therapies is found in behavioral medicine and psychology. Critiques of studies in which investigators have used specific relaxation therapies provide an excellent perspective on these interventions (Borkovec & Sides, 1979; Hillenberg & Collins, 1982; Lehrer & Woolfolk, 1984; Snyder, 1984).

Outcomes of the therapies rather than specific relaxation therapies were chosen for organizing studies for review. The number of studies in which investigators used a particular therapy was usually very small and, in some studies, the effectiveness of several therapies was compared. Comfort, improvement in physiological status, improvement in psychological status, and improvement in both physiological and psychological status were the four outcomes selected. The overall focus of the research was the determining factor for placing a study in a particular outcome section.

A computer search of nursing literature from 1970 to 1986 was done to identify studies in which progressive muscle relaxation, meditation, biofeedback, imagery, or autogenic training has been used as relaxation therapies. Those studies identified in the search that were done in nursing or by nurses were reviewed. In addition, several studies were identified through the references cited in the articles being reviewed. A total of 24 studies are reviewed. Although studies on relaxation therapies from other disciplines were not reviewed, findings from selected studies were used for comparison.

DEFINITIONS OF RELAXATION THERAPIES

Consensus about the definitions of many of the relaxation interventions was lacking. Modifications of techniques were made to fit particular situations. Therefore, brief descriptions of the relaxation therapies reported in the nursing studies reviewed are provided for clarification.

Autogenic therapy is a method of autosuggestion for achieving mental and physiological equilibrium (Luthe, 1969; Schultz, 1953).

The individual is provided with a series of phrases to repeat; the phrase serves to suggest to the person that certain physiological sensations are occurring, for example, "my left arm is heavy."

In *biofeedback*, electronic equipment is used to assist the person to gain control over involuntary or unfelt physiological events. Functions such as heart rate, temperature, or muscle contraction are controlled by manipulating the data on the monitor (Fischer-Williams, Nigl, & Savine, 1981).

Imagery is the formation of a mental representation of an object that is usually only perceived through the senses. A person can use imagery to understand and control patterns of thinking, to gain access to emotion and experience it more deeply, and to assist in controlling autonomic nervous system functions (Sodergren, 1985).

In *meditation*, stimulus input is limited by directing the person's attention to a single unchanging or repetitive stimulus (Carrington, 1978, 1984). This stimulus may be a word, mantra, or sound.

Progressive muscle relaxation is the tensing and relaxing of successive muscle groups to achieve overall relaxation. The person's attention is focused on discriminating between the feeling experienced when the muscles are tensed and when they are relaxed (Jacobson, 1938).

OUTCOME MEASURES

Comfort

In three nursing studies investigators explored the effect that relaxation therapies had on lessening postoperative pain (Flaherty & Fitzpatrick, 1978; Horowitz, Fitzpatrick, & Flaherty, 1984; Wells, 1982). Although the therapies used in the studies differed, reduction in discomfort was noted in the treatment groups in the three studies. Wells used a combination of techniques: meditation, biofeedback, and an adaptation of Jacobson's progressive relaxation.

Flaherty and Fitzpatrick (1978) used a portion of Jacobson's progressive relaxation technique, the relaxation of throat and jaw muscles. A comparison of the effectiveness of a localized relaxation technique that included relaxation of the jaw and throat muscles and the relaxation response, which the investigators termed a general relaxation technique, was made in the study by Horowitz, Fitzpatrick, and Flaherty (1974). Patients taught the relaxation response had significantly less pain and distress than the control group or local relaxation group. In addition to self-reports on distress scales, the investigators determined the effect relaxation therapies had on other variables such as vital signs, use of analgesics, and muscle relaxation; these indices were proposed as indicators of pain.

There was no consistency across the three studies in the effects produced. A number of factors such as environment, differences in the mechanisms of action of the therapies taught, and the types of surgical procedures may have contributed to this lack of congruency. Only in the Flaherty and Fitzpatrick study (1978) did patients who were taught relaxation use significantly fewer narcotics postoperatively than the control group. However, subjects in the experimental group in Wells's study used fewer analgesics than the control group. The small size of each group ($n = 6$) made it difficult to establish statistical significance.

In a laboratory study Geden, Beck, Hauge, and Pohlman (1984) examined the effects on reducing pain associated with childbirth of pleasant imagery, pleasant imagery plus relaxation, sensory transformation, sensory transformation plus relaxation, neutral imagery, neutral imagery plus relaxation, combined strategies, and no treatment. After subjects had received a 1-hour training session on the particular technique, laboratory methods for producing painful stimuli were implemented. Although subjects in all treatment groups showed some decrease in pain as measured by a pain thermometer (Chaves & Barber, 1974), subjects receiving sensory transformation demonstrated the greatest treatment response. However, the therapies produced no significant changes in objective relaxation measurements. This study was unique in the nursing studies reviewed because of its sophisticated design and control of variables. However, caution is needed in comparing results from studies of pain induced in a laboratory setting with those done in clinical areas because subjects in the former can exert control over the situation.

The findings from the four studies in which relaxation therapies were used for reduction of pain provided evidence that a variety of interventions may be effective. In studies outside of nursing, these therapies have been found to be effective in the treatment of numerous conditions such as tension headaches (Silver & Blanchard, 1978) and chronic pain (Korn, 1983). The relatively short period in the nursing studies for teaching the technique and the absence of practice sessions for mastering the specific intervention did not prevent patients from experiencing some efficacy from the therapy. In the two studies (Geden et al., 1984; Wells, 1982) in which EMG measurements were taken to verify the degree of muscle relaxation achieved, patients had not achieved relaxation of specific muscle groups. Therefore, the effects of the interventions appeared to be due to factors other than muscle relaxation.

Improved Physiological Status

The effect of relaxation therapies on the improvement in physiologic status was explored in five nursing studies. The investigators hypothesized that the resulting lessened anxiety from the use of relaxation therapies would have a positive impact on physiological parameters. Samples studied included persons with chronic obstructive pulmonary disease (COPD), surgical patients, persons receiving chemotherapy, and women in childbirth. In one study on urinary incontinence, the purpose of the biofeedback therapy was retraining rather than lessening of anxiety.

Sitzman, Kamiya, and Johnston (1983) determined that use of biofeedback training resulted in a decrease in respiratory rate and an increase in tidal volume from pretraining levels in three of four patients with chronic obstructive pulmonary disease. The small sample size prohibited generalizations, but the investigators stated that the findings provided guidance for continued study on the use of biofeedback in this population. Another factor lacking in the study was a control group that would have served to differentiate the impact the investigator may have had on the outcome.

Two other studies were designed for the use of biofeedback to improve physiological parameters (Britt, 1981; Sugar, 1983). Using audio biofeedback with women during labor, Britt found no significant differences between the control and experimental groups on diastolic blood pressure, respiratory rate, pulse rate, or electromyographic scores. Findings for the experimental group, however, showed greater relaxation of the frontalis muscle according to electromyographic measurements than was present in the control group. Britt did not begin biofeedback training until the early stages of labor and only used a 10-minute training session. Subjects, therefore, may not have had an adequate knowledge about the technique. Sugar reported employing biofeedback for bladder training with an adolescent with enuresis. One-year follow-up confirmed that urinary continence had been maintained.

Although a number of studies have been designed to look at relaxation therapies that would reduce anxiety in preoperative patients, few investigators evaluated the impact of heightened anxiety on physiologic parameters. In one of the earliest nursing studies in this area, Aiken and Henrichs (1971) used the muscle relaxation portion of the systematic desensitization technique (Wolpe & Lazarus, 1966) to effect variables that they believed were associated with stress. Although significant difference was found between the treatment and control groups on anesthesia time, cardiopulmonary bypass time, units of blood required, and degrees of hypothermia, one questions whether the use of relaxation therapy could have accounted for these differences. The comparison group was selected from open-heart surgical patients from prior years; the advancement in technology present for the experimental group may have contributed to the findings.

Cotanch (1983) explored the effect that Surwit's relaxation program (1980) had on decreasing nausea and vomiting in patients receiving chemotherapy. Subjects had been identified as having considerable trouble with nausea and vomiting despite the use of antiemetic medications. Nine patients reported a decrease in nausea and vomiting and an increase in food intake. The study design did not include a control group. Furthermore, the effect of investigator bias was not known.

Although the number of studies was small in which relaxation therapies were used for their impact on physiological indices, the outcomes suggested that continued explorations with these populations might be useful. Nurses often assume prime responsibility for interventions with problems such as nausea and vomiting and difficulty in breathing. Verification of the effectiveness of the interventions would be valuable for improved patient care.

Improved Psychological Status

Many of the studies conducted by nurses to investigate the efficacy of relaxation therapies included both psychological and physiological indices to determine the effectiveness of the therapy in reducing anxiety. Because disparity between physiological and psychological measurements of anxiety have been common in studies on the effectiveness of relaxation therapies, measurements of both were made frequently. Emphasis on the effect that the therapies had on psychological indices was noted, however, in a number of studies reviewed. A variety of instruments were used for measuring the psychological effect of the relaxation therapies, making comparison across studies difficult.

Investigators have commented on the presence of high levels of anxiety in persons who have had myocardial infarctions (Bengtsson, Hallstrom, & Tibblin, 1973; Thiel, Parker, & Bruce, 1973). Researchers outside of nursing have found that relaxation therapies were effective in lessening anxiety in patients with cardiac problems (Benson, Rosner, Marzetta, & Klemchuck, 1974; Borkovec, Grayson, & Cooper, 1978). Bohachick (1984), a nurse, investigated the effect of progressive relaxation on anxiety in cardiac patients. Subjects who were taught Goldfried and Davison's technique (1976) of progressive relaxation showed a significant decrease in somatization, interpersonal sensitivity, anxiety, and depression scale scores of the Symptom Checklist-90 Revised (Derogatis, 1977) as compared to the control group. Likewise, a significant difference between the treatment and control groups was found for scores on the State Anxiety Inventory (Spielberger, Gorsuch, & Lushene, 1970). Although the investigator did not detail the procedure used, it was noted that training was done during three weekly sessions. The number of sessions may have allowed many of the subjects to master the technique and, thus, have contributed to the positive effect.

High levels of anxiety have been found in patients undergoing diagnostic procedures (Sime & Libera, 1985). Rice, Caldwell, Butler, and Robinson (1986) used a form of muscle relaxation, relaxation-via-letting go, with patients undergoing cardiac catheterization. Patients who used the technique did not have lower state anxiety scores, manifestations of distress, or self-reported distress scores than the control group. Although the majority of patients reported using the technique during the cardiac catheterization procedure, the investigators hypothesized that the lack of significant findings may have resulted from patients not having mastered the technique prior to its use during the procedure. Paul and Trimble (1970), in a study comparing live and taped relaxation instructions, found that persons receiving live instructions achieved better treatment results than persons taught via tape-recorded instructions. Other inconsistencies between methods of instruction may have influenced the findings.

Nurse investigators used relaxation therapies in two studies with psychiatric populations (Sheer, 1980; Tamez, Moore, & Brown, 1978).

Medications are prescribed commonly to lessen anxiety in this population; in these two investigations nurse researchers explored the effectiveness of alternatives to medications for reducing anxiety. In the Sheer study, patients' anxiety as measured by the Adjective Check List (Zuckerman, 1960) decreased on the days on which patients participated in progressive relaxation sessions. Sheer did not control for variables such as medications and prior relaxation training. Thus, the results were suspect. Progressive relaxation also was used by Tamez and colleagues to determine if it would be effective in lessening the use of pro re nata (p.r.n.) tranquilizers. No significant difference was found between the control and treatment groups in the Tamez et al. (1978) study. The investigators suggested that this outcome may have resulted because all of the patients experienced lessened anxiety when they found themselves in the safe, protective atmosphere of the hospital.

Improved well-being in patients with epilepsy was studied by Snyder (1983). Patients were taught the Bernstein and Borkovec progressive muscle relaxation technique (1973) in an attempt to improve psychosocial functioning. No difference in psychosocial functioning as measured by the Washington Psychosocial Seizure Inventory (Dodrill, Batzel, Queissen, & Temkin, 1980) was found between the control and experimental groups, nor between pretreatment and posttreatment scores for either group. The investigator suggested that a time period longer than 6 months may be needed to change psychosocial functioning. The Snyder study points to problems encountered in doing longitudinal studies—a large attrition of subjects occurred. Although longitudinal studies are needed to determine the long-term effects of relaxation therapies, mechanisms to promote continued participation of subjects in the study are critical to valid data.

Several of the studies by nurse investigators included use of relaxation therapies with nonpatient populations (e.g., Donovan, 1979; Fehring, 1983). Nurses working with oncology patients were identified by Donovan (1979) as being involved in high-anxiety-producing situations. Her sample included nurses from hospital oncology units and home care agencies that provided care to cancer patients. Subjects in the experimental group were taught relaxation along with guided imagery. The only significant finding was the durability of the reduction on the depression scale of the short form of the Symptom Checklist-90 (Derogatis, 1977). In the design of the study the researcher tried to account for some of the effects that participation and completion of instruments could have on the results. Difficulty in analyzing data was encountered because of a lack of homogeneity.

Fehring (1983) studied the effects that several relaxation therapies had on state anxiety as measured by the State Anxiety Inventory (Spielberger, Gorsuch, & Lushene, 1970) and the Profile of Mood States (McNair, Lorr, & Droppleman, 1971). Healthy college students were placed in one of three groups: those taught the Benson relaxation response (1975), those taught biofeedback in addition to the Benson relaxation response, or a control group. Students taught biofeedback in addition to the relaxation response had significantly lower scores on state anxiety and profile of mood states after the 8-week teaching-practice period than did those students who only received training on the Relaxation Response or no training. These findings were consistent with the view of Smith (1985), who advocated allowing patients to combine elements from several relaxation therapies. One could not conclude from the Fehring study whether biofeedback alone would have achieved the same results.

Only one study conducted by nurses included the use of relaxation therapies with children. Lack of relaxation studies with this population was striking in that teaching children ways to lessen anxiety could have a profound impact on their future health. LaMontagne, Mason, and Hepworth (1985) taught muscle relaxation skills and imagery to second-graders. Stories, instead of specific instructions on how to relax, were used to induce relaxation. Although a significant decrease in anxiety as measured by the Gills Child Anxiety Scale (Gills, 1980) was not found between the experimental and control groups, children who were taught relaxation manifested a decrease in anxiety scores.

Improved Psychological and Physiological Status

In a number of the studies attention was given to both physiological and psychological indices for measuring the effectiveness of relaxation therapies. The findings from the studies by nurses were consistent with those in other disciplines in that frequently congruency between the physiological and psychological indices was absent (Reinking & Kohl, 1975). Davidson and Schwartz (1976) hypothesized that these differences occur because relaxation therapies vary in the dimensions of anxiety on which they have an impact.

Murphy (1983) compared the effects of biofeedback, progressive muscle relaxation, and self-relaxation training on lessening the stress experienced by subjects (nurses) who did not have serious cardiovascular problems. Scores on the Trait Anxiety Inventory (Spielberger et al., 1970) were lowered significantly from pretraining levels in all three groups. Subjects in the biofeedback group displayed a greater increase in hand temperature than did the subjects in the other two groups. Subjects in the progressive muscle relaxation group demonstrated the greatest reduction in tension of the frontalis muscle. In a follow-up questionnaire, 88% of the respondents indicated they were using the skills to help them relax 3 months after the training session ended. These results are unusual in that the majority of the participants did not continue to practice the techniques on a daily basis after the study was terminated. According to Bernstein and Borkovec (1973), relaxation is a learned skill and continued practice is necessary if the technique is to be effective.

Bowles, Smith, and Parker (1979) compared the effectiveness of biofeedback training and progressive muscle relaxation. Subjects included nursing students and nursing faculty members. Electromyogram levels and state anxiety measurements revealed that biofeedback used in conjunction with progressive muscle relaxation was superior to the use of progressive muscle relaxation. A notable finding was that the degree of muscle relaxation did not continue over time. Persons taught relaxation by biofeedback may become dependent on the biofeedback machine and thus not acquire the skills necessary to achieve relaxation without the technology.

Kogan and Beaton (1984) carried out a large evaluation study to determine the effectiveness of biofeedback and stress counseling for clients in a model nursing clinic established to assist patients in handling adverse responses to stress. Clinic patients presented an array of stress-related conditions including tension headaches, chronic muscle tension, pain, anxiety, gastrointestinal complaints, essential hypertension, Raynaud's disease, and migraine headache. Psychological measurements administered included the Symptom Checklist-90 and the Personal Opinion Survey (Coan & Fairchild, 1974). Electromyogram, digital temperature, and skin conductance were used to measure physiological parameters. Significant improvement over time was noted on both the psychological and physiological indices of stress. Almost half of the clients, 120 out of 258, participated in a 6-month follow-up to determine the effectiveness over time. Almost all showed retention of the skills gained.

Kogan and Beaton's findings (1984) included evidence to support usefulness of relaxation therapies in clinic settings. The investigators reported that their dropout rate was only 18%, as compared to a dropout rate of 34% from a traditional clinic in the same setting. A major factor for this may have been the interest and attention provided to the clients by the investigative team.

Banks (1981) studied the effects of progressive muscle relaxation combined with biofeedback training on anxiety in obese patients. The therapies resulted in a significant reduction in state anxiety, but there was no correlation between degree of relaxation and the amount of weight lost, although subjects did lose weight. Anxiety was the only psychological variable measured; establishing the presence or absence of other factors would have provided valuable information regarding a mutiplicity of variables that may have influenced weight loss. Subjects were placed into groups according to their age in order to control for age-related metabolic differences. Because all groups received treatment, the impact of the therapist could not be determined.

Benson, Rosner, Marzetta, and Klemchuck (1974) were instrumental in drawing the public's attention to the role that the relaxation response could have in reducing blood pressure in persons with hypertension. Investigators have explored the effectiveness of other relaxation therapies in reducing blood pressure. Only one study was found in which a nurse explored the effects of relaxation therapy on blood pressure. Pender (1984) taught the Bernstein and Borkovec (1973) technique of progressive muscle relaxation to 22 subjects with hypertension. The mean decrease in systolic pressure was 8mm Hg over the period of instruction and at the 4-month follow-up; this result was a significantly greater change than that found in the control group. However, there was no significant decrease in the diastolic blood pressure. Although the results do not provide conclusive evidence for the use of relaxation therapies for controlling hypertension, particularly because the alterations in diastolic pressure did not occur, the fact that decreases persisted over time and that subjects continued to use the relaxation technique was encouraging. Further research is needed to explore whether the decreases in blood pressure produced by relaxation therapy occur at times other than at the training sessions; this finding would be essential if relaxation was to be used in place of medications for reducing diastolic and systolic pressures.

Pender (1985) also examined the effect that progressive relaxation had on anxiety and locus of control. Scores on both subscales of the State-Trait Inventory showed significant decreases in the treatment group. Locus of control (Wallston, Wallston, & DeVellis, 1978), like trait anxiety, has been considered to be a personality trait. Experimental group subjects' scores on the Health Locus of Control Scale (Wallston et al., 1978) shifted to reflect increases in internal locus of control responses. Instructions were provided over a 3-week period of time, and the subjects were followed on a weekly basis for 6 weeks. Home practice also was stressed. This intensive training may have helped subjects to master the technique to such a degree that the relaxation had a significant impact.

DISCUSSION AND DIRECTIONS
FOR NURSING RESEARCH

This review of nursing research on the use of relaxation therapies revealed a visible lack of research programs. Only one group of investigators conducted more than one study in this area; the second study was an expansion of the first investigation (Flaherty & Fitzpatrick, 1978; Horowitz, Fitzpatrick, & Flaherty, 1984). Although nurse investigators made reference to studies done by other nurses, replication or building on previous studies often was lacking. Failure to use standardized procedures, employment of the same therapy procedure with a sample drawn from a different population, or use of different measurement tests for the dependent variables were noted. Because many studies were characterized by small sample sizes, the need for replication is important so that directions for application in the clinical area can be established.

One problem hindering replication was that adequate descriptions of the therapy and teaching sessions were often absent in the published reports. Numerous techniques exist for each of the relaxation therapies reviewed. Two reviews of literature (Borkovec & Sides, 1979; Lehrer, 1982) have been done to determine the efficacy of the various techniques for progressive relaxation. The latter reported that Jacobson's original technique was more powerful than the modifications in reducing physiological activity and symptoms of stress.

Variations in the methods for teaching and using progressive relaxation are common. Seven different techniques were employed in the studies by nurses in which progressive relaxation was used. Altering a technique to fit a particular environment or sample may be indicated, but the researcher needs to be explicit about the modifications made so that replication is possible.

Other variables involved in the teaching of relaxation therapies need to be specifically detailed in reports. Instruction by tapes or instructor, group or individual sessions, and length of session can influence the effectiveness of the therapies. Designing studies to explore further the impact of these variables is warranted. While Borkovec and Sides (1979) found that multisession live training produced the most beneficial results, little attention has been given to the effect of group versus individual teaching sessions. Determination of the efficacy of groups would be important in today's cost-conscious health care system.

In many of the studies of progressive relaxation, the number of teaching sessions used was less than the number advocated by the developer of a specific technique. Borkovec and Sides (1979) found that in studies in which significant results were found, at least four teaching sessions were used. Mastery in relaxing muscle groups is also important to the success of progressive relaxation; sessions should be held until the person achieves relaxation of the muscle group. Electromyography is frequently used for determining mastery. Pender (1984) used electromyography, but she did not note whether additional teaching sessions were held if EMG readings indicated lack of mastery. Several investigators (Rice, Caldwell, Butler, & Robinson, 1986; Snyder, 1983) suggested that lack of success by patients may have resulted from the subjects' lack of mastery. Determination of muscle relaxation should be incorporated into research studies so that the results truly reflect whether progressive muscle relaxation is effective.

Controversy exists over whether relaxation therapies produce an overall relaxation response or if the various therapies induce specific effects. Benson (1975) supported the general effect theory, but Davidson and Schwartz (1976) hypothesized that some therapies are more effective for reducing anxiety related to somatic stimuli, whereas other techniques are more appropriate for anxiety generated by cognitive sources. In several studies investigators tested this hypothesis, but findings to date have been inconclusive (Norton & Johnson, 1983; Schwartz, Davidson, & Goleman, 1978). Continued research in this area is needed; nurse investigators could be instrumental in helping to determine whether specific relaxation therapies are effective for treating particular types of anxiety.

Obtaining data on personality characteristics of the subjects would assist in establishing characteristics of persons for whom a particular relaxation therapy would be the therapy of choice. Davidson and Schwartz (1976) suggested that attention needs to be given to the fit between subject preferences and the technique used. Findings from longitudinal studies indicate that many subjects do not continue to use the relaxation therapy after the teaching sessions are completed. A number of factors may contribute to the therapy not being used. One factor requiring consideration is suitability of a particular intervention for an individual. Assessment tools need to be developed that would help in establishing the appropriateness of specific therapies for an individual.

The majority of study designs precluded a determination of the effect that contact with the therapist may have had on the outcome. The therapist may have a major impact on the outcomes achieved from the therapy (Woolfolk & Lehrer, 1984). Borkovec, Johnson, and Block (1984) state that therapist bias and therapist characteristics represent a key but often ignored variable in relaxation research. However, constructing designs to circumvent the effect of the therapist is difficult; it has been shown that better results are obtained from live instructions than from taped instructions. Possible approaches include using multiple therapists or using therapists who are biased toward the therapy that the investigator has predicted to be inferior.

In an extensive review of relaxation therapies, Lehrer and Woolfolk (1984) concluded that a combination of therapies tends to produce better outcomes than the use of a single therapy. Several nurse investigators compared the effectiveness of a combination of therapies. Additional studies are needed to examine the incremental effects of combining therapies.

Longitudinal studies on relaxation therapies are uncommon both in nursing and in other disciplines. In most instances in which relaxation therapies are taught, continued use by the clients is necessary for the maintenance of the effects. Therefore, studies over time are needed to determine whether this is occurring. Burish, Hendrix, and Frost (1981) stressed the importance of assessing the effectiveness of relaxation therapies during stressful situations. Results obtained during teaching sessions may vary considerably from those that occur during life situations.

Relaxation therapies have often been viewed as having no adverse effects. Research conducted by investigators from other disciplines has provided evidence that relaxation therapies, such as progressive relaxation, may not be as benign as generally was believed. Heide and Borkovec (1984) reported the possibility of relaxation-induced anxiety resulting from practice of progressive muscle relaxation. Precautions also are needed in the use of medications in persons being taught relaxation techniques. A trophotropic state resulting from being relaxed may potentiate the dosage of a medication resulting in drug overdosage (Everly & Rosenfeld, 1981). These are only two of the possible adverse reactions that can result from the use of relaxation therapies. Researchers need to be alert to these in planning studies. Reporting adverse reactions will assist other researchers and practitioners in developing protocols.

Research findings in nursing and other disciplines are beginning to indicate conditions for which specific therapies or combinations are effective in reducing symptoms. However, considerable research is still needed to determine the specific effects and mechanisms of action. Quality studies by nurses can provide a unique perspective within this area of inquiry.

REFERENCES

Aiken, L. H., & Henrichs, T. F. (1971). Systematic relaxation as a nursing intervention technique with open heart surgery patients. *Nursing Research, 20*, 212–217.

Banks, J. (1981). The effects of relaxation training and biofeedback on the weight of black, obese clients. Unpublished doctoral dissertation, The Catholic University of America, Washington, DC.

Bengtsson, C., Hallstrom, T., & Tibblin, G. (1973). Social factors, stress experience and personality traits in women with ischemic heart disease, compared to a population sample of women. *Acta Medica Scandinavica, 549*, 82–92.

Benson, H. (1975). *The relaxation response.* New York: Avon Press.

Benson, H., Rosner, B. A., Marzetta, B. R., & Klemchuk, H. M. (1974). Decreased blood pressure in pharmacologically treated hypertensive patients who regularly elicit the relaxation response. *Lancet, 1*, 289–291.

Bernstein, D. A., & Borkovec, T. D. (1973). *Progressive relaxation training.* Champaign, IL: Research Press.

Bohachick, P. (1984). Progressive relaxation training in cardiac rehabilitation: Effect on psychologic variables. *Nursing Research, 33*, 283–287.

Borkovec, T. D., Grayson, J. B., & Cooper, K. M. (1978). Treatment of general tension: Subjective and physiological effects of progressive muscle relaxation. *Journal of Consulting and Clinical Psychology, 46*, 518–528.

Borkovec, T. D., Johnson, M. C., & Block, D. L. (1984). Evaluating experimental designs in relaxation research. In R. L. Woolfolk & P. M. Lehrer (Eds.), *Principles and practice of stress management* (pp. 368–403). New York: Guilford Press.

Borkovec, T. D., & Sides, J. K. (1979). Critical procedural variables related to the physiological effects of progressive relaxation: A review. *Behavior Research and Therapy, 17*, 119–125.

Bowles, C., Smith, J., & Parker, K. (1979). EMG biofeedback and progressive relaxation training: A comparative study of two groups of normal subjects. *Western Journal of Nursing Research, 1*, 179–189.

Britt, S. (1981). Audio biofeedback and level of stress in the minimally prepared gravida during labor. Unpublished doctoral dissertation, University of Alabama in Birmingham.

Burish, T. G., Hendrix, E. M., & Frost, R. O. (1981). Comparison of frontal EMG biofeedback in several types of relaxation instruction in reducing multiple indices of arousal. *Psychophysiology, 18*, 594–602.

Carrington, P. (1978). *Clinically standardized meditation (CSM) instructor's kit.* Kendall Park, NJ: Pace Educational Systems.

Carrington, P. (1984). Modern forms of meditation. In R. L. Woolfolk & P. M. Lehrer (Eds.), *Principles and practice of stress management* (pp. 108–141). New York: Guilford Press.

Chaves, J., & Barber, T. X. (1974). Cognitive strategies, experimental modeling, and expectations in the attenuation of pain. *Journal of Abnormal Psychology, 83*, 356–363.

Coan, R., & Fairchild, M. (1974). *The Personal Opinion Survey.* Unpublished manuscript.

Cotanch, P. H. (1983). Relaxation training for control of nausea and vomiting in patients receiving chemotherapy. *Cancer Nursing, 6*, 277–282.

Davidson, R. J., & Schwartz, G. E. (1976). The psychobiology of relaxation and related states: A multi-process theory. In D. Mostofsky (Ed.), *Modification and control of physiological activity* (pp. 399–442). Englewood Cliffs, NJ: Prentice Hall.

Davis, M., McKay, M., & Eshelman, E. R. (1980). *The relaxation and stress reduction workbook.* Richmond, VA: New Harbinger Publications.

Derogatis, L. E. (1977). *Symptom Checklist (SCL) — 90 Manual-R.* Baltimore, MD: Johns Hopkins University, Clinical Psychometrics Unit.

Dodrill, C. B., Batzel, L. W., Queissen, H. R., & Temkin, N. R. (1980). An objective method for the assessment of psychological and social problems among epileptics. *Epilepsia, 21*, 123–135.

Donovan, M. I. (1979). Assessment of the impact of relaxation with guided imagery on the reduction of stress among cancer nurses. Unpublished doctoral dissertation, University of Pittsburgh, PA.

Everly, G. S., & Rosenfeld, R. (1981). *The nature and treatment of the stress response.* New York: Plenum Press.

Fehring, R. J. (1983). Effects of biofeedback-aided relaxation on the psychological stress symptoms of college students. *Nursing Research, 32*, 362–366.

Fischer-Williams, M., Nigl, A. J., & Savine, D. L. (1981). *A textbook of biological biofeedback.* New York: Human Sciences Press.

Flaherty, G. G., & Fitzpatrick, J. J. (1978). Relaxation technique to increase comfort levels of postoperative patients: A preliminary study. *Nursing Research, 27*, 352–355.

Geden, E. A., Beck, N., Hauge, G., & Pohlman, S. (1984). Self-report and psychological effects of five pain-coping strategies. *Nursing Research, 33*, 260–265.

Gills, J. S. (1980). *Child anxiety scale.* Champaign, IL: Institute for Personality and Ability.

Goldfried, M. R., & Davison, G. C. (1976). *Clinical behavior therapy.* New York: Holt, Rinehart, & Winston.

Heide, F. J., & Borkovec, T. D. (1984). Relaxation-induced anxiety: Mechanisms and theoretical implications. *Behavior Research and Therapy, 22,* 1–12.

Hillenberg, J. B., & Collins, F. L. (1982). A procedural analysis and review of relaxation training research. *Behavior Research and Therapy, 20,* 251–260.

Horowitz, B. F., Fitzpatrick, J. J., & Flaherty, G. G. (1984). Relaxation techniques for pain relief after open heart surgery. *Dimensions of Critical Care Nursing, 3,* 364–371.

Jacobson, E. (1938). *Progressive relaxation.* Chicago: University of Chicago Press.

Kogan, H. N., & Beaton, R. (1984). Blending of a conceptual model and nursing practice. In *Accommodation to self-determination: Nursing's role in the development of a health care policy* (ANA Publication No. G-153). Kansas City: American Nurses' Association.

Korn, E. R. (1983). The use of altered states of consciousness and imagery in physical and pain rehabilitation. *Journal of Mental Imagery, 7,* 25–34.

LaMontagne, L. L., Mason, K. R., & Hepworth, J. T. (1985). Effects of relaxation on anxiety in children: Implications for coping with stress. *Nursing Research, 35,* 289–292.

Lehrer, P. M. (1982). How to relax and how not to relax: A re-evaluation of the work of Edmund Jacobson (Part I). *Behavior Research and Therapy, 20,* 417–428.

Lehrer, P. M., & Woolfolk, R. L. (1984). Are stress reduction techniques interchangeable, or do they have specific effects?: A review of the comparative empirical literature. In R. L. Woolfolk & P. M. Lehrer (Eds.), *Principles and practice of stress management* (pp. 404–477). New York: Guilford Press.

Luthe, W. (1969). *Autogenic therapy* (6 vols.). New York: Grune & Stratton.

McNair, D. M., Lorr, M., & Droppleman, L. F. (1971). *Profile of mood states.* San Diego: Educational and Industrial Testing Service.

Murphy, L. R. (1983). A comparison of relaxation methods for reducing stress in nursing personnel. *Human Factors, 25,* 431–440.

Norton, G. R., & Johnson, W. E. (1983). A comparison of two relaxation procedures for reducing cognitive and somatic anxiety. *Journal of Behavior Therapy and Experimental Psychiatry, 14,* 209–214.

Paul, G. L., & Trimble, R. W. (1970). Recorded versus "live" relaxation training and hypnotic suggestion: Comparative effectiveness for reducing physiological arousal and inhibiting stress response. *Behavior Therapy, 1,* 285–302.

Pender, N. J. (1984). Physiologic responses of clients with essential hypertension to progressive muscle relaxation. *Research in Nursing and Health, 7,* 197–203.

Pender, N. J. (1985). Effects of progressive muscle relaxation training on anxiety and health locus of control among hypertensive adults. *Research in Nursing and Health, 8,* 67–72.

Reinking, R. H., & Kohl, M. L. (1975). Effects of various forms of relaxation training on physiological and self-report measures of relaxation. *Journal of Consulting and Clinical Psychology, 43,* 595–600.

Rice, V. H., Caldwell, M., Butler, S., & Robinson, J. (1986). Relaxation training and response to cardiac catheterization: A pilot study. *Nursing Research, 35,* 39–43.

Schultz, J. (1953). *Das autogene training.* Stuttgart, Germany: Georg-thieme Verlag.

Schwartz, G. E., Davidson, R. J., & Goleman, D. J. (1978). Patterning of cognitive and somatic processes in the self-regulation of anxiety: Effects of meditation versus exercise. *Psychosomatic Medicine, 40*, 321–328.

Sheer, B. (1980). The effects of relaxation training on psychiatric patients. *Issues in Mental Health Nursing, 2*(6), 1–15.

Silver, B. V., & Blanchard, E. B. (1978). Biofeedback and relaxation training in the treatment of psychophysiological disorders: Or, are the machines really necessary? *Journal of Behavioral Medicine, 1*, 217–239.

Sime, A. M., & Libera, M. B. (1985). Sensation information, self-instruction, responses to dental surgery. *Research in Nursing and Health, 8*, 41–47.

Sitzman, J., Kamiya, J., & Johnston, J. (1983). Biofeedback training for reduced respiratory rate in chronic obstructive pulmonary disease: A preliminary study. *Nursing Research, 32*, 218–223.

Smith, J. C. (1985). *Relaxation dynamics.* Champaign, IL: Research Press.

Snyder, M. (1983). Effects of relaxation on psychological functioning of persons with epilepsy. *Journal of Neurosurgical Nursing, 15*, 250–254.

Snyder, M. (1984). Progressive relaxation as a nursing intervention: An analysis. *Advances in Nursing Science, 6*(3), 47–58.

Sodergren, K. M. (1985). Guided imagery. In M. Snyder, *Independent nursing interventions* (pp. 103–124). New York: Wiley.

Spielberger, C. D., Gorsuch, R. L., & Lushene, R. E. (1970). *Manual for the State-Trait Anxiety Inventory.* Palo Alto, CA: Consulting Psychologist Press.

Sugar, E. (1983). Bladder control through biofeedback. *American Journal of Nursing, 83*, 1152–1154.

Surwit, R. (1980). *Relaxation training program.* Durham, NC: Duke University Press.

Tamez, E. G., Moore, M. J., & Brown, P. L. (1978). Relaxation training as a nursing intervention versus pro re nata medications. *Nursing Research, 27*, 160–164.

Thiel, H. G., Parker, D., & Bruce, T. A. (1973). Stress factors and the risk of myocardial infarction. *Journal of Psychosomatic Research, 17*, 43–57.

Wallston, K. A., Wallston, B. S., & DeVellis, R. (1978). Development of multidimensional health locus of control (MHCC) scales. *Health Education Monographs, 6*, 160–170.

Wells, N. (1982). The effect of relaxation on postoperative muscle tension and pain. *Nursing Research, 31*, 236–238.

Wolpe, J., & Lazarus, A. A. (1966). *Behavioral therapy techniques.* New York: Pergamon Press.

Woolfolk, R. L., & Lehrer, P. M. (1984). Clinical stress reduction: An overview. In R. Woolfolk & P. Lehrer, *Principles and practice of stress management* (pp. 1–11). New York: Guilford Press.

Zuckerman, M. (1960). The development of an affect adjective check list for the measurement of anxiety. *Journal of Consulting Psychology, 24*, 457–462.

PART II

Research on
Nursing Care Delivery

Chapter 6

Variable Costs of Nursing Care in Hospitals

MARGARET D. SOVIE
SCHOOL OF NURSING
UNIVERSITY OF ROCHESTER
STRONG MEMORIAL HOSPITAL

CONTENTS

Each patient has unique and varying needs for nursing care. Yet the concept of variable costs of nursing care was not introduced in hospitals until the early 1970s and then was implemented in only a few scattered institutions. Instead, the prevailing practice, continuing today as the industry's norm, is that hospital nursing costs are assigned to occupied beds and fixed. Nursing costs are included as a part of the established daily room rate, which varies with the patient's assignment to either a regular patient care unit or an intensive care unit. In each of

The author gratefully acknowledges the contributions of Meg Johantgen, R.N., M.S., Surgical Clinician II, Strong Memorial Hospital, University of Rochester Medical Center, Rochester, NY, to the literature search.

131

these locations the patient is charged a fixed daily room rate regardless of the amount of nursing resources consumed.

In this era of consumer activism and patients' rights, it is reasonable that patients expect to pay for the care they receive and to know the basis on which charges for services are made. Furthermore, in a hospital payment system based on per case reimbursement, it is important to identify the costs of services provided to individual patients. Burik and Duvall (1985) have defined a service item as "any distinct and measurable consumption of resources that can be associated with a specific patient" (p. 26). Costs for these services can be classified as variable when the measurable activities in providing the services change based on individual patients' needs. The latter is clearly the case for nursing care, that is, patients receive varying amounts of the service — nursing care — based on their individual needs.

The predominant management technique for allotting and monitoring the utilization of nursing care resources in hospitals has been and continues to be the statistic of *nursing care hours per patient day.* The concept of nursing care hours per patient day is one of fixed hours and fixed nursing costs per occupied bed, and is based on an assumption that all patients on a unit are equal in terms of nursing care requirements. Nursing care hours per patient day are gross monitors of nursing resource utilization and nursing productivity and do not reflect the variations that exist when the unit of measurement is the individual patient rather than the occupied bed.

In their 1940 study Pfefferkorn and Rovetta had as one of their objectives to develop methods and criteria to enable valid comparisons of nursing costs between and among institutions. These early investigators acknowledged many institutional and personnel variables that influenced total bedside nursing time requirements in different institutions and in different units in the same institution. Interestingly, however, the individual patient having a unique response to illness and unique needs for nursing care was not mentioned. Cost was defined "as the sum of all expenses allocated to a particular unit, such as a meal, a pound of steam, or an hour of nursing service" (p. 8). The focus was the institution, the unit, and not the patient.

Connor (1961) identified this problem of lack of focus on the individual patients. His pioneering work with the Johns Hopkins Operations Group was directed toward problems of matching personnel resources, particularly nursing, to patient needs. Connor and his group developed a patient classification system to determine the direct care work load for nursing staff. One major contribution of those investigators was the finding that individual patient needs were the determinants of demand for nursing care, and not the occupied bed per se. It was unfortunate that their methodology did not include ways of capturing and retaining the information permanently as it related to specific patients because their work was a major influence on the subsequent developments in patient classification. Twenty-eight years later, a vast majority of hospitals still have not captured or retained patient-specific nursing patient classification data permanently.

The national movement to case-based and capitated payments to hospitals by third party payers provides a compelling motivation for hospital managers to want to know the costs associated with providing care to individual patients. Prospective payment systems based on Diagnostic Related Groups (DRGs) are strong external forces driving hospitals to systems of product-line accounting. Both national and state policymaking groups are taking action to support the creation of separate revenue and cost centers within institutions for direct nursing care (Institute of Medicine, 1983, p. 18; Maine's 42 hospitals, 1985; Prospective Payment Assessment Commission, 1985). In addition, hospital cost control is receiving increasing priority as a result of growing competition in providing health services, sparked by the prudent buyers in health maintenance organizations and preferred provider arrangements.

THE LITERATURE SEARCH

The computerized files of *Index Medicus* and *International Nursing Index* were searched to identify material for this chapter. Journals written in English and published between 1979 and 1985 were targeted for review. Subject headings included: economics-nursing; case mix; diagnostic related groups; direct service costs; cost allocation; fees and charges. As yet, no entry has been provided entitled *costs of nursing care*. Other references searched included the *Medical Care Review, Abstracts of Health Care Management Studies*, the citations in published manuscripts, and selected books.

With the exception of references included for historical relevance, the following criteria were used to determine eligibility of studies for inclusion in this review: (a) nursing care was treated as a discrete and measurable service that is provided to individual patients based on varying needs; (b) patient-specific data were collected and used in the determination of nursing resource utilization; (c) the investigators described the approach used to allocate variable nursing care hours or costs to specific patients in the sample; and (d) the study hospitals were located in the United States of America.

PATIENT CARE HOURS AND
COST ALLOCATION METHODOLOGIES

Clinical care units, relative intensity measures, and patient classification systems are the three approaches used by the investigators to allocate nursing care hours or costs to patients. Patient classification systems within nursing constitute the predominant approach.

Clinical care units refers to a nursing cost allocation measurement that represents the amount of care delivered to patients, based on their diagnosis and day of stay. Poland, English, Thornton, and Owens (1970) developed an assessment system (PETO), with nursing care units as the basic unit of hospital service to the patient. They recognized the potential utility of billing patients based on nursing care units instead of days of care. With such a system in place, patients would pay for nursing care based on the amount of care delivered. Wood (1982) took their ideas and transformed them into a unique application at the Massachusetts Eye and Ear Infirmary. Clinical care units at this specialty hospital were predetermined on the basis of extensive case studies of the nursing care requirements for patients with particular diagnoses.

Arndt and Skydell (1985) studied an adaptation of the Infirmary's clinical care units system at five metropolitan general hospitals. Each hospital used the GRASP[1] patient classification system within nursing. Arndt and Skydell defined nursing care requirements to include indirect as well as direct care expressed in hours rather than clinical care units. Daily patient classification data plus the uniform hospital discharge data set were collected on over 30,000 patients between October 1983 and June 1984. Financial data came from the

---

[1] GRASP is a registered trademark and a division of FCG Enterprises, Inc., P. O. Box 1854, Morgantown, NC 28655.

Medicare cost report and were adjusted to approximate 1984 costs. Their findings confirmed the heterogeneity of DRGs relative to nursing care requirements and costs. Mean total nursing costs were reported, including direct and indirect costs. The numbers of patients for the DRGs were not provided, and this absence was one limiting factor in evaluating the results.

Relative intensity measures were developed by Caterinicchio (1984) as a client-focused, case-mix-sensitive measure of resource use for the allocation of inpatient general nursing costs. The measures were based on a sample of 2660 patients in eight acute-care New Jersey hospitals. Data were collected between 1979 and 1981. A maximum sampling period of 32 days for any study patient was a criterion used in the data collection methodology; consequently, length of stay outliers beyond this point were excluded. Caterinicchio observed the critical importance of variation in staff mix relative to patient care activities and created a registered-nurse-equivalent unit of service index to adjust for differences. Relative intensity measures were based on 13 nursing service isoresource categories created from the 23 major diagnostic categories within the DRG prospective payment system. The isoresource categories were based on similar patterns of nursing resource use and were used to cluster patients into the "best" classes. Caterinicchio's approach caused concern because the isoresource categories were created from the DRG system, which has been demonstrated consistently as heterogeneous from a nursing resource utilization perspective. Furthermore, relative intensity measures were client-focused rather than client-specific, that is, based on isoresource categories instead of the daily, variable nursing requirements of patients. Consequently, the measures were not sensitive to the uniqueness of individual patients' responses to illness and therapy.

Patient classification systems that were dependent on the daily classification of patients according to nursing intensity or acuity have been the most common approach to allocating variable costs of nursing care to individual patients. In those systems, patients were assigned to categories of nursing intensity by one of two approaches: the fit with a typical description of patient characteristics in each category; or, more commonly, the sum of weights assigned to selected indicators descriptive of patients' needs or nursing care requirements (Giovannetti, 1979). Nursing care hours were assigned to each of the categories of intensity based on hospital-specific studies, and the assumption was made that the respective category assignment reflected the average number of nursing care hours provided to the patients during the 24-hour period. A number of different patient classification systems have been developed. Use of those systems for allocating nursing care costs to patients has required demonstrated validity and reliability and an established audit trail in the patient's record. Such an audit trail included a requirement that the summary statistic—the category of nursing intensity, or the completed patient classification instrument—be retained in the individual patient's record.

Holbrook (1972) described a specific billing system for nursing charges, separate from room and board charges, that was established in 1967 at Deaconess Hospital in Great Falls, Montana. When first established, the charge was based on nursing care hours per patient day, which was essentially an occupied bed concept. However, a study of 1970 historical data was used to establish nursing hours standards in a system with four categories for floor care plus an intensive care unit category. As a historical benchmark, it was noted that nursing care costs per category ranged from $0.75 per hour to $2.55 per hour; the semiprivate and intensive care room rates were $14 and $26 respectively.

Patient classification systems within nursing were developed and used by other hospitals for staffing purposes, but retaining and using patient-specific data for determining the variable costs of nursing had a slow start in the 1970s. Acceleration began in the 1980s, catalyzed by prospective payment systems and the need to know the price of hospital products.

METHODOLOGICAL APPROACHES, INCONSISTENCIES, AND CONCERNS

In the studies that follow, investigators contribute knowledge about the approaches that have been used to determine costs of nursing care in hospitals. They also illustrate methodological inconsistencies that should be addressed to strengthen future research, facilitate data comparisons, advance knowledge, and contribute to the formulation of health policy at the state and national level. These inconsistencies include: (a) variations in the definitions of similar terms and confusion in the use of selected concepts; (b) differences in the numbers of categories considered essential to depict the range of nursing intensity; (c) variations in the type of provider classifying the patients; (d) variations in both the elements and the methods used for determining assigned costs; (e) inconsistent reporting of descriptive information that facilitates data interpretation and utilization, such as the mix of nursing staff and the organizational system for nursing practice in the participating hospitals; and (f) differences in the type of data and statistics reported in the various studies. To advance knowledge and contribute to policy formulation, it is important to have a minimum set of uniformly defined data elements that each investigator uses and reports as a part of study results.

Higgerson and Van Slyck (1982) advanced the application of the concept of variable billing for nursing care with their description of the classification, staffing, and billing system developed at St. Luke's Hospital Medical Center in Phoenix, Arizona. A patient classification instrument called the nursing care record—a permanent part of the patient's record—was completed each shift by the staff member caring for the patient. At the end of the 24-hour hospital day, a nurse summed the points assigned to each selected item on the record, thereby determining the patient's classification (acuity) level. Seven levels of acuity were used, with levels 1 through 5 in use on regular patient care units, and levels 6 and 7 reserved for intensive care units. Although the practice modality of team nursing was specified, there was no mention of the nursing staff mix, and registered nurses (RNs) were not differentiated from licensed practical nurses (LPNs) on a scheduling matrix. Nursing care charges were determined by the required staffing and supplies used by patients in each acuity level and were summarized on the patient's bill by number of days at particular acuity levels. The inclusion of patient supplies in a nursing care charge obscured the identification of actual nursing costs.

Riley and Schaefers (1983) defined nursing costs as all costs under the nursing department operating budget and direct nursing costs as those associated with all aspects of nursing care provided to a patient. The head nurse was excluded from direct nursing care hours and costs. However, according to those definitions, the head nurse, support personnel such as unit clerks, and patient care supplies were included in deriving the total nursing cost figures. Such compounded cost data are one argument for using nursing care hours as the data element for comparisons among different studies rather than nursing care costs. St. Paul-Ramsey Medical Center in St. Paul, Minnesota, a 418-bed tertiary hospital, was the site for data collection, which occurred in 1982 on a proportionate random sample of 98 patients in four DRGs. Neither staff mix nor the type of patient classification system was specified. However, reference was made to a system with values ranging from 1 (low) to 8. Reported results included average nursing care hours, direct and total nursing costs, and length of stay for each of four DRGs.

Walker (1983) reported on an exploratory study that included descriptions of the separation of the costs of nursing care from the all-inclusive room rate. The sample was comprised of Level 3 patients in an adult intensive care unit (ICU) at Stanford University Hospital in Palo Alto, California, a 668-bed university-owned teaching hospital with a predominantly RN staff. Data were collected on 30 patients, five patients in each of six disease categories, over a 1-month period. The patient classification system consisted of five levels of nursing care, with one representing the lowest. Level 3 patients received one-on-one care. The results included comparisons of nursing care costs with other hospital charges embedded in the room rate. Unfortunately, similar entities, that is, costs to costs or charges to charges, were not compared. With that serious limitation noted, the major result reported was that the total nursing care cost was approximately 55% of the per diem ICU charge. It was difficult to evaluate the data or the results because little information was given on the cost allocation methodology and the data provided on the sample were meager. Unit managers, clerks, and equipment technicians were included in the direct nursing care costs. However, there were no specifics about how many of these employees were on the staff of the adult ICU used as a study site.

The range in levels of nursing care or patient classification categories, as well as the inconsistency in how levels of care were represented, was illustrated in the case study reported by Staley and Luciano (1984). The patient classification system used in their project resulted in the assignment of the patient to one of six levels of care, with Level 1 as the highest level and requiring 24 hours of care per patient day. Direct nursing care costs were defined as salary expenses and supply costs. The latter included patient nourishment, supplies, and equipment maintenance.

Lagona and Stritzel (1984) reported on 35 patients with myocardial infarctions (DRG 121 and DRG 122) who were studied at a 547-bed community teaching hospital. This Rochester, New York hospital had a nursing staff mix of 58.7% RNs, 14.6% LPNs, 17.7% nursing assistants, and 9% nursing support personnel. Their results included the average nursing care hours and direct nursing costs for these two DRGs. For some unstated reason, these investigators did not sum the nursing care hours required by all patients in the DRG and divide by the number of patients in the DRG to obtain average hours and costs per DRG. Instead, the method they used to quantify the average amount of nursing care consumed per DRG was to multiply the average length of stay by the average hours of nursing care consumed per day by each patient.

Variable nursing care costs have been calculated from the approximate amount of nursing care time that specific patients receive. McClain and Selhat (1984) investigated the actual amounts of direct and indirect nursing care delivered to 20 patients within three DRGs at a 265-bed general hospital in Philadelphia. The nursing staff mix was reported as 50% professional nursing staff with the remainder nonprofessional caregivers. Data were collected through retrospective record reviews, and the daily nursing patient classification level was transformed into hours of nursing care using the O'Leary and Associates Patient Classification System[2]. Results included average nursing care hours and nursing costs. The nursing costs were based on total nursing department budget and included salaries of ward clerks as well as supervisory personnel.

Mitchell, Miller, Welches, and Walker (1984) used a patient classification system to determine average nursing care hours and costs for four DRGs at Stanford University Hospital. Data were collected prospectively from March to August 1983 on four nursing units with selected admission diagnoses as study entry criteria. The classification system had a "unit constant" figure to represent care planning, charting, report, and other activities of the caregivers. Including care planning in the unit constant, rather than attributing the activity to individual patients as a variable, seems unique and worthy of note. The mix of nursing staff on the study units was not disclosed. However, the investigators noted that calculation of costs took into account the ratio of RNs to nursing assistants. The results included average hours of nursing care and average direct nursing costs. The direct nursing costs were considered the variable portion of the nursing costs and the remainder were considered fixed and calculated on a patient-day basis. This approach to allocating fixed costs was quite common across the studies reviewed but was not the sole method used, a finding that illustrated the importance of knowing cost allocation methodology in order to make meaningful comparisons. The study results also dem-

---

[2] For additional information contact O'Leary and Associates, 331 Lowella Ave., Wayne, PA.

onstrated the heterogeneity of DRGs when used to reflect nursing resource utilization. These investigators also compared nursing costs to hospital charges but noted the problem of inconsistency and the need to compare costs with costs.

Schaefers (1985) used a patient classification system to study the costs of nursing for the 25 most frequent DRGs at St. Paul-Ramsey Medical Center. Only RNs and LPNs were included as the direct caregivers. All other staff, including head nurses, charge nurses, nursing assistants, and ward secretaries, were considered noncaregivers and constant, that is, their numbers did not vary based on patient acuity. The latter group was included in the costs for indirect nursing support services, which were calculated by multiplying length of stay by an established cost per day. Schaefers described this as the benefits-available concept. Certain supply items, such as forms and stethoscopes, also were considered part of the costs of nursing, as were the expenses of the nurse epidemiologists in the hospital. These types of cost inclusions illustrate again the extreme variability of cost allocation approaches and underscore the extreme limitations of cost data for interhospital comparative purposes. Schaefers's cost calculations were unit-specific and not hospital-wide; that is, there were direct and support service costs that varied for each unit, with nursing administration support services as the only constant costs across all units. Data from the Schaefers' study included 1725 cases from 1982 and 613 cases from 1984, and comparisons of the data were made between the two years.

Schaefers (1985) compared the 1982 data for 16 DRGs with data from the same 16 DRGs that were reported by Sovie, Tarcinale, Van-Putte, and Stunden (1985). Both studies were based on a patient classification system that consisted of critical indicators of care to assign patients to categories of acuity. Each system included nursing care hours per category of acuity developed for each nursing unit. Because cost allocation methodologies differed, comparisons were limited to average nursing care hours and average length of stay per DRG. Schaefers also reported mean total nursing costs for some of the DRGs.

Sovie et al. (1985) reported the most comprehensive data on nursing care hours, costs, and DRGs. The study was conducted at the University of Rochester's Strong Memorial Hospital, a 741-bed teaching hospital in Rochester, New York, with a nursing staff mix of 92% RNs and 8% LPNs, NAs, and technicians. These investigators sought to (a) identify the nursing care hours required to meet patients' care needs according to category of acuity; (b) combine DRGs, a medical classification system, with a patient classification system; and (c) use the combination of data to predict nursing resource utilization. Data from 24,879 patients were studied. The patient classification system had four categories of acuity with specific nursing care hour assignments for each category on each of 34 patient care units.

The time study component of the Sovie et al. (1985) investigation included two partitions of patient-assignable time — direct time and other. Direct time was defined as all patient-centered activity carried out directly with the patient or family; other time was time spent away from the patient or family, but in preparation for or completion of patient-specific direct care. All unit-assigned nursing staff as well as the head nurse were included in the nursing acuity category time assignments. Costs of services were computed using the Medicare step-down methodology, and all data comparisons were performed using cost figures. Direct nursing care costs consisting solely of actual salaries and benefits for RNs, LPNs, and NAs were computed using a hospital-wide rather than a unit-specific determined average hourly rate for a nursing care hour. Unit secretarial costs were excluded. Four categories of nursing acuity, with unit-specific assignment of nursing care hours, were sufficient to represent accurately the nursing resource need and utilization on all patient care units, including intensive care units. Regretfully, these investigators were not consistent in including in their first published tables the number of patients in each DRG reported, a critical element for data interpretation. In addition, the narrative describing the data reported for the top 22 DRGs on a medical unit was extremely sparse and did not make it clear that patient days spent on other units, such as ICUs, were excluded from this one table. The results demonstrated the heterogeneity of DRGs from a nursing resource utilization perspective. In addition, Sovie et al. identified the extreme limitations of reported data for comparative analyses among studies because of differences in definitions and methodologies.

The American Nurses' Association study of the relationship between nursing care costs and DRG reimbursement was conducted by McKibbin, Brimmer, Galliher, Hartley, and Clinton (1985a,b). Data were collected in 1984 on the 21 most common DRGs in two 400-bed hospitals — Mt. Sinai Medical Center in Milwaukee and Waukesha Memorial Hospital in Waukesha, Wisconsin. Two versions of the Medicus patient classification system were used to collect nursing intensity data, a four-level and a five-level version. McKibbin et al. used the costs for all nursing personnel in each hospital to calculate nursing costs, including what they termed indirect care employees such as secretaries and monitoring aides. However, they noted that personnel costs for each care unit were divided by hours actually worked to calculate the average hourly nursing cost per unit. Nursing staff mix at the study hospitals was not disclosed, but there must have been wide variation, given that they reported a range of hourly nursing costs from $13 in an intermediate care unit to $22 in an intensive care unit. Another caution in reviewing these data was that length of stay and cost outliers were excluded.

Mowry and Korpman (1985) used a patient classification system to examine variations in acuity levels within five DRGs and determine the average costs of nursing services of these DRGs. Data were collected in 1983 in a 425-bed acute-care hospital in a Los Angeles suburb, using the St. Luke's (Phoenix) Hospital Medical Center's patient classification system with seven acuity levels. Average direct nursing care costs were determined using unit-specific salary and benefit figures. No details were provided on mix of nursing staff or on types of personnel costs included in the determination of nursing care costs. Nursing care hours were not reported. Instead, full-time equivalents were reported per acuity level in an acuity conversion table, and mean nursing labor costs were given.

Another variation in methodology was reflected in the study conducted by Reschak, Biordi, Holm, and Santucci (1985) at a 500-bed teaching hospital in the Chicago metropolitan area. The study was designed to determine the total cost of nursing care (direct and indirect) for two DRGs. Data were collected prospectively over a 4-month period in 1984 using a patient classification instrument that was completed by the head nurse or designee each day. Direct nursing care costs were based on unit-specific wages and benefits, and average indirect nursing care costs were calculated per patient day.

Bargagliotti and Smith (1985) studied four DRGs at a 345-bed acute-care urban hospital in northern California. These investigators used a patient classification system designed by Quantitative Health System Inc., in which indicators were summed and converted by computer program into hours of nursing care for each patient. The hours per paid patient day for each case were retrieved from nursing administration records. Costs specific to each unit were used in determining nursing care costs. The ICU, with an all-RN staff, had a cost per hour of $21, compared to a range of $14 to $15 per hour for the medical-surgical unit with a staff of 70% RNs and 30% LPNs. Costs of head nurses and unit secretaries were included in indirect costs. In this study, nursing costs again were compared to hospital charges, but recognition was given to the limitations of the comparison.

Dahlen and Gregor (1985) used a revised version of a patient classification system designed by Lawrence J. Donnelly. This system of five levels was used to study the costs of nursing care with an all-RN staff at Meridian Park Hospital, a 150-bed acute-care facility in Tualatin, Oregon. A separate classification system was used for ICU and recovery room patients. The 10 most common DRGs at that hospital were used to test the hypothesis that the cost of an all-RN nursing care was no higher a percentage of the patient's total hospital bill than mixed-staff nursing care. In their cost allocation methodology, the costs of pharmacy nurses were included in nursing costs because those individuals administered routine medications and intravenous fluids on the general nursing units. The nurse epidemiologist and the enterostomal therapist also were included in indirect nursing costs. Unit-specific salary and benefit expenses were used to determine direct hourly costs. Indirect nursing costs were calculated using a constant patient day amount. The average for the nursing costs for the ten DRGs came to 14% of the total patients' bills and compared favorably with other reports of 17 to 20% of total hospital bills. Average nursing care hours for each of the ten DRGs were not reported. Cost data were reported with direct nursing, pharmacy nursing, and indirect nursing as the components of total nursing costs.

deMars Martin and Boyer (1985) described the product line costing system methodology developed at Children's Memorial Hospital in Chicago. Costs of utilized services and procedures were accumulated at the level of the individual patient diagnosis (ICD-9-CM). Because nursing generated 36% of the hospital revenues, it was given priority for costing procedure development and implementation. The patient acuity level was defined as the unit of care in nursing, and nursing costs were compiled by patient acuity level on each nursing unit. The patient classification system incorporated four levels of acuity. Each nursing unit had unique direct care hours per patient day assigned to each acuity level. The methodology was illustrated with one ICU baby with a diagnosis of Tetralogy of Fallot and an operative procedure of systemic pulmonary arterial shunt. The costs of the nursing services for this 9-day length of stay were $3421.

Trofino (1986) used a patient classification system, entitled Reality Based System, to determine the average hours and costs of direct nursing care for DRGs at Riverview Medical Center in Red Bank, New Jersey and compared data based on this system to that collected in six other New Jersey hospitals. In this patient classification system, 1 hour of nursing care was called a nursing care unit and 1 hour of required patient care was equal to one patient care unit. The method described for allocating nursing costs was based on the derivation of an average price per patient unit, but no cost figures were given. Average patient care units were reported for two DRGs from three hospitals that each had similar staff mixes — approximately 57% RNs, 14% LPNs, and 29% NAs and clerks.

The final study in this review was conducted by Wolf, Lesic, and Leak (1986), who used the variable costing of nursing care to demonstrate support for the cost-effectiveness of primary nursing in comparison to team nursing. Using a 474-bed acute-care community hospital with a 70% RN staff mix, those investigators compared length of stay, daily acuity, and nursing care costs over a 6-month period on two 28-bed medical-surgical units — one with primary nursing and the other with team nursing. Patient classification instruments were completed daily by the assigned nurses, resulting in placement of patients into one of four levels of acuity. Each level of acuity was given a relative weight that represented the amount of nursing care required. This latter amount was labeled the relative index of workload (RIW), and each RIW equaled 3.6 hours of care. Total direct nursing care costs were calculated by multiplying 3.6 by the average hourly salary for direct caregivers by the number of RIWs accumulated over the patient's length of stay. These costs then were linked with the DRG assigned to the patient at discharge. The final sample included 190 patients representing 34 DRGs. Total acuity for patients on the primary nursing unit was 28% greater than for patients on the team nursing unit; the primary unit staff included 82% RNs, compared to 76% RNs on the team unit. Patients' average length of stay was 24% longer on the primary nursing unit. The average daily cost per patient per DRG was $1.30 less per patient on the primary nursing unit than on the team nursing unit.

RESULTS AND RESTRICTIONS
ON COMPARISONS

The majority of investigators reported their findings on the variable costs of nursing care for patients according to DRGs. Forty-three of a total of 467 DRGs, or 9.2% of the DRGs, were included in two or more studies in which nursing care hours or cost data were reported. The extent of the comparisons was limited because of the methodological issues and concerns identified earlier. Because of the different cost allocation methodologies, as well as regional wage and salary differences, the mean nursing costs reported offer little comparative information. The mean nursing hours were of greater utility, even though still limited. For example, in order to interpret the findings, the reader needed to know the mean length of stay and whether patients were included whose stay was either extremely short or long. In addition, the mix of nursing staff and the organizational system for nursing practice were important. Yet, some investigators did not report these descriptive facts.

A patient classification system was the most commonly used approach to identify variable costs for nursing care. However, these systems are not identical in design, and there were variations in the number of patient classification categories considered necessary to represent nursing intensity or patient acuity. Interestingly, those studies in which the researcher reported use of a patient classification system with unit-specific assignment of nursing care hours per category of intensity more frequently were based on four levels of nursing acuity, with one representing the lowest. However, the representation of Level 1 was not consistent, and Staley and Luciano (1984) used that category for reporting the highest level of acuity. In those patient classification systems designed with more than four categories, the categories 5 to 8 frequently were reserved for describing nursing acuity of intensive care unit patients. If there was consistency in the number of categories of nursing intensity, comparisons of distribution of acuity levels also would be possible.

Consistency in the definition of data elements, as well as the particular set of data elements themselves, would contribute significantly to advancing knowledge about nursing needs of patients and nursing costs. Securing solid data on nursing hours and costs is of critical importance for refining DRG cost allocations as well as informing policy and decision makers on the cost benefits of professional nursing care. Wolf et al.'s (1986) approach is excellent.

Investigators do nothing to advance knowledge when illogical comparative data are used to illustrate nursing's costs. Comparing nursing costs to hospital charges or reporting nursing costs as a percentage of particular charges is an example of this point.

Of serious concern is the mixture of patient supply costs and nursing care costs. The buyer of hospital care should be able to identify the products being purchased. Linen costs, housekeeping, and routine supplies can be a part of the hotel costs, or identified separately, but should not be bundled with nursing care costs. Of equal concern is the inclusion of unit managers and unit clerks as components of the nursing care costs. Again, unit management can be identified as a distinct cost center, and these costs should be separated from the nursing care costs. Nurse epidemiologists' costs as well as enterostomal therapists' costs also should be separated and identified in different cost centers.

Several researchers provided evidence on the relationship between length of stay and nursing care hours by DRG. This finding was expected and obvious because patients received nursing care each day they were in a hospital. However, as length of stay was shortened, nursing intensity and nursing hours increased (Schaefers, 1985). The majority of the investigators demonstrated the wide range of nursing hours and nursing costs in each of the DRGs and provided support for the conclusion that DRGs are not homogeneous for nursing resource utilization.

The trend of collecting and retaining patient-specific nursing acuity and cost data is the single greatest contribution signaled by these studies. Nurses have been collecting and recording patient data for use by others and have neglected their own professional needs for information and research data.

The relevance of reporting staff mix and organization systems for nursing practice as factors contributing to total required nursing resources is another strength emanating from these works. The RN is the best-prepared provider to assess and meet the nursing care needs of patients. One only can speculate on the differences in quality of patient care when essentially the same hours of care are delivered to two groups of patients, one group with a 93% RN staff and the other with a 57% RN staff.

The lack of data on the quality of the nursing care provided during these reported hours of nursing care is one of the serious weaknesses in all the studies. Effectiveness as well as efficiency is an important variable in product costing, and energies should be devoted to designing quality of care measurements that can be applied systematically across institutions.

The lack of consistency in categories of nursing acuity as well as the meaning of the designated levels was another weakness. Use of four to eight categories of acuity with ICU patients treated uniquely in many patient classification systems has inhibited generation of a national data base. In addition, there was inconsistency in the method of assigning nursing hours to designated levels of acuity. The majority of investigators used hours of nursing care. However, Mowry and Korpman (1985) used full time equivalents (FTEs). Yet, they did not report the worked hours for these FTEs, and without such information it was impossible to convert them to comparable nursing care hours.

Another major weakness is the variety of cost allocation methodologies and the diversity of elements included in nursing care costs. These deficiencies are identified in the reviews of the studies.

Reporting inconsistencies is a major weakness that easily is remedied. Certainly, fellow professionals should expect to find number of subjects, along with standard deviations, when central tendency statistics are reported. In addition, a standard unit of measurement, such as nursing care hours, should be agreed upon and reported. Editors and journal reviewers can assist by insisting on the inclusion of common data elements in manuscripts reporting nursing research on variable costs of nursing care in hospitals.

RECOMMENDATIONS FOR FUTURE RESEARCH

The establishment of a nursing minimum data set (NMDS) (Werley, Lang, & Westlake, 1986; Werley & Lang, in press) would advance the potential for significant research on nursing practice and the costs of nursing care. The use of a NMDS would facilitate multihospital studies with findings that are generalizable. Terms describing data elements in a NMDS would have standardized definitions, and data would be comparable across studies.

National consensus building regarding data elements for study, as well as their definitions, along with agreement on acceptable methodological approaches, is needed and of paramount importance. Nurses could agree on such basics as the essential data output to be obtained from a patient classification system, for example, the number of hours of nursing care received by each patient over a hospital length of stay. This statistic, then, could be incorporated into the uniform hospital billing data set requirements that are used to establish and monitor DRG relative weights and payments. Other third party payers, as well as different regulators and administrators, would have a meaningful statistic that describes nursing care resource utilization by patient and by groups of patients. If nurses also could agree on measurable quality care indicators, these variables could serve the profession and policymakers as well.

The most important DRGs from a nursing information perspective also need to be identified and studied. Currently limited nursing hours and cost data from multiple studies are available on approximately 9% of the possible DRGs. Valid, comparable data are needed on the most common DRGs that constitute the discharge diagnoses from multiple hospitals.

The identification and retention of patient-specific acuity and cost data are steps in the right direction. Establishing nursing as a revenue center as well as a cost center would provide the economic accountability required to complement the professional care accountability that nurses have now. The studies included in the review are the initial efforts, and national collaborative studies in these areas would provide the evidence necessary to advance knowledge of the variable costs of nursing care.

REFERENCES

Arndt, M., & Skydell, B. (1985). Inpatient nursing services: productivity and cost. In F. A. Shaffer (Ed.), *Costing out nursing: Pricing our product* (pp. 69–84). New York: National League for Nursing.

Bargagliotti, L. A., & Smith, H. (1985). Patterns of nursing costs with capitated reimbursement. *Nursing Economics, 3*(5), 123–130.

Burik, D., & Duvall, T. J. (1985). Hospital cost accounting: Strategic considerations. *Healthcare Financial Management, 39*(2), 19–28.

Caterinicchio, R. P. (1984). Relative intensity measures: Pricing of inpatient nursing services under diagnosis-related group prospective hospital payment. *Health Care Financing Review, 6*(1), 61–70.

Connor, R. J. (1961). Effective use of nursing resources: Research report. *Hospitals, 35*(9), 30–39.

Dahlen, A. L., & Gregor, J. R. (1985). Nursing costs by DRG with an all RN staff. In F. A. Shaffer (Ed.), *Costing out nursing: Pricing our product* (pp. 113–122). New York: National League for Nursing.

deMars Martin, P., & Boyer, F. J. (1985). Developing a consistent method for costing hospital services. *Healthcare Financial Management, 39*(2), 30–37.

Giovannetti, P. (1979). Understanding patient classification systems. *Journal of Nursing Administration, 9*(2), 4-9.

Higgerson, N. J., & Van Slyck, A. (1982). Variable billing for services: New fiscal direction for nursing. *The Journal of Nursing Administration, 12*(6), 20-27.

Holbrook, F. K. (1972). Charging for level of nursing care. *Hospitals, 46*(16), 80-88.

Institute of Medicine. (1983). *Nursing and nursing education: Public policies and private actions.* Washington, DC: National Academy Press.

Lagona, T. G., & Stritzel, M. M. (1984). Nursing care requirements as measured by DRG. *The Journal of Nursing Administration, 14*(5), 15-18.

Maine's 42 hospitals, obeying a unique new law, begin to charge their patients for nursing care. (1985). *American Journal of Nursing, 85*, 1166-1167.

McClain, J. R., & Selhat, M. S. (1984). Twenty cases: What nursing costs per DRG. *Nursing Management, 15*(10), 27-34.

McKibbin, R. C., Brimmer, P. F., Galliher, J. M., Hartley, S. S., & Clinton, J. (1985a). *DRGs and nursing care.* Kansas City, MO: American Nurses' Association.

McKibbin, R. C., Brimmer, P. F., Galliher, J. M., Hartley, S. S., & Clinton, J. (1985b). Nursing costs & DRG payments. *American Journal of Nursing, 85*, 1353-1356.

Mitchell, M., Miller, J., Welches, L., & Walker, D. D. (1984). Determining costs of direct nursing care by DRGs. *Nursing Management, 15*(4), 29-32.

Mowry, M. M., & Korpman, R. A. (1985). Do DRG reimbursement rates reflect nursing costs? *Journal of Nursing Administration, 15*(7,8), 29-35.

Pfefferkorn, B., & Rovetta, C. A. (1940). *Administrative cost analysis for nursing service and nursing education.* New York: National League of Nursing Education. (Published jointly with the American Hospital Association, Chicago)

Poland, M., English, N., Thornton, N., & Owens, D. (1970). PETO — A system of assessing and meeting patient care needs. *American Journal of Nursing, 70*, 1479-1482.

Prospective Payment Assessment Commission. (1985). *Report and recommendations to the secretary, U.S. Department of Health and Human Services (technical appendixes)* (NCHSR 85-87). Rockville, MD: National Center for Health Services Research and Health Care Technology Assessment.

Reschak, G. L. C., Biordi, D., Holm, K., & Santucci, N. (1985). Accounting for nursing costs by DRG. *Journal of Nursing Administration, 15*(9), 15-20.

Riley, W., & Schaefers, V. (1983). Costing nursing services. *Nursing Management, 14*(12), 40-43.

Schaefers, V. (1985). A cost allocation method for nursing. In F. A. Shaffer (Ed.), *Costing out nursing: Pricing our product* (pp. 69-84). New York: National League for Nursing.

Sovie, M. D., Tarcinale, M. A., VanPutte, A. W., & Stunden, A. E. (1985). Amalgam of nursing acuity, DRGs and cost. *Nursing Management, 16*(3), 22-42.

Staley, M., & Luciano, K. (1984). Eight steps to costing nursing services. *Nursing Management, 15*(10), 35-38.

Trofino, J. (1986). A reality based system for pricing nursing service. *Nursing Management, 17*(1), 19-24.

Walker, D. D. (1983). The cost of nursing care in hospitals. *The Journal of Nursing Administration, 13*(3), 13-18.

Werley, H., Lang, N., & Westlake, S. (1986). Brief summary of the nursing minimum data set conference. *Nursing Management, 17*(7), 42–45.

Werley, H., & Lang, N. (In press). *Identification of the Nursing Minimum Data Set.* New York: Springer Publishing Co.

Wolf, G. A., Lesic, L. K., & Leak, A. G. (1986). Primary nursing: The impact on nursing costs within DRGs. *Journal of Nursing Administration, 16*(3), 9–11.

Wood, C. T. (1982). Relate hospital charges to use of services. *Harvard Business Review, 60*(2), 123–130.

PART III

Research on Nursing Education

Chapter 7

Psychiatric–Mental Health Nursing Education

MAXINE E. LOOMIS
COLLEGE OF NURSING
UNIVERSITY OF SOUTH CAROLINA

CONTENTS

The review of research related to psychiatric nursing education contained in this chapter includes studies published between 1963 and 1986. Although admittedly arbitrary, 1963 was selected as the beginning review date because of its historical relevance to mental health practitioners in general. The Community Mental Health Centers Act was passed by Congress in 1963 and eventually led to the deinstitutionalization movement, which persists at the time of this writing. As federal funds for mental health services have declined steadily over the ensuing 20 years, deinstitutionalization has come to represent a withdrawal of treatment and even care and support services for the mentally ill.

The Community Mental Health Centers Act also had a significant impact on psychiatric nursing practice and education. Specifically, National Institutes of Mental Health (NIMH) funds were allocated to prepare generic and graduate-level psychiatric–mental health nurses to provide comprehensive community mental health services. This legislation underscored the importance of psychiatric–mental health nursing within the nursing curriculum, and one would expect this importance to be reflected in research conducted on the preparation of psychiatric–mental health nursing students. This review indicated that such was not the case.

Studies included in this review were obtained through an ERIC search of nursing education and psychiatric nursing and a personal review of *Nursing Research, Research in Nursing and Health, Western Journal of Nursing Research, Journal of Nursing Education, Perspectives in Psychiatric Care,* and *Journal of Psychosocial Nursing and Mental Health Services.* Research is presented within the major categories of (a) predicting success on the State Board Test Pool Examination, (b) characteristics of students and graduates, and (c) the impact of curriculum on students.

Research included is descriptive, correlational, and experimental and has been conducted within all levels of programs preparing basic and advanced practitioners. The lack of subsequent studies or programmatic research might suggest that students are a convenient population for meeting degree requirements and that psychiatric nursing education research has suffered from a lack of replication and extension.

PREDICTING SUCCESS ON THE STATE BOARD
TEST POOL EXAMINATION

Twelve studies designed to predict success on the State Board Test Pool Examination were published in *Nursing Research* ($n = 8$) and *Nursing Outlook* ($n = 4$) from 1966 through 1978. Predictor variables most frequently examined were theory and practice grades (Baldwin, Mowbray, & Taylor, 1968; Bell & Martindill, 1976; Brandt, Hastie, & Schumann, 1966; Miller, Feldhusen, & Asher, 1968; Muhlenkamp, 1971; Shelley, Kennamer, & Raile, 1976) and National League for Nursing (NLN) Achievement Test scores (Baldwin et al., 1968; Bell & Martindill, 1976; Brandt et al., 1966; Deardorff, Denner, & Miller, 1976; Mueller & Lyman, 1969; Muhlenkamp, 1971; Papcum, 1971; Wolfle & Bryant, 1978). Demographic variables (Miller et al., 1968; Mueller & Lyman, 1969; Reed & Feldhusen, 1972), high school class rank (Backman & Steindler, 1971; Baldwin et al., 1968; Miller et al., 1968; Reed & Feldhusen, 1972), and Scholastic Achievement Test (SAT) scores (Backman & Steindler, 1971; Miller et al., 1968; Muhlenkamp, 1971; Reed & Feldhusen, 1972; Wolfle & Bryant, 1978) also were examined as predictor variables with some regularity. Natural and social science test scores (Brandt et al., 1966), preentrance examination scores (Baldwin et al., 1968), high school grades (Miller et al., 1968), intelligence tests (Backman & Steindler, 1971), anxiety test scores (Miller et al., 1968), memory test scores (Miller et al., 1968), aptitude tests (Mueller & Lyman, 1969), personality tests (Mueller & Lyman, 1969), and college grade point average (GPA) (Muhlenkamp, 1971; Wolfle & Bryant, 1978) were included only sporadically as predictor variables.

Associate degree graduates were subjects in six of the studies (Backman & Steindler, 1971; Deardorff et al., 1976; Miller et al., 1968; Papcum, 1971; Reed & Feldhusen, 1972; Wolfle & Bryant, 1978), diploma graduates in three studies (Baldwin et al., 1968; Mueller & Lyman, 1969; Shelley, Kennamer, & Raile, 1976), and baccalaureate graduates in the remaining three studies (Bell & Martindill, 1976; Brandt et al., 1966; Muhlenkamp, 1971). Because of the lack of consistency in the predictor variables used and the diverse nature of the methodologies and research reports, it was impossible to draw any conclusions regarding differences related to level of educational preparation. What did seem reasonable was a summary of the findings that related to psychiatric nursing education.

Wolfle and Bryant (1978) developed and then tested a causal model of nursing education and State Board Examination (SBE) scores. The data used to test the model were obtained from all graduates of an associate degree nursing program in southwest Virginia from 1970 through 1976. The researchers found that SBE performance on the medical, surgical, and obstetric tests depended primarily on mastery of the subject matter, whereas performance on the pediatric and psychiatric tests depended to a large extent on ability acquired prior to entering the nursing program. They proposed that SBE scores in pediatric and psychiatric nursing did not measure mastery of a medically technical subject matter but rather a competent ability to adapt, adjust, or deal with individuals and situations. Intellectual ability and GPA were equal in importance to mastery of the subject matter in predicting SBE performance in pediatric and psychiatric nursing. It was unclear from this study how the nature of the content of the SBE or the nature of the examination influenced these findings.

In general, psychiatric nursing grades have not contributed significantly or consistently as predictors of overall SBE performance. Brandt et al. (1966) found that grades received in the various nursing theory courses correlated positively with SBE tests of baccalaureate graduates with the exception of psychiatric nursing. They suggested that a different type of ability was needed for doing well in psychiatric as opposed to maternal–child or medical–surgical nursing.

Muhlenkamp (1971) reported low and negative correlations between grades in psychiatric nursing practice and all five licensure tests, including psychiatric nursing. There was a positive correlation ($r = .412$) between psychiatric nursing theory and practice grades in this study of baccalaureate graduates. Also, the combination of SAT Verbal score and psychiatric nursing theory grades was the best predictor of success on the SBE psychiatric nursing score ($r = .57$). Similar findings are reported by Backman and Steindler (1971) in their study of associate degree graduates from 1959 through 1964. Scores on the information, vocabulary, and picture completion scales of the Wechsler Adult Intelligence Scale (Wechsler, 1958) as well as verbal SAT scores and high school rank were correlated significantly with SBE scores in psychiatric nursing.

As factor-relating research, the above studies offer little empirical explanation for the questions they leave unanswered. Are psychiatric nursing theory and practice different from those of other nursing specialties? If so, how are they different and what are the implications of these differences for generic-level psychiatric nursing education?

Data for these studies were collected on nursing graduates from 1957 through 1976. There have been no subsequent attempts to examine the impact of integrated curricula on student performance, on psychiatric nursing grades, or on SBE scores. This is a crucial area of neglect, given the concerns expressed by graduate faculty regarding the impact of integrated curricula on enrollments in psychiatric nursing specialty programs (Martin, 1985).

CHARACTERISTICS OF STUDENTS AND GRADUATES

Basic students, practicing nurses, and graduate students in psychiatric–mental health nursing have been the subjects of a limited number of studies. The primary dependent variables in these studies have been: (a) attitudes toward mental patients (Meyer, 1973), subsequent specialty preference and work activity (Stauffacher & Navran, 1968), and personality characteristics (Canter & Shoemaker, 1960) of basic students; (b) personality structure (Navran & Stauffacher, 1957, 1958) and clinical expertise (Davis, 1972, 1974) with practicing psychiatric nurses; and (c) personality characteristics (Gilbert, 1975; Lukens, 1965; Miller, 1965) with graduate student subjects.

Between 1954 and 1960 Stauffacher and Navran (1968) administered the Edwards Personal Preference Schedule (EPPS) (Edwards, 1954) to 680 nursing students during their psychiatric nursing affiliation. The researchers obtained responses to 5-year follow-up questionnaires from 453 of the original sample to determine the specialty area in which subjects had the most experience and their preferred work area. They concluded that personality factors as measured on the EPPS were not related to the predominant type of nursing experience in the first 5 years of work, nor did the EPPS discriminate among the subspecialty practice groups. They did find that subjects who preferred psychiatric nursing initially scored lowest on Achievement and Order and were the highest group on intraception.

Meyer (1973) examined the differences between junior and senior baccalaureate nursing students and their university peers on the Opinions About Mental Illness Scale (Cohen & Struening, 1963). Nursing students differed from their university peers on only two of the five subscales: They were lower on Authoritarianism and higher in Interpersonal Etiology. Further, senior nursing students were significantly lower than junior nursing students on the Interpersonal Etiology subscale, but not on the Authoritarianism subscale, following a junior-level course in psychiatric nursing completed by both groups. These results are of concern in light of the Canter and Shoemaker (1960) results that demonstrated a significant relationship between authoritarian personality tendencies and a negative or fearful attitude toward mental illness among diploma nursing students during their psychiatric affiliation.

Practicing psychiatric nurses have been the subjects of relatively few investigations. The classic studies of Navran and Stauffacher (1957, 1958) were included in this review because of the historical perspective they provided on the personality structure of psychiatric nurses. In their original work, Navran and Stauffacher (1957) administered the EPPS to 196 psychiatric staff nurses of unreported educational backgrounds and found that they were significantly different from college women in general. They had higher scores on Order, Deference, Endurance, and Aggression and lower scores on Autonomy, Affiliation, and Exhibition. The researchers concluded that the best psychiatric nurses as ranked by their chief nurses were relatively less timid and more warm in their interpersonal relationships, more stable, and more capable of leadership than the less highly rated nurses.

Navran and Stauffacher (1958) followed with a study comparing psychiatric and general medical–surgical nurses, again using the EPPS. They found that psychiatric nurses scored higher on Aggression, Introception, and Heterosexuality and scored lower on Abasement. They concluded that general medical–surgical nurses were more work-oriented than people-oriented. It should be noted that both of these studies were conducted before the renaissance of psychiatric nursing in the 1960s, and no replication has been reported in the published literature.

Davis (1972, 1974) conducted two studies of the relationship between educational preparation and clinical expertise as measured by paper-and-pencil responses to five patient situations developed by Verhonick, Nichols, Glor, and McCarthy (1968). Davis (1972) found that the quantity and quality of patient care responses written by psychiatric clinical nurse specialists were significantly better as compared to those written by baccalaureate-prepared psychiatric nurses. Further, additional education was correlated with maintenance of quality and quantity of responses after 3 to 5 years of clinical experience. Results of the Davis (1974) replication were similar. In addition, she found that diploma-prepared nurses performed less well than baccalaureate-prepared nurses and that medical–surgical nurses performed highest on both medical–surgical and psychiatric functions.

Finally, personality characteristics of graduate students selecting psychiatric nursing as opposed to other specialty programs have been examined in three studies. Miller (1965) investigated personality characteristics of graduate nursing students using the Strong Vocational Interest Blank for Women (Strong, 1959), the California Psychological Inventory (Gough, 1957), two brief attitude questionnaires, and life history interviews. Her subjects were 61 graduate students enrolled in medical–surgical, public health, maternal–child, and psychiatric nursing clinical majors at the University of California, San Francisco, School of Nursing during 1960–1961. Data showed the psychiatric nursing majors to be more forceful and highly independent, rebellious toward rules and restrictions, with broad and varied interests similar to those of creative individuals. They were also highly preoccupied with personal conflicts.

Lukens (1965) compared 238 psychiatric and medical–surgical nursing graduate students from six programs in the East and Midwest using the Stern Activities Index (Stern, 1959), the Poe Inventory of Values (Poe, 1954), an open-ended question related to occupational values, an investigator-developed intraception scale, Sharaf's Self-Deception Scale (Sharaf, 1959), and a scale designed to measure authoritarianism or dogmatic stands on social issues. The researcher concluded that the personality patterns of medical–surgical and psychiatric nursing students were indeed different. The psychiatric students (a) had higher needs for emotionality and reflectiveness, (b) were more psychologically minded and more willing to acknowledge socially undesirable and value-violating feelings and motivations, (c) scored lower on religious and humanitarian values, and (d) scored higher on valuing the type of work setting and type of nurse–patient relationship expected in their field.

Gilbert (1975) compared 30 medical–surgical and psychiatric nursing graduate students from the metropolitan Chicago area using the California Psychological Inventory (CPI) and the Managerial Key for the CPI (Gough, 1957), thus adding leadership ability to the variables previously reported. She found no significant difference between the two groups in leadership potential, and the psychiatric nursing group was significantly different on only one personality variable, that of responsibility. There appeared to be a marked similarity between the two groups of students not demonstrated in the earlier studies. One could speculate that the 10 years between 1965 and 1975 might somehow account for the difference in findings; however, no subsequent researchers have replicated these studies or explained the disparate results.

IMPACT OF CURRICULUM ON STUDENTS

Only nine reports were located that dealt with the impact of psychiatric–mental health learning experiences on nursing students. In addition, a study of the development of empathy in beginning associate degree nursing students (Kalisch, 1971) was included in this review because of the relevance of its content and its frequent citation in the psychiatric nursing literature. These 10 studies were grouped for review according to the independent variables of (a) psychiatric nursing clinical experiences and (b) interactional group experiences.

Psychiatric Nursing
Clinical Experiences

The experience of diploma students in psychiatric nursing rotations or affiliations has been studied by Morris (1964), Johannsen, Redel, and Engel (1964), and Mealey and Peterson (1974). Morris (1964) examined attitude change, using a modified version of the Opinions About Mental Illness Scale (Cohen & Struening, 1963), as a function of the psychiatric nursing experience with 56 students. She concluded that authoritarian attitudes were modified as a result of the psychiatric nursing experience but that mental hygiene ideology was not changed, perhaps because of its correlation with education, occupation, and social class. The researcher also found significant positive correlations between mental hygiene ideology and total NLN Achievement Test scores and scores on the NLN psychiatric nursing test.

Johannsen, Redel, and Engel (1964) measured personality and attitudinal changes before and after psychiatric affiliation using the Opinions About Mental Illness Scale (Cohen & Struening, 1963), the Custodial Mental Illness Scale (Gilbert & Levinson, 1956), and the California Psychological Inventory (Gough, 1957). Their design included 96 diploma students affiliating at either public or private psychiatric hospitals and a control group of 39 hospital students with no psychiatric affiliation. The researchers found that changes in the Achievement via Independence scale of the California Psychological Inventory were most stable. Students tended to change in the direction of more forcefulness, maturity, dominance, independence, and self-reliance during their psychiatric nursing affiliation. On the Custodial Mental Illness Scale they demonstrated increasing liberal treatment attitudes and a decrease in authoritarianism on the Opinions About Mental Illness Scale, results that were consistent with findings of other studies. There was surprisingly little change in mental hygiene ideology on the Opinions About Mental Illness Scale. The researchers concluded that their subjects possessed benevolent and paternalistic attitudes toward their patients that increased during their psychiatric affiliation.

Mealey and Peterson (1974) used the Personal Orientation Inventory (Shostrom, 1966) in an attempt to measure self-actualization in diploma nursing students before and after their course in psychiatric nursing. The students demonstrated significant improvement on the inner-directedness factor and some improvement on the remaining 11 factors, leading the researchers to conclude that changes that occurred during a psychiatric nursing course could be identified and measured.

Swain (1973) conducted a laboratory experiment with diploma and baccalaureate students to measure attitudes toward mental illness before and after their psychiatric nursing course. This study was unique because of the researcher's use of two distinct study conditions (perceived normal partners and perceived ex-mentally ill partners) in a standardized laboratory procedure. The researcher found an overall improvement in negative attitudes toward mental illness following the course as rated on a self-report questionnaire; however, that change was accounted for statistically by the diploma students. The baccalaureate students demonstrated no difference in attitudes following their psychiatric nursing course. The researcher suggested that this may reflect a relatively less positive rating more than it reflected an actual negative rating.

Finally, Walsh (1971) conducted pre- and posttest comparisons of anxiety and Opinions About Mental Illness scores for baccalaureate students from five programs in the New York City area. She found that anxiety for the total group was reduced significantly following instruction in psychiatric nursing. Scores on authoritarianism and social restrictiveness decreased, while scores on benevolence, mental hygiene ideology, and interpersonal etiology increased, as has been demonstrated with other populations.

Interactional Group Experience

Sensitivity training (Thompson, Lakin, & Johnson, 1965), group dynamics courses (Garner & Lowe, 1965), empathy training (Kalisch, 1971), and interactional group experiences (Adams, 1971, 1972) have been studied with all levels of clinical nursing students. Although the Kalisch (1971) research on empathy training was not directed specifically at psychiatric nursing education, it has become a point of reference in the field and is the only one of this group of studies that included standardized measures. When viewed collectively, these studies are less than conclusive.

Thompson et al. (1965) found that baccalaureate student participants in a sensitivity training group reported a decrease in self-concept, particularly in self-ratings of "how I think others see me." Garner and Lowe (1965) concluded that psychiatric and maternal–child health master's students reported (a) a moderate decrease in cooperation with colleagues, (b) a moderate increase in cooperation with superiors, (c) a decrease in dependency on superiors, and (d) a general increase in awareness of hostile tendencies following a one-semester, nondirective group experience.

The study of empathy training by Kalisch (1971) was well-designed, well-executed, and included a range of standardized objective and subjective measures that included student, faculty, and patient ratings of student empathy. The researcher demonstrated that the experimental method of teaching empathy was effective on the student's self-evaluation of empathy and clinical instructor evaluation of student empathy, as well as on the posttest of predictive empathy with a patient. No change was reported on patient evaluations of student empathy, a predictive empathy test with a classmate, and predictive empathy with a generalized other.

Adams's (1971) initial study of diploma students' evaluation of an interactional group experience indicated that participants found the experience worthwhile, although they expressed the need for a better understanding of the purpose of the group. Three to fifteen-month follow-up questionnaire responses from this same sample (Adams, 1972) indicated the participants felt they had changed along a variety of personal dimensions and wanted to continue changing. This alteration included a reported and desired increase in the expression of negative feelings. Adams (1972) also added an immediate response group (students who just completed a group experience) of 32 baccalaureate students who reported positive changes on 7 of 10 personal dimensions: openness, warmth and closeness, influence on others, participation in group interaction, helpfulness to others, taking risks in the group, and empathy. No change was reported in their sense of responsibility for group interaction, expression of positive feelings, or expression of negative feelings.

Although these studies of the impact of psychiatric nursing clinical experiences and interactional group experiences are inconclusive and at times flawed by methodological problems, the investigators are to be commended for their attempts to quantify and explain important aspects of psychiatric nursing education. Unfortunately, such work appears to have disappeared from the published literature since 1974, and there is no record of replication conducted in psychiatric nursing education for the past decade.

SUMMARY AND RESEARCH DIRECTIONS

Research included in this review has been reported in three major categories. The 12 studies designed to predict success on State Board Test Pool Examinations provide evidence that psychiatric nursing grades have not contributed significantly or consistently as predictors overall to SBE performance. It is important to note that data for these studies were collected between 1957 and 1976 and do not reflect adequately the impact of integrated curricula on psychiatric nursing course grades, NLN Achievement Test scores, or SBE scores.

Studies of the characteristics of students and graduates in psychiatric–mental health nursing have included a variety of personal and attitudinal variables. Results of these investigations were not consistent and have provided only speculation and little direction for psychiatric–mental health nursing educators. Again, there has been no programmatic research that might document any changes as a result of integrated curricula or advancement of the specialty practice area in the past 15 years.

Researchers studying the impact of psychiatric nursing courses and interactional group experiences have provided evidence of a variety of changes in students' attitudes, anxiety, opinions about mental illness, and ability to relate to self and others. Because the dependent variables in these studies were measured by self-report and paper-and-pencil tests, there was no way to examine the practice behavioral change or patient outcome consequences of psychiatric–mental health educational experiences.

In 1975 NIMH mandated that funding for mental health educational programs had to be relevant to and derived from the manpower needs of unserved and underserved populations: children, youth, the aged, the chronic mentally ill, minorities, and women. It was clear from the published research literature that psychiatric nursing educators were never able to make the required adjustment from the examination of test scores, personality characteristics of students, and educational experiences to documentation of the impact of their programs on patient care. Although the causal link between an educational program and improved patient outcomes was a difficult one to prove, it did not appear that psychiatric–mental health nursing educators even attempted to meet the challenge.

Project directors of training grants are required to report the impact that students and faculty have on patients during their generic and graduate educational experiences as well as the impact of program graduates. Differences must be documented in terms of increased productivity of patients, access to care, and economic and reimbursement issues. Lego (1980) challenged the specialists in psychiatric–mental health nursing to explore and document how the one-to-one relationship is different in psychiatric nursing from that of the other mental health disciplines. Fagin (1983) addressed a future for psychiatric–mental health nursing based on competition and substitution among professions. The politics of practice legislation and reimbursement mandate documentation of the impact of educational programs in psychiatric–mental health nursing.

Finally, research is essential for the development of innovative models for delivery of psychiatric–mental health nursing care. Mitsunaga (1982) and Martin (1985) have advocated holistic, primary care approaches in educating psychiatric–mental health nurses. Their admonitions present a challenge at a time in which the majority of NIMH funding for mental health research is being directed at biomedical interventions. However, the survival of nursing education and practice specialty could hinge on how researchers, educators, clinicians, and students respond to the need to demonstrate an impact on the mental health needs of society.

REFERENCES

Adams, J. (1971). Student evaluations of an interactional group experience. *Journal of Psychiatric Nursing and Mental Health Services, 9*(4), 28–36.

Adams, J. (1972). A quantitative follow-up study of nursing student reactions to an interactional group experience. *Journal of Psychiatric Nursing and Mental Health Services, 10*(5), 11–14.

Backman, M. E., & Steindler, F. M. (1971). Prediction of achievement in a collegiate nursing program and performance on State Board Examinations. *Nursing Outlook, 19*, 487.

Baldwin, J. P., Mowbray, J. K., & Taylor, R. G., Jr. (1968). Factors influencing performance on State Board Test Pool Examinations. *Nursing Research, 17*, 170–172.

Bell, J. A., & Martindill, C. F. (1976). A cross-validation study for predictors of scores on State Board Examinations. *Nursing Research, 25*, 54–57.

Brandt, E. M., Hastie, B., & Schumann, D. (1966). Predicting success on State Board Examinations: Relationships between course grades, selected test scores, and State Board Examination results. *Nursing Research, 15*, 62–69.

Canter, F. M., & Shoemaker, R. (1960). The relationship between authoritarian attitudes and attitudes toward mental patients. *Nursing Research, 9*, 39–41.

Cohen, J., & Struening, E. L. (1963). Opinions about mental illness, mental hospital occupational profiles and profile clusters. *Psychology Reprints, 12*, 111–124.

Davis, B. G. (1972). Clinical expertise as a function of educational preparation. *Nursing Research, 21*, 530–534.

Davis, B. G. (1974). Effects of levels of nursing education on patient care: A replication. *Nursing Research, 23*, 150–155.

Deardorff, M., Denner, P., & Miller, C. (1976). Selected National League for Nursing Achievement Test scores as predictors of State Board Examination scores. *Nursing Research, 25*, 35–38.

Edwards, A. L. (1954). *Manual for the Edwards Personal Preference Schedule.* New York: Psychological Corporation.

Fagin, C. M. (1983). Concepts for the future: Competition and substitution. *Journal of Psychosocial Nursing and Mental Health Services, 21*(3), 36–40.

Garner, G. S., & Lowe, A. (1965). Group dynamics in graduate education of nurses. *Nursing Research, 14*, 146–150.

Gilbert, D. C., & Levinson, D. J. (1956). Ideology, personality, and institutional policy in the mental hospital. *Journal of Abnormal and Social Psychology, 53*, 263–271.

Gilbert, M. A. (1975). Personality profiles and leadership potential of medical-surgical and psychiatric nursing graduate students. *Nursing Research, 24*, 125–130.

Gough, H. G. (1957). *Manual for California Psychological Inventory.* Palo Alto, CA: Consulting Psychologist Press.

Johannsen, W. J., Redel, Sister M. C., & Engel, R. G. (1964). Personality and attitudinal changes during psychiatric nursing affiliation. *Nursing Research, 13*, 342–345.

Kalisch, B. J. (1971). An experiment in the development of empathy in nursing students. *Nursing Research, 20*, 202–211.

Lego, S. (1980). The one-to-one nurse–patient relationship. *Perspectives in Psychiatric Care, 18*, 67–89.

Lukens, L. G. (1965). Personality patterns and choice of clinical nursing specialization. *Nursing Research, 14*, 210–221.

Martin, E. J. (1985). A specialty in decline? Psychiatric–mental health nursing, past, present, and future. *Journal of Professional Nursing, 1*, 48–53.

Mealey, A. R., & Peterson, T. L. (1974). Self-actualization of nursing students resulting from a course in psychiatric nursing. *Nursing Research, 23*, 138–143.

Meyer, L. M. (1973). Comparison of attitudes toward mental patients of junior and senior nursing students and their university peers. *Nursing Research, 22*, 242–245.

Miller, C. L., Feldhusen, J. F., & Asher, J. W. (1968). The prediction of State Board Examination scores of graduates of an associate degree program. *Nursing Research, 17*, 555–558.

Miller, D. I. (1965). Characteristics of graduate students in four clinical nursing specialties. *Nursing Research, 14*, 106–113.

Mitsunaga, B. K. (1982). Designing psychiatric/mental health nursing for the future: Problems and prospects. *Journal of Psychosocial Nursing and Mental Health Services, 20*(12), 15–21.

Morris, K. D. (1964). Behavioral change: A concomitant of attitude change in nursing students. *Nursing Research, 13*, 132–138.

Mueller, E. J., & Lyman, H. B. (1969). The prediction of scores of the State Board Test Pool Examination. *Nursing Research, 18*, 263–267.

Muhlenkamp, A. F. (1971). Prediction of state board scores in a baccalaureate program. *Nursing Outlook, 19*, 57.

Navran, L., & Stauffacher, J. C. (1957). The personality structure of psychiatric nurses. *Nursing Research, 5*, 109–114.

Navran, L., & Stauffacher, J. C. (1958). A comparative analysis of the personality structure of psychiatric and nonpsychiatric nurses. *Nursing Research, 7*, 64–67.

Papcum, I. (1971). Results of achievement tests and state board tests in an associate degree program. *Nursing Outlook, 19*, 341.

Poe, W. A. (1954). *Differential value patterns of college students.* Unpublished doctoral dissertation, University of Nebraska, Lincoln.

Reed, C. L., & Feldhusen, J. F. (1972). State Board Examination score prediction for associate degree nursing program graduates. *Nursing Research, 21*, 149–153.

Sharaf, M. R. (1959). *An approach to the theory and measurement of intraception.* Unpublished doctoral dissertation, Harvard University, Cambridge, MA.

Shelley, B., Kennamer, D., & Raile, M. (1976). Correlation of NLN achievement test scores with State Board Test Pool Examination scores. *Nursing Outlook, 24*, 52–55.

Shostrom, E. L. (1966). *EITS manual for the Personal Orientation Inventory.* San Diego, CA: Educational and Industrial Testing Service.

Stauffacher, J. C., & Navran, L. (1968). The prediction of subsequent professional activity of nursing students by the Edwards Personal Preference Schedule. *Nursing Research, 17*, 256–260.

Stern, G. G. (1959). *The Stern Activities Index: Scoring instructions and college norms.* Syracuse, NY: Psychological Research Center, Syracuse University.

Strong, E. K., Jr. (1959). *Manual for Strong Vocational Interest Blank for Men and Women.* Palo Alto, CA: Consulting Psychologists Press.

Swain, H. L. (1973). Nursing students' attitudes toward mental illness. *Nursing Research, 22*, 59–65.

Thompson, V. D., Lakin, M., & Johnson, B. S. (1965). Sensitivity training and nursing education: A process study. *Nursing Research, 14*, 132–137.

Verhonick, P. J., Nichols, G. A., Glor, B. A., & McCarthy, R. T. (1968). I came, I saw, I responded: Nursing observation and action survey. *Nursing Research, 17*, 38–44.

Walsh, J. E. (1971). Instruction in psychiatric nursing, level of anxiety, and direction of attitude change toward the mentally ill. *Nursing Research, 20*, 522–529.

Wechsler, D. (1958). *The measurement and appraisal of adult intelligence* (4th ed.). Baltimore: Williams & Wilkins.

Wolfle, L. M., & Bryant, L. W. (1978). A causal model of nursing education and State Board Examination scores. *Nursing Research, 27*, 311–315.

Chapter 8

Community Health
Nursing Education

BEVERLY C. FLYNN
SCHOOL OF NURSING
INDIANA UNIVERSITY

CONTENTS

The research included in this review was focused on education for community health nursing (CHN). The content of this chapter includes several areas: criteria and procedures for conducting the review, methodological issues, research on basic education, research on graduate education, trends, and recommendations for future research.

CONDUCTING THE REVIEW

A broad conceptual definition of CHN was employed in conducting the review. Authors contributing in previous reviews clearly indicated that there is a lack of conceptual clarity within the field of CHN (Highriter, 1984; Sills & Goeppinger, 1985). This problem caused some difficulty in the retrieval of research because the terminology in the field has continued to change over the years. This review is consistent with the approach taken by Highriter (1984), in which the retrieval of research was guided by the inclusive American Nurses' Association (ANA) (1980) definition of CHN. The ANA's definition broadly referred to professional nurses working in the community (Anderson & Meyer, 1985). The selection of research, however, was guided by the American Public Health Association's (APHA) (1980) definition of public health nursing, which emphasized population groups at risk to health problems in the community. Because previous reviews of research on the topics of clinically oriented primary care and continuing education in nursing were included in recent issues of *The Annual Review of Nursing Research* (ARNR), those topics were eliminated from this analysis (Kuramoto, 1985; Shamansky, 1985). This chapter is focused on formal basic preparation for CHN practice in certificate, undergraduate, and graduate programs.

An examination of the operational details of the research reviewed was attempted. However, many of the researchers did not present enough information about the study methods for the analysis to occur in a systematic way. There were particular inconsistencies in the reporting of sample size, reliability or validity of data, and data analyses. When such information was clearly reported it was noted in the review; otherwise, the reader can assume it was not addressed by the investigators in their reports.

Several approaches to retrieving information were employed. The bibliographies of studies bearing on the topic of interest provided previously cited research. Several computerized searches were conducted to retrieve research for the 16-year period of 1970 through 1985 (inclusive): MEDLINE, MEDLARS, ERIC, Dissertation Abstracts, and CATLINE. The following key words were used: community health nursing, public health nursing, research, nursing education, and curriculum. Because of the dearth of studies found, a manual search was conducted in the *Cumulative Index to Nursing and Allied*

Health (1970–1985) in order to avoid deleting any relevant research. Manual searches were also conducted in journals relevant to the topic of inquiry: the *International Journal of Nursing Studies* (1980–1985); *International Nursing Review* (1980–1985); *Public Health Nursing* (1984–1985); and *Nurse Educator* (1977–1985). The actual information sources included dissertations, published research, and published reports. The rationale for including dissertation research was that there were few studies in the field and many of the published studies had conceptual and methodological problems. The intent was to review as much research in the field as possible.

One criterion for inclusion of research for review was the requirement that studies be reported in English. Studies were data-based, thus excluding conceptual, opinion-based, or descriptive reports of experiences. Because CHNs have been prepared in schools of public health as well as schools of nursing, studies conducted in schools of public health were included if nurses were reported in the samples. A total of 45 studies met these criteria and were included in the review. Thirty-seven of the studies were authored or coauthored by nurses; 32 were conducted in the United States, 8 in the United Kingdom, 2 in Israel, 1 in Nigeria, 1 worldwide study, and 1 study in a number of developing countries. Although the process used to select studies was systematic and comprehensive, some studies inadvertently may have been omitted.

Perhaps most intriguing is the question, Why are there so few studies that met the criteria for inclusion? A historical perspective might provide some insight on this issue (Roberts & Heinrich, 1985). Curricula in CHN are relatively new in schools of nursing. Nursing programs in the late 1950s and early 1960s were encouraged by the National League for Nursing (NLN) to integrate CHN concepts and clinical experiences formerly taught in schools of public health. There were few prepared CHN faculty to meet the new demands. Young nurses minimally qualified and with little work experience were employed as faculty by schools of nursing to help set up these programs. With such changes faculty had to focus their attention on program needs and had little time or skill to conduct research. Often these faculty viewed CHN as "out of hospital" nursing rather than community-focused practice. Curricula in the 1960s and 1970s were focused mostly on the individual and family. In 1980 the ANA and APHA defined CHN and public health nursing practice, which suggested some confusion in the field (ANA, 1980; APHA, 1980).

METHODOLOGICAL ISSUES

Serious conceptual and methodological issues were apparent in much of the identified research. Because of the limitations of the studies reviewed, caution must be used in the application of findings to educational programs.

Community health nursing involves the synthesis of public health and nursing sciences. It was evident that, to date, neither public health science nor nursing science provided an integrated theory useful in CHN education research. It is understandable that investigators studying CHN education research have had conceptual difficulties.

Often the authors' messages were unclear about the methodology employed. Of the 45 reports reviewed, 11 did not include clear descriptions of the methods used in the studies. Although the studies often could be categorized under more than one research design, most commonly used were the cross-sectional and the quasi-experimental designs in which two or more groups were compared. Although 26 studies were categorized as using cross-sectional design, 12 of these studies showed overlap with the quasi-experimental design. Investigators employed a case study methodology in 8 studies and a retrospective design in 4; 15 studies were longitudinal, and 2 were phenomenological.

The studies varied by level of analysis and sample size, one was a worldwide survey; six were nationwide surveys, and the remaining studies were either program-specific or incorporated a convenience sample of subjects. Researchers reported random assignment in four studies, with a matched comparison group for one study. Stratified random samples were used in two of the five projects.

Thirty-seven of the forty-five studies incorporated researcher-made instruments. Pilot-testing or assessments of the reliability or validity of the data were reported only for 12 studies. Also noteworthy was the fact that investigators used more than one instrument to collect information about any one group in only 13 of the studies.

Consistent with these methodological limitations, the data were analyzed using very simple techniques. For one of the national surveys, researchers reported limitations in the data analysis because of the extensive use of open-ended questions. In 34 of the studies, simple descriptive statistics were used, that is, frequencies and percents; the Chi Square statistic was reported in 8 studies, and other inferential statistics such as correlations, the *t*-test, and analysis of variance in 13.

BASIC EDUCATION

Selection of Students

Selection of students was the focus of six studies, and all were international studies, perhaps because CHN education was postbasic education in most countries other than the United States and, therefore, a practical problem for research. In the United Kingdom, investigators in four studies used standardized tests and correlated preprogram results with final examination scores that included testing of knowledge and practice skills (M.E. Davies & Khosla, 1974; Dellar, 1981; Hack, 1983; Jarvis & Gibson, 1981). In health visitor training, M. E. Davies and Khosla (1974) and Dellar (1981) used the Progressive Matrices Scale and Mill Hill Vocabulary Scale (Raven, 1962) at preprogram, and Dellar added preprogram results from the Eysenck Personality Measure (Eysenck, 1964), two essays, and an interview. M. E. Davies and Khosla, in their study of 150 students, concluded that the Mill Hill Vocabulary and the Progressive Matrices Scales were useful discriminators in initial screening of candidates and in predicting success on the final examination. Although Dellar found the Mill Hill Scale to show a more positive relationship to the final examination than the Progressive Matrices Scale, none of the standardized testing results were related significantly to examination scores.

Hack (1983) studied cognitive and noncognitive differences between high and low achievers among 42 students in a health visiting course. The Eysenck Personality Inventory (Eysenck, 1964), the Conservatism Scale (Wilson & Patterson, 1970), an intelligence test, and an essay test graded by the teacher were administered at preprogram. The most effective predictor of success in formal written examinations was the subjectively assessed essay that formed part of the selection process. The next most effective predictor was the fact that younger students achieved higher marks on the written examination, a finding also reported by Dellar (1981). Hack (1983) found that none of the preprogram tests discriminated between high and low achievers in clinical practice.

Dellar (1981) and Jarvis and Gibson (1981) studied the effects of Ordinary "O" level passes in the British General Certificate of Education testing on program success; these were similar to the achievement of basic education skills in the United States. Dellar found "O" level passes to have a more significant relationship to final examination scores than the Advanced "A" level examination scores that were taken prior to college or university education in England. Advanced "A" level examinations are somewhat like college entrance examinations in the United States, but taken in content areas. Jarvis and Gibson, who also included two other standardized tests at preprogram for their sample of 100 students, concluded that none of the preprogram factors provided an adequate basis for selection of district nurses.

In Israel, Bergman (1972, 1973) compared demographic and professional data on students admitted to a postbasic baccalaureate program, of which CHN was a part, with like data on nurses employed in positions similar to those held by students prior to admission. One objective of the longitudinal study of 75 students and the comparison group of 122 nurses was to evaluate the criteria used in selecting students. A five-part instrument with reported reliability and validity was administered; it included personal data, the California Psychological Inventory (Gough, 1956), and knowledge and judgment testing in a number of professional areas. Bergman concluded that the regular university criteria were not as useful in the selection of nursing students as the preprogram nursing test; the latter she reported as being in need of further research and development.

Classroom Coursework

Integration of CHN Concepts.   Three studies, two in the United States and one in England, were focused on the integration of CHN concepts in the curriculum (Holt, 1970; Knollmueller, White, & Yaksich, 1979; Owen, 1977; C. White, Knollmueller, & Yaksich, 1980). Holt's (1970) study was one of the earliest and provided a historical perspective. In a survey of 13 baccalaureate programs in New England, Holt found that theory and practice were taught concurrently in all programs during a period of time in the senior year. Although five programs provided structure for some integration of CHN concepts, five others offered no experience in CHN during the first 2 years.

A more recent national survey of 526 service agencies providing student experiences in CHN and 140 NLN-accredited schools of nursing indicated that the majority of respondents in schools and agencies reported integrated CHN curricula (Knollmueller et al., 1979; C. White et al., 1980). Over half of the respondents in service agencies and schools of nursing endorsed an integrated curriculum with exposure to CHN at all levels in the baccalaureate program. Problems in this research were related to the extensive use of open-ended responses to questions, making data analysis cumbersome and often incomplete.

In England, Owen (1977) compared two groups of health visiting students, one from an integrated baccalaureate program of six courses ($n = 57$) and the other from the traditional 3-year program for state-registered nurses, including a 1-year health visiting course ($n = 63$). The groups were matched and given the Occupational Values and Stereotypes Inventories (Rosenberg, 1957; Singh & Mac Guire, 1971). The integrated course group was significantly more likely to select an ideal job based on prestige, being helpful, and gaining adventure and could differentiate more clearly the roles of the nurse and the health visitor. Owen (1977) also included responses on a pilot-tested questionnaire from 149 chief nursing officers; two-thirds of them rated the students in the integrated course higher than the other group.

Concepts and Competencies. Five studies were focused on the inclusion of selected concepts and competencies in the curriculum, three from the United States and two international studies. In the United States, Blank (1985) described the CHN concepts and competencies that faculty believed were essential in baccalaureate nursing education. A pretested questionnaire was sent to persons responsible for the CHN component in 339 NLN-accredited baccalaureate nursing programs. The concepts found most essential were family-centered care, holism, health maintenance and promotion, levels of prevention, continuity of care, community, home health care, and self-care. Competencies receiving the greatest emphasis in the curricula included family assessment, health education, referral, physical assessment, home care, community assessment, and collaboration. The results indicated that emphasis appeared to be placed on practice-oriented concepts rather than on more abstract conceptual areas, indicating a greater consensus on clinical skills for professional practice than on CHN content.

Simson and Wilson (1985) surveyed 131 NLN-accredited baccalaureate nursing programs to determine the extent to which the curricula covered content in the areas of disease prevention, health promotion, and aging. Questionnaires were mailed to program directors ($n = 74$), and 94 school catalogues were evaluated using content analysis. Over three-fourths of the school catalogues were found to contain courses on prevention. Consistent with the catalogues, 90% of the directors reported that courses in health promotion, disease prevention, and aging were required. This recent research gave evidence that key CHN concepts were being used in the majority of nursing curricula.

Brown (1976) conducted a survey of 40 NLN-accredited baccalaureate programs to determine the occupational health nursing content in the curricula. She reported that over half of the 27 participating schools included the most content on the effects of work on health and the influence of health on work. Seventy percent of the content was taught in CHN courses.

One of the two international studies was a survey of chief nurses in countries throughout the world (Jaeger-Burns, 1981). A pretested questionnaire translated into four languages was sent to chief nurses worldwide to study the inclusion in the curriculum of primary health care, as defined by the World Health Organization (1978). Although community health and primary health care were integrated into the curricula in a majority of the 54 countries for which data were provided, a definite response bias was noted by the investigator that limited the generalizability of the results. In Nigeria, Okunade (1980) surveyed 8 CHN training schools and concluded that nurses were not being prepared adequately in the area of screening for handicaps in children.

Teaching Methods.   Only one study was focused on teaching methods (Shaffer & Pfeiffer, 1978). The investigators developed and tested a videotape designed to teach baccalaureate students the nursing process as related to CHN home visits, and comparisons were made to the traditional lecture-discussion method. Although there were no reported significant differences in cognitive learning, students preferred the classroom session using the videotape.

Course Evaluations.   Two studies were related to CHN course evaluations (Holzemer, Kelly, & Ohlson, 1979; Wilson, Vaughan, & Gaff, 1977). In one the further development of the Adjective Rating Scale (Kelly, 1978) was reported, with the conclusion that further testing of the scale on age and sex of respondents was needed (Holzemer et al., 1979). The second study was focused on evaluating a baccalaureate program for registered nurses and gave some evidence of the effectiveness of the early integration of CHN concepts in the curriculum (Wilson et al., 1977). The first three classes of students

($N = 135$) were interviewed after their first year. The students reported changes in their professional attitudes, with a broader recognition of preventive aspects of health care, the importance of becoming familiar with the client's community environment, and approaches for dealing with health problems within the family context.

Clinical Experiences

Clinical Sites.   The studies related to clinical sites were focused on arrangements between service agencies and schools and the types of sites used for CHN practice, with several studies on community nursing centers. Investigators in two surveys compared the views held by respondents from schools of nursing and from CHN service agencies on the clinical arrangements for CHN practice (Carotenuto, 1981; Knollmueller et al., 1979; C. White et al., 1980). As reported in a large national survey, many agency personnel were involved heavily in student learning and were instrumental in providing the experiences (Knollmueller et al., 1979; C. White et al., 1980). Faculty were involved in supervising and evaluating students and teaching through lectures and clinical conferences. Personnel in almost all of the schools and agencies reported that written contracts existed between the two organizations. Although the majority reported ongoing exchange of ideas and information between personnel in agencies and schools, major deterrents to collaboration were insufficient opportunities for communication and perceived deficiencies in the education and preparation of agency personnel and faculty. Evidence from Carotenuto's (1981) study in one Northeastern state indicated that although faculty and supervisors had similar graduate educational preparation, the faculty had less CHN staff nursing experience than the supervisors, suggesting different career tracks for the two groups of nurses.

Graham and Gleit (1981) studied a stratified random sample of NLN-accredited baccalaureate programs ($N = 108$) by geographical areas of the country to identify the types of clinical sites used in these programs. Eighty percent of clinical usage was in secondary care settings, homes, and health departments. Although most nursing programs used 10 sites, 70% extensively used only three or fewer clinical sites.

In three studies investigators reported evaluations of community nursing center experiences for CHN students; this type of setting was relatively new in the literature (Barger, 1985; Hauf, 1977; Ossler, Goodwin, Mariani, & Gillis, 1982). Senior nursing students randomly assigned to a nursing center were matched with students assigned to public health agencies in the state (Hauf, 1977). Used to compare the two groups were several data collection instruments, including preceptor evaluation, student self-evaluation, teacher-made tests, and a standardized achievement examination that was not specified. The investigator reported no significant differences between the student groups, indicating similar levels of achievement.

In two studies with methods not reported clearly, investigators indicated that baccalaureate students had a limited range of clinical experiences in nursing centers (Barger, 1985; Ossler et al., 1982). Ossler et al. (1982) conducted a retrospective record audit over 2 years and found that the majority of clients visited at home were over 50 years old, female, widowed, and under medical supervision with multiple chronic illnesses. Barger (1985) found that about one-third of the time spent by undergraduates was in observing and screening in the center and by the graduate students in screening, teaching, and direct care. The investigator reported that faculty evaluations of students were lower than the faculty had expected.

Abuse During Home Visiting.   Three studies were concerned with students' views of aspects of abuse encountered during their home visiting experiences (Castles & Keith, 1971; Edwards, Eyer, & Kahn, 1985; Keith & Castles, 1976; Lawrence, 1982). Castles and Keith (1971; Keith & Castles, 1976) compared nursing students ($N = 53$) and staff nurses ($N = 106$) in official and nonofficial governmental community health agencies on their preferences for various kinds of protection. The students preferred protection that would enhance their autonomy, decrease peer visibility, and preserve the one-to-one nurse–patient relationship. The type of agency was not associated significantly with preferences for various kinds of protection.

Lawrence (1982) conducted a retrospective survey to determine the incidence and types of abuse CHN students experienced while making home visits. A pretested questionnaire was mailed to 80 NLN-accredited schools of nursing in cities, and 691 responses were obtained from students. A total of 133 separate incidents that were frightening or unpleasant were reported by about 16% of the students, and some of the incidents involved two or three types of abuse. The most common incident was labeled "other threatening" circumstances in which students were not harmed or harassed but were suspicious of acts of others; verbal harassment was the second most common type. Type of sponsoring agency and escort service were related significantly to abuse. Students under the auspices of mental health agencies and students accompanied by someone else reported more incidents, suggesting the possible influence of setting characteristics.

Edwards et al. (1985) examined baccalaureate nursing students' views of partners in home visiting. A questionnaire with reported reliability and content validity was administered to 132 generic and registered nurse students enrolled in a baccalaureate program. Students viewed the partner relationships in making home visits to have positive benefits in the areas of support, safety, and collaboration. Although there were no statistically significant differences between generic students and registered nurse students, younger students were significantly more likely to report that a partner increased their safety than those 25 years or older. Students with clinical practice in city agencies were significantly more likely to report that their partners provided increased safety.

Student Achievement.   In two studies there were differences between faculty and supervisors as to whether new graduates were prepared for entry-level positions in CHN (Carotenuto, 1981; Knollmueller et al., 1979; C. White et al., 1980). Faculty indicated that the students were prepared in CHN; yet supervisors in home health agencies did not agree and were likely to require that new graduates have experience prior to employment in their settings. Carotenuto (1981) noted differences in how supervisors and faculty would assign cases to new graduates. There were also significant differences between the two groups on whether or not graduates could establish priorities in giving individual care and how much experience in management of a caseload the graduates had had as students. The faculty thought the graduates had had this experience, and the supervisors did not.

In the United Kingdom Milne (1981) examined students' case management skills by comparing 16 general practitioners, 16 health visitors, 16 district nurses, and 16 social workers (all students) on their abilities in interviewing families. The health visitor and district nurse students were less skilled in questioning than general practitioners and social work students. The CHN students gave information, advice, or service rather than establishing and relating to the expressed needs of clients.

In another study conducted in the United Kingdom, Dingwall (1976) used a qualitative approach for describing 260 health visitor student visits and their associated record entries. A difference was found between information obtained on home visits and records. Although the health visitors recorded their visits, information in the records met organizational requirements rather than the practice needs of the health visitors.

Client ($n = 108$) views of students' ($n = 40$) home visits were requested following the students' last home visits (Formolo, 1979). Although the majority of responses were very positive, 14% of the respondents identified areas with which students could have used more instructor help, predominantly in child care.

Porter and Faller (1979) focused on the overall effectiveness of two types of clinical experiences in CHN, massed and distributive clinical practicums. Massed clinical practicum involved concentrated clinical time over 8 weeks, whereas distributive clinical practicum occurred over 16 weeks. Senior nursing students were assigned randomly to either massed ($n = 49$) or distributive clinical practicums ($n = 42$). Five data collection instruments were administered. Two instruments were the NLN Achievement Examinations in medical–surgical nursing and CHN and the State Board Test Pool Examinations, which have established reliability and validity. The other three instruments were questionnaires, and content validity and reliability were reported on one. Although statistical significance was not established on most of the results, the findings indicated that students in distributed experiences were able to make more effective application of CHN concepts and also improved in self-confidence.

Student Evaluation of Experiences. Two evaluation studies were conducted by faculty on students' views of their field experiences, one conducted in Switzerland (Chafetz & Gaillard, 1978) and the other in England (M. J. Davies, 1977). In Switzerland, two groups of postbasic public health nursing students ($N = 38$) were interviewed (Chafetz & Gaillard, 1978). Students' verbatim comments were analyzed to determine their reactions to conducting home visits to families with health problems but without the need for physical nursing care. Students reported a great deal of initial stress related to fears of intruding on and exploiting families and some concern about the need for the visits when physical nursing care was not required.

M. J. Davies (1977) monitored four community care courses over 6 years. A reportedly reliable and valid questionnaire was administered to 831 students enrolled in the courses. The investigator noted students' positive attitude changes and discussed the value of the community care courses after the students returned to hospital nursing.

GRADUATE EDUCATION

Master's Curricula

Several investigators reported on the CHN content in master's programs (Hickman, 1982; Kornblatt, Goeppinger, & Jagger, 1985; Ulin, 1978). Hickman (1982) surveyed baccalaureate nurses working in CHN in the United States ($n = 428$) and in developing countries ($n = 39$) to determine their perceived educational needs for master's work. The investigator reported that over half of the nurses indicated the following subjects to be very important: physical assessment of adults and children, community needs assessment, program planning, health education methods, family counseling, gerontology, nutrition therapy, and current issues and trends. Ulin's (1978) survey of 22 former students provided support for the importance of many of these subjects. Hickman (1982) also found differences in educational needs perceived by the two groups of nurses, but caution should be taken in generalizing from the findings because of the vast differences in sample sizes. However, the data confirmed that the educational needs of CHNs reflected the different contexts of practice.

In another study Kornblatt et al. (1985) surveyed the epidemiology content in 60 NLN-accredited master's programs in CHN. Two-thirds of the programs offered an epidemiology course, and about half required students to take such a course. The most frequent requirement was a three-credit epidemiology course, usually within a school of nursing. Content areas usually included were morbidity, mortality, incidence, and prevalence. Least frequent was content in screening and epidemics, important areas in CHN practice.

Pittman (1972) studied attitudes toward various role sets of graduate CHN students between 1964 and 1969. Students who were either in supervision, teaching, or school nursing completed a semantic differential scale with reported reliability. The teaching students gave the concept of supervision a low rating, and all three groups rated the concept of patient lower than any other concept in the role set. The latter finding was unexpected, suggesting a need for additional research on nurses' attitudes about patients.

Two studies were reports of evaluation of graduate curricula (Anderson, Gottschalk, Grimes, Ives, & Skrovan, 1977; Ulin, 1978). One comprehensive case study of an innovative community-based nursing program in a school of public health gave evidence that all evaluations, using a wide range of data collection methods, were supportive of the educational program (Anderson et al., 1977). In the second study Ulin (1978) found that 22 former students said that their program did not prepare them for the realities of CHN. The CHN seminars lacked pertinent content and were unrelated to practical problems.

Graduates' Employment

Because substantial numbers of CHNs have obtained graduate degrees in schools of public health, two studies on nurses graduating from schools of public health were reviewed (Goldston & Padilla, 1975; P. E. White et al., 1976). Goldston and Padilla (1975) conducted a national survey of 4,459 graduates from 11 schools of public health during the years 1961 to 1967. Nurses were the second largest professional group (15.0%) after physicians (19.4%) to graduate from these schools. In a previous survey of graduates from a stratified sample of schools of public health for the years 1956 through 1972, P. E. White et al. (1976) indicated that nurses comprised only about 8% of the respondents. In both studies the majority of nurses selected public health nursing for specialization. It was interesting to note that in a review of existing records of a more current master of public health (M.P.H.) extended degree program, 40 of the 94 students matriculating for the degree were nurses (Wainwright, Peterson, & Farrier, 1984). The most important reasons reported by graduates specializing in public health nursing for attending a school of public health were to update public health knowledge, develop an ability to recognize trends and predict needs, and understand contemporary health policy and planning issues (P. E. White et al., 1976).

Variables associated with occupational positions of master's graduates were studied by a number of investigators (Anderson, 1983; Balint, Menninger, & Hurt, 1983; Ostrand & Willis, 1978; Ray & Flynn, 1985; Segall & McKay, 1984; P. E. White et al., 1976). In a nationwide study, Anderson (1983) surveyed CHN practitioners ($n = 105$), educators ($n = 109$), and administrators ($n = 91$) to determine their perceptions related to 50 validated community-focused functions, categorized by the steps of the nursing process. Although each group indicated that the functions were important, educators placed a higher degree of importance on them than the other two groups. Administrators perceived the functions as more important than did practitioners and were viewed as having the major responsibility for performing the functions, which probably was consistent with their job requirements.

Ray and Flynn (1985) reported on a pilot-tested questionnaire sent to 387 graduates from 10 master's programs in CHN. The respondents were mostly white, female, married, and employed in administrative and instructor positions, with a median age of 35 years and a median salary of $21,000. None of the unemployed CHNs were looking for work. Although the graduates generally were satisfied with their work, administrators, supervisors, educators, and consultants were the most satisfied. P. E. White et al. (1976) also reported graduates' satisfactions with their employment. Ray and Flynn (1985) reported graduates' dissatisfactions as including opportunity to do research, opportunity to move up in the organization, organizational policy and administration, opportunity to work with community groups, and administrative details of the work. The most important reasons for selecting a position were professional and personal interests. Graduates' roles as women influenced the particular employment they selected, but not the position. The investigators reported that graduates were prepared adequately, both didactically and clinically, and were able to carry out community-based nursing practice. Graduates in positions of administration, supervision, education, and consultation were more likely to focus their practice on the community.

Another national study by Ostrand and Willis (1978) was conducted to determine if MPH programs prepared nurses for teaching in schools of nursing. Nurse faculty ($n = 142$) who were graduates from 14 schools of public health and deans ($n = 70$) who were responsible for CHN curricula in schools of nursing were surveyed. The faculty believed that their greatest skills were their relationships with personnel in community agencies, their clinical field teaching, and their seminars and clinical conferences. Deans reported that these faculty had the greatest expertise in public health or CHN content, field teaching in CHN, and interpersonal skills. Both groups agreed that the faculty were less skilled in research, curriculum development, student evaluation, and classroom teaching; and about half rated faculty with the M.P.H. degree as better or as good as the M.S.N.-prepared faculty.

Investigators in one university surveyed 43 graduates and 30 of the graduates' supervisors (Segall & McKay, 1984). The respondents indicated that the required clinical content on family, group, and community was the most valuable in relation to their job performance. The graduates were dissatisfied with their preparation in the areas of supervision, administration, and consultation. The supervisors agreed with the graduates that they demonstrated leadership, teaching ability, and skills in application of the nursing process.

There seems to be agreement among investigators on the positions held by master's graduates of CHN programs and employment openings. In one study (Balint et al., 1983) investigators examined the job market for master's-prepared nurses by recording information on 6,661 positions for 3 years in 26 nationally circulated American nursing journals. Each year close to half of the positions were in schools of nursing, with the majority as faculty. Most openings were in medical–surgical nursing, followed by psychiatric–mental health, community health, and maternal–child nursing. Between 7% and 11% were administrative positions in public health departments or visiting nurse associations. The researchers found that the percentage of faculty positions open to master's prepared graduates was decreasing, whereas the positions open to doctorally prepared graduates were increasing.

TRENDS

In spite of the methodological and substantive deficiencies in the research, recognizable patterns were found. The research related to the selection of students in CHN programs indicated that there were international differences in nursing education. In the United States baccalaureate education has included basic preparation in CHN, whereas this has not been the case in most other countries. In many other countries nurses were prepared in CHN following their basic education, and these programs appropriately were called postbasic programs. Although the selection of students in CHN was not an issue in basic education in the United States, the research experiences of other countries in which faculty selected students to specialize in the field could be applicable to American graduate education in CHN. Unfortunately, the international studies provided inconclusive evidence on what predicted success in CHN programs. Several investigators reported that standardized tests were not convincing predictors of success. Younger students and selected, subjectively assessed, preprogram tests were reported consistently as factors useful in predicting program success. These findings suggested that younger students might have been more successful because they were accustomed to studying and taking tests in that they had continued their education within a shorter time frame than the older students. It is also possible that there were more younger students in the programs and that faculty had geared their subjective preprogram tests to program outcomes. Also, possibly, students who scored well at preprogram might have achieved some of the program goals prior to admission through work experiences.

The majority of research related to classroom coursework has been focused on concepts and competencies in basic CHN education. Over the years content and experiences in CHN appeared to be integrated into the curricula rather than found in a single or separate CHN course. There was some evidence that students in an integrated curriculum more clearly differentiated their roles and scored higher on practice evaluations than their counterparts in a nonintegrated course of study. Several investigators found that more emphasis was placed in basic CHN curricula on practice-oriented competencies such as family-centered care, health promotion, disease prevention, and health maintenance. There was less agreement on the more abstract, theoretical content.

The greatest proportion of investigators focused on students' clinical experiences, indicating the complexities and difficulties in providing appropriate experiences for students. There was evidence of considerable involvement in CHN student learning by agency personnel as well as faculty. Faculty and agency personnel perceived deficiencies in the educational preparation and experiences of each other as well as of students completing nursing programs. These findings supported the age-old dilemma of the schism between nursing service and nursing education. Schools of nursing were using a variety of community-based settings, and students and their clients were satisfied with their clinical experiences. However, students who spent longer periods of time in the community made more effective applications in CHN. There were conflicting reports on the usefulness of community nursing centers as clinical sites. Some of the research gave evidence that students who traveled in teams for home visits were more likely to report abusive incidents. More information was needed to identify the variables inherent in such situations.

There were some trends based on students' or potential students' perceived educational needs in master's education. Reported needs were found in the areas of physical assessment, health promotion, gerontology, community health assessment, planning, and management. One comprehensive study indicated positive evaluations of a curriculum preparing students for community-based practice.

The research on master's graduates' employment was concentrated on characteristics of graduates and their occupational positions. Many nurses had been enrolled or graduated from schools of public health, with the majority majoring in public health nursing. These graduates appeared to have different expertise than graduates from schools of nursing, with nurses from schools of public health having less skill in research and in teacher education. The majority of CHN graduates were employed in positions in education, administration, and supervision. Although graduates generally were satisfied with their employment, graduates in positions in education, administration, and supervision were more satisfied and more likely to carry out community-based nursing practice. Reasons for selecting positions were professional and personal, yet the graduates' roles as women influenced the particular employment they selected but not the position. For the most part graduates were prepared adequately for their jobs, a finding confirmed in two studies of the graduates and their administrators.

RECOMMENDATIONS FOR
FUTURE RESEARCH

Recommendations for future research include conceptual, methodological, and substantive considerations. Perhaps most important, future research in CHN education needs to be related to a conceptual base. Investigators could apply and modify conceptual frameworks that have been found useful in health services or educational research. Such application would enhance the organization of knowledge in research on CHN education and encourage appropriate generalizations across studies.

The existing research on CHN education reflects a lack of attention to the application of sound principles of social science and nursing research. Many of the studies were evaluations, aimed at obtaining pieces of information deemed valuable to a particular educational program. Sound principles of basic research can be applied in evaluation research, which requires a higher level of skills than research performed in controlled settings (Weiss, 1972). Nursing is a practice profession and is in need of sound evaluation research aimed at problems rising out of the practice environment and the utilization of research findings for decision making about future nursing practice.

Although many of the recommendations in this section relate to quantitative issues in research, it is obvious that results of naturalistic inquiry have rarely been reported. Such methods should be encouraged and, where appropriate, applied along with quantitative approaches.

Only a small proportion of the investigators used comparison groups, a practice that limited the generalizability of the results. Although many researchers reported vast sample sizes, perhaps careful attention to alternative sampling procedures could have been made. In future research randomization, stratification, or matching groups could be used for the study or control of selected intervening variables.

There is a need to build on previous research experiences, including methodologies and findings. Rarely were the same or similar instruments used, even when common concepts were studied. The great majority of investigators used researcher-made instruments, mainly questionnaires. Replication of studies in different settings would facilitate the establishment of instrument reliability and validity.

A particular need is for the use of more than one indicator of the identified conceptual variable. This practice would enhance the reliability and validity of the data and help to build a systematic body of knowledge in the field. Researchers could facilitate this process by reporting clearly what was done in their studies.

The results of this review of research give evidence that there is more of a collage than a clear picture of basic and graduate education in CHN. Many of the recommendations for future research could be incorporated into a single study or into cluster studies in which similar phenomena are investigated using different designs or methodologies.

In other countries research has been focused on the selection of students. What is needed in the United States is marketing research to help in the attraction of potential students to the field of nursing. Nursing is a diverse profession, and CHN offers expanding and often untapped opportunities for practice. Traditional agencies may not be the major employers of graduates in the future. Marketing research can help potential students match their career desires with opportunities that exist or can exist in CHN. As enrollments in schools of nursing decline, shortages in the profession are likely to escalate. Marketing research can provide important information to potential students, faculty, and potential employers.

Very little research on innovations in educational programs has been reported, including the areas of content, teaching methods, and clinical experiences. Research needs to be done on home visiting with and without escorts to determine if there are differences in CHN students' achievements and expertise. Alternative community field experiences should be studied, such as comparing students working in traditional CHN agencies with students working in nursing centers administered by schools of nursing and with students working in neighborhoods involving a variety of community agencies. Research on computer applications in CHN education is a priority. As faculty in schools of nursing grapple with expanding curricula in nursing education, time-saving CHN learning experiences are needed. Computer-assisted technologies in the areas of community assessment, case finding, and case management are a few examples needing development and testing.

Although there was some consistency in the perceived educational needs of master's students, the scope of these needs is, at best, beyond the feasibility of any one educational program. For example, physical assessment skills and skills in community-based nursing practice are distinctly different and require different educational preparation (Williams, 1977). As basic educational programs are updated to include physical assessment skills, there may be less need for this preparation at the master's level. Research is needed to focus on both basic and graduate education so that educational trends and changes in curricula can be documented. This review did not include research on doctoral programs with majors in CHN because none was reported. Future research on doctoral education in CHN is important.

As stated earlier in this chapter, CHN is concerned with population groups at risk to health problems in the community. To date, research on the educational preparation of CHNs has not been linked clearly to the health of population groups and the community. What is needed is policy research because it is in the policy arena that the health of populations often is best addressed. Consistent with the recommendations of the Cabinet on Nursing Research (ANA, 1985), there is a need for evaluation research to document the effectiveness of CHN graduates by levels of education in employment settings. Only then can educators gain confidence in their curricula and be assured that the gap between education and service is being narrowed.

REFERENCES

American Nurses' Association. (1980). *A conceptual model of community health nursing* (ANA Publication No. CH-10 2M 5/80). Kansas City, MO: Author.

American Nurses' Association. (1985). *Direction for nursing research: Toward the twenty-first century* (ANA Publication No. D-79 2M 5/85). Kansas City, MO: Author.

American Public Health Association. (1980). *The definition and role of public health nursing in the delivery of health care: A statement of the public health nursing section.* Washington, DC: Author.

Anderson, E. T. (1983). Community focus in public health nursing. Whose responsibility? *Nursing Outlook, 31*, 44–48.

Anderson, E. T., Gottschalk, J., Grimes, D., Ives, J., & Skrovan, C. (1977). *The development and implementation of a curriculum model for community nurse practitioners* (DHEW Publication No. HRA 77-24). Hyattsville, MD: Division of Nursing, U.S. Department of Health and Human Services.

Anderson, E. T., & Meyer, A. T. (1985). *Consensus conference on the essentials of public health nursing practice and education.* Rockville, MD: Division of Nursing, U.S. Department of Health and Human Services. (NTIS Accession HRP 0906582)

Balint, J., Menninger, K., & Hurt, M. (1983). Job opportunities for master's prepared nurses. *Nursing Outlook, 31*, 109–114.

Barger, S. E. (1985). Evaluating a nurse-managed center. *Nurse Educator, 10*(4), 36–39.

Bergman, R. (1972). Evaluation of the Tel Aviv University post-basic baccalaureate nursing programme—I. *International Journal of Nursing Studies, 9*, 211–223.

Bergman, R. (1973). Evaluation of the Tel Aviv University post-basic baccalaureate nursing programme—II. *International Journal of Nursing Studies, 10*, 21–32.

Blank, J. J. (1985). *An evaluation of baccalaureate public health/community health nursing curricula in relation to essential concepts, competencies, and professional definitions.* Unpublished doctoral dissertation, University of Illinois, Chicago.

Brown, E. M. (1976). Summary of a descriptive study of the occupational health nursing content in baccalaureate curricula of selected schools of nursing. *Occupational Health Nursing, 24*(10), 9–12.

Carotenuto, R. P. (1981). *Congruence between expectations of baccalaureate nursing faculty and community agency supervisors about baccalaureate graduates' ability to function as beginning community health nurses.* Unpublished doctoral dissertation, Columbia University, New York, NY.

Castles, M. M., & Keith, P. M. (1971). Correlates of environment fear in the role of the public health nurse. *Nursing Research, 20*, 245–249.

Chafetz, L., & Gaillard, J. (1978). The impact of a therapeutic nurse–family relationship on post graduate public health nursing students. *International Journal of Nursing Studies, 15*, 37–49.

Davies, M. E., & Khosla, T. (1974). Predictive value of two intelligence tests as a criteria of success in a health visitor examination. *Nursing Times, 70*(48), 109–112.

Davies, M. J. (1977). A 6 year survey of community care courses for basic nursing students. *Journal of Advanced Nursing, 2*, 597–608.

Dellar, C. J. (1981). The selection of students for health visitors training courses. *Journal of Advanced Nursing, 6*, 111–115.

Dingwall, R. (1976). The social organization of health visitor training 2. The practical side of health visiting. *Nursing Times, 72*(8), 29–32.

Edwards, L. H., Eyer, J., & Kahn, E. H. (1985). The use of partners in undergraduate public health nursing. *Public Health Nursing, 2*, 213–221.

Eysenck, H. J., & Eysenck, S. B. G. (1964). *Manual of the Eysenck Personality Inventory*. London: University of London Press.

Formolo, R. (1979). Client response to student visits. *Nursing Outlook, 27*, 458–461.

Goldston, S. E., & Padilla, E. (1975). The professional public health worker. *American Journal of Public Health, 65*, 831–836.

Gough, H. (1956). *California Psychological Inventory*. Palo Alto, CA: Consulting Psychologists Press.

Graham, B. A., & Gleit, C. J. (1981). Clinical sites used in baccalaureate programs. *Nursing Outlook, 29*, 291–294.

Hack, K. (1983). Differences between high and low achievers on a health visiting course. *Health Visitor, 56*, 370–371.

Hauf, B. J. (1977). An evaluative study of a nursing center for community health nursing student experiences. *Journal of Nursing Education, 16*(8), 7–11.

Hickman, M. J. (1982). *An analysis of master's educational needs perceived by baccalaureate educated community health nurses working in developed and developing areas*. Unpublished doctoral dissertation, Ball State University, Muncie, IN.

Highriter, M. E. (1984). Public health nursing evaluation, education, and professional issues: 1977 to 1981. *Annual Review of Nursing Research, 2*, 165–189.

Holt, F. A. (1970). Public health nursing concepts in the basic curriculum. *The Journal of Nursing Education, 9*(1), 15–21.

Holzemer, W. L., Kelly, E. F., & Ohlson, V. M. (1979). Factorial validation of a measure of attitude toward public health nursing courses. *Evaluation and the Health Professions, 1*(5), 110–120.

Jaeger-Burns, J. (1981). The relationship of nursing to primary health care internationally. *International Nursing Review, 28*, 167–175.

Jarvis, P., & Gibson, S. J. (1981). An investigation into the validity of specifying 5 'O' levels in the general certificate of education as an entry requirement for the education and training of district nurses. *Journal of Advanced Nursing, 6*, 471–482.

Keith, P. M., & Castles, M. (1976). Community health nurses preferences for systems of protection. *Nursing Research, 25*, 252–255.

Kelly, E. F. (1978). The development and use of the Adjective Rating Scale: A measure of attitude toward courses and programs. *Journal Supplement Abstract Services: Catalogue of Selected Documents, 8*, 19. Washington, D.C.: American Psychological Association.

Knollmueller, R. M., White, C., & Yaksich, S. (1979). *Preparation for community health nursing in baccalaureate programs*. Washington, D.C.: American Public Health Association, Public Health Nursing Section.

Kornblatt, E. S., Goeppinger, J., & Jagger, J. (1985). Epidemiology in community health nursing education: Fit or misfit? *Public Health Nursing, 2*, 104–108.

Kuramoto, A. M. (1985). Research on continuing education in nursing. *Annual Review of Nursing Research, 3*, 149–170.

Lawrence, J. T. (1982). *Safety of community health nursing students in large cities: A survey of the incidence and types of abuse and factors related to abuse.* Unpublished doctoral dissertation, Temple University, Philadelphia, PA.

Milne, M. A. (1981). Community enquiry techniques. *Midwife, Health Visitor and Community Nurse, 17*, 237–241.

Okunade, A. O. (1980). Screening for handicaps in children: Are Nigerian nurses equipped? *International Journal of Nursing Studies, 17*, 181–187.

Ossler, C. C., Goodwin, M. E., Mariani, M., & Gillis, C. L. (1982). Establishment of a nursing clinic for faculty and student clinical practice. *Nursing Outlook, 30*, 402–640.

Ostrand, L., & Willis, W. (1978). Faculty preparation: An MPH or MSN degree? *Nursing Outlook, 26*, 637–640.

Owen, G. M. (1977). Curriculum integration in nursing education: A concept or a way of life? A study of six courses integrating basic nursing education and health visiting in a single course. *Journal of Advanced Nursing, 2*, 443–460.

Pittman, R. J. (1972). Attitudes toward their role set of graduate students preparing for school nursing or teaching or supervision in community health nursing. *International Journal of Nursing Studies, 9*, 33–41.

Porter, K. K., & Feller, C. M. (1979). The relationship between patterns of massed and distributive clinical practicum and student achievement. *Journal of Nursing Education, 18*(8), 27–34.

Raven, J. C. (1962). *Guide to using the Mill Hill Vocabulary Scale with the Progressive Matrices Scale.* London, England: Lewis & Co.

Ray, D. W., & Flynn, B. C. (1985). Graduate education in public health nursing: Evaluation and recommendations. *Public Health Nursing, 2*, 82–92.

Roberts, D. E., & Heinrich, J. (1985). Public health nursing comes of age. *American Journal of Public Health, 75*, 1162–1172.

Rosenberg, M. (1957). *Occupations and values.* Glencoe, IL: Free Press.

Segall, M., & McKay, R. (1984). Evolution of an aggregate-based community health curriculum. *Nursing Outlook, 32*, 308–312.

Shaffer, M. K., & Pfeiffer, I. L. (1978). Videotape as a method for staff development of nurses. *The Journal of Continuing Education in Nursing, 9*(6), 19–24.

Shamansky, S. L. (1985). Nurse practitioners and primary care research: Promises and pitfalls. *Annual Review of Nursing Research, 3*, 107–125.

Sills, G. M., & Goeppinger, J. (1985). The community as a field of inquiry in nursing. *Annual Review of Nursing Research, 3*, 3–23.

Simson, S., & Wilson, L. B. (1985). Disease prevention, health promotion and aging: Curricular trends. *Nurse Educator, 10*(3), 10–13.

Singh, A. J., & Mac Guire, J. M. (1971). Occupational values and stereotypes in a group of trained nurses. *Nursing Times, 67*(42), 165–168.

Ulin, P. R. (1978). What master's students want to know. *Nursing Outlook, 26*, 629–632.

Wainwright, R. B., Peterson, M. L., & Farrier, J. M. (1984). Feasibility of an extended MPH degree program for fully employed practicing health professionals. *American Journal of Public Health, 74*, 1258–1262.

Weiss, C. H. (1972). *Evaluation research.* Englewood Cliffs, NJ: Prentice-Hall.

White, C., Knollmueller, R., & Yaksich, S. (1980). Preparation for community health nursing: Issues and problems. *Nursing Outlook, 28*, 617–623.

White, P. E., Richardson, A. H., Bright, M., Gottfredson, L. S., McQueen, D., Sanders, B., & Vlasak, G. J. (1976). *Graduates of American schools of public health: A survey of graduates 1956–1972*. Washington, D.C.: Association of Schools of Public Health.

Williams, C. A. (1977). Community health nursing—What is it? *Nursing Outlook, 25*, 250–254.

Wilson, G. D., & Patterson, J. R. (1970). *Manual for the Conservatism Scale*. Windsor, England: National Foundation for Educational Research.

Wilson, H. S., Vaughan, H. C., & Gaff, J. G. (1977). The second step model of baccalaureate education for registered nurses: The students' perspective. *Journal of Nursing Education, 16*(6), 27–35.

World Health Organization. (1978). Primary health care. *Report of the International Conference on Primary Health Care*. Geneva, Switzerland: Author.

PART IV

Research on
the Profession of Nursing

Chapter 9

Men in Nursing

LUTHER P. CHRISTMAN
COLLEGE OF NURSING
RUSH UNIVERSITY

CONTENTS

Professional nurses, along with a few other professionals such as occupational therapists and dietitians, are imbedded in strongly sex-segregated professions. Men constitute 3.3% of the nursing profession (Division of Nursing, United States Department of Health and Human Services, 1984) even after over 20 years of affirmative action and dramatic changes in the gender composition of most of the professions. Research is necessary to ascertain if nurses have adopted an attitude of passive resistance to the democratization of membership within their ranks, whether there exists a variety of structural variables that impedes the attainment of a more socially representative profession, or whether complex forces external to the profession serve to maintain the present status of men and minorities in nursing. Certainly, the fact that professional nurses are 90% white female so long after the civil rights legislation of 1964 and the President's Executive Order of 1965 raises questions that merit investigation. In a society that is growing rapidly in greater complexity, the investigation of structural variables that constrain the achievement of true equal opportunity appears to be an essential scientific activity in order to mirror accomplishments in the other major professions. This chapter contains an analysis of studies on men in nursing; it does not include research on other minorities.

HISTORICAL OVERVIEW

The present sex-segregated motif has been a strong contrast to the early development of nursing care as a societal need. In his analysis of the Hippocratic Collection, Levine (1971) concluded that the first formally trained nurses appeared during the Hippocratic period. Furthermore, most nursing care "was undoubtedly performed chiefly by men and almost always under the supervision of men" (Levine & Levine, 1965, p. 87). The supervisors of care, according to Hippocrates, were physicians (Levine & Levine, 1965).

Various historians (Dolan, 1973; Jameson, 1966; Kauffman, 1976, 1978) have portrayed the amount of nursing care by men during the Middle Ages and the Renaissance period. The fanning of religious fervor in combination with the Crusades was a strong stimulus to the formation of male nursing orders. Thus, men were committed intensely to provide a humane service of quality and of insightful concern for the health of the populations they served.

The present distribution of gender within the nursing profession appeared to be tied closely to the Industrial Revolution. The demand for men workers for heavy industry along with the normative expectation that men had to be the chief economic providers for their families sharply lessened the entry of men into the field. In addition, the militancy of finding careers for women, as displayed by Florence Nightingale and others, in all likelihood contributed to a de-emphasis on men in the profession. The decrease of men as nurses probably went unnoticed in the social changes of the times. Science and technology, then as now, had a strong base in economic progress. Specific divisions of labor and the refinement of knowledge have been associated closely with and have been shaped to a great extent by economic resources.

In 1901, the act of Congress that created the Army Nurse Corps for women automatically barred men from serving their country as nurses. The contribution of the Knights Hospitallers, Teutonic Knights, and other male nursing organizations was glossed over (Kalisch & Kalisch, 1976). This action led to a near depletion of the number of men entering the nursing profession during World War II. Because men could not serve in the Nurse Corps of the various armed services, they were not granted educational deferments. Schools were reluctant to accept them as students. Despite a nurse shortage in the various services during the war years, male nurses who had been drafted were assigned to activities that had no relation to health care (Kalisch & Kalisch, 1976).

After World War II, the rapid growth of the women's movement, as measured by rate of change in the previous history of the nation, was focused sharply on adjusting sex imbalances in the professions dominated by men. Compliance with guidelines and policies to remove gender imbalance may have been treated differently in the professions dominated by men than in those dominated by women. The present corrections of sex imbalance percentages are one indicator that enforcement probably has differed. Gender stereotypes prevailed within both groups and in only the male-dominated professions has substantial adjustment taken place.

Studies of men in the nursing profession have been approached in three general ways. These are: (a) survey research; (b) focused interview; and (c) use of standardized test batteries to assess personality, intelligence, and attitudes.

SURVEY RESEARCH

One of the early studies was done by Mannino (1963), a male nurse, as his doctoral dissertation. At the time of the study, men comprised only 1% of the total registered nurse population. He cited as a comparison that women then were about 6.5% of the nation's physicians. Mannino endeavored to ascertain why men chose nursing as a career; he also documented some of the characteristics of male nurses. The data were obtained from questionnaires. Five hundred forty-three questionnaires were mailed to nurses in 33 states and three foreign countries. Of these, 394 were sent to graduates of the Pennsylvania Hospital School of Nursing for men as one means of determining how many graduates had remained in the profession. Subjects responded that they chose to be nurses because (a) they liked people and enjoyed helping them; (b) they wanted to enter medicine but were financially unable; (c) they wanted to improve their status in life; (d) they wanted to enter a field of service in which they could give the greatest contribution to help fulfill the needs of humanity; and (e) they wanted security for themselves and their families. The findings from a second questionnaire showed that most of the men (70.8%) were married, and 73.2% had wives who were nurses. A majority would have recommended nursing as a career (73.6%); and 57.3% reported membership in a professional group. From his analysis Mannino concluded that after men entered the profession, they tended to remain as nurses or to enter a related field, such as hospital administration or medicine. Only 19 men in the sample dropped from the status of nurse to a nonprofessional status.

Vaz (1968) surveyed 506 senior high school boys by means of an attitude questionnaire. The findings showed that, of seven occupations, high school boys viewed nursing as the least suitable masculine occupation for men. Men who chose a career in nursing were perceived by the study sample as violating sex role vocational choices.

Schoenmaker and Radosevich (1976) studied male nursing students at the University of Iowa. Thirty-five men and a stratified random sample of 58 women from a population of 478 students formed the sample. They found that men of lower social and economic background were more apt than other students to oppose the usual baccalaureate emphasis on the theoretical over the practical. Schoenmaker and Radosevich (1976) concluded from the sample responses that men entered the field for the more pragmatic reasons of job security and steady income than did women. As a minority group, the male students experienced some of the same problems that long have plagued minority groups in general. These included a lack of social support, guarded acceptance, and not enough significant others in the environment with whom to relate.

Rogness (1976) surveyed his male classmates in nursing at the University of California at San Francisco. Nine juniors and six seniors returned the questionnaire. All questions were open-ended and required short descriptive answers. Most respondents stated that they were given more respect than women and that more was expected of them. Rogness concluded that male students had to cope with isolation, loneliness, and a lack of adequate behavioral models and were forced to deal with others' ignorance and stereotypes.

Studying the attitudes of female nurses toward male nurses, Fottler (1976) hypothesized that (a) female nurses held generally positive attitudes toward the male nurse; and (b) more positive attitudes toward the male nurse were held by younger, single, better educated, urban-socialized nurses, those employed in a higher-level position outside a hospital, and those having extensive contact with male nurses. Questionnaire data were collected anonymously from 126 female nurses who were drawn at random from the files of the New York State Nurses Association, District 1.

About 75% of the nurses who responded to the survey (Fottler, 1976) indicated positive attitudes and no desire to exclude males. Among the other 25%, most of the negative attitudes clustered around perceptions of real or potential favoritism toward male nurses. No significant differences were noted in the attitudes of nurses in different employing organizations, different positions, and different clinical areas. The negative attitudes seemed to be held by younger nurses, those without much exposure to male nurses, or those who perceived employer discrimination in favor of the male. One can speculate that where competition was perceived as playing a strong role negative attitudes toward competitors more easily could be formed. The investigator cautioned that the data were attitudinal rather than behavioral. He concluded that the reason for the gender segregation of the nursing profession may have emanated from the traditional social, cultural, and economic values of society and the nature of the nursing role itself. As Vaz (1968) pointed out, the nature of the nursing role is consistent with a nurturing female role but inconsistent with the traditional male image and role.

McCarragher (1984) studied the question of stigmatization of male nurses within the nursing profession. In this study stigma was conceived as a negative by-product of the need to assess a stranger expediently and develop a generalization or category for the stranger that would influence future interactions with him. The sample was drawn from the membership of the Ohio Nurses' Association. Questionnaires were mailed to all 104 male members and to 208 randomly selected female members. Respondents were asked to state their degree of agreement with 10 statements; the study appeared to be a replication of the study by Fottler (1976).

Two of the three hypotheses in the study were rejected, and one was accepted. The hypothesis that female nurses held generally positive attitudes toward male nurses was rejected. The hypothesis that male nurses held generally positive attitudes toward the male as a nurse was supported. A third hypothesis that more positive attitudes toward the male nurse were held by younger, single, better educated, urban-socialized nurses, those employed in a higher-level position outside a hospital, and those having extensive contact with male nurses was rejected. McCarragher concluded from these data that the question of stigma associated with men in nursing remained nebulous and poorly defined.

These investigators employed survey methods in their research. A general criticism of not having any means of validating attitudinal responses holds for all of the studies. It is difficult to obtain reliable data on intraprofessional attitudes when only questionnaires are used. These forms of data would have to be correlated with observed behavioral data to ensure reliability. Prejudice is not a socially acceptable value; hence, questionnaire responses can be biased to a considerable extent. Any list of single questions about complex phenomena will yield data of uncertain reliability. Furthermore, the response rates or poorly constructed samples can result in sampling bias and incomplete knowledge of the phenomenon under study. These studies represent emotional approaches; they do not lend direction to the research effort.

FOCUSED INTERVIEW

In a preliminary investigation designed to examine role strain in men in the nursing profession, Greenberg and Levine (1971) used a sample of 15 men. By means of a focused interview, they gathered data on the way men perceived their status. The subjects ranged in age from 25 to 65 years. The men in the sample ran the gamut of diverse role assignments from staff nurse to director of nursing. The investigators concluded that male nurses perceived role strain as an adjustment problem. All 15 respondents stated that most men tended to gravitate to such clinical areas as urology, anesthesiology, and psychiatry as well as to supervision and administration as a partial means of reducing this strain. The respondents all stated that these areas demanded less intimate care and, thus, minimized role conflict and resulting role strain. Intimate care was defined in the study as care that required direct contact between patient and nurse. The "touching specialties" were considered more appropriate for a female nurse who served as a mother figure. Teaching and management were considered less intimate.

Bush (1976) carried out focused interviews of white males, students and graduate nurses, at a midwestern university. Two each of the students were sophomores, juniors, seniors, and graduate students. The other two men were in active employment; one was employed in a school of nursing and the other in a university hospital. Seven of the ten were married. Early in the interviews Bush concluded that she was not getting consensus data and thus treated all subjects as informants. Based on the interview data, she concluded that (a) most of the overt pressure to dissuade men from entering the profession came from parents, particularly the father; (b) their college friends were either supportive or unconcerned; (c) men usually had some associated work experience or a "significant other" who influenced their decisions; (d) men had to develop coping skills to deal with cultural pressures, especially the attribution of homosexuality; (e) men stated that they were as responsive as women in the affect area; and (f) men tended to select specialty areas in which potential conflict with the societal role of men would be reduced.

In each of these studies the sample size was quite small and nonrepresentative of the general population. Additionally, there was no reported effort to validate the interview content by gathering data from relevant others or employers. Reservations about the validity of the content are justified without a system of rigorous checking on subjective data and with a very unrepresentative and inadequate sample. Both studies could be classified as scouting expeditions at best.

USE OF STANDARDIZED TEST BATTERIES

Aldag and Christiansen (1967) explored the personality characteristics of male nursing students. The sample consisted of 29 male students of nursing, 29 female students of nursing, 29 female junior college students, and 29 male junior college students. To obtain a gross index of profile similarity between groups, rank order correlations of scores on the short form of the Minnesota Multiphasic Personality Inventory scale were calculated (Hathaway & McKinley, 1951) with exclusion of scale M_f (masculinity–femininity). The investigators found that the personality profile of the male nursing students was more similar to female nursing students than was the profile of male junior college students to their counterpart female group.

Over 500 men who were enrolled as nursing students in English hospitals in 1968 were studied by Brown and Stones (1972). To collect data on intelligence and personality, the Mill Hill Vocabulary Test (Raven, 1962) and the Raven Progressive Matrices Test (Raven, 1960) were administered to 456 men, and the Eysenck Personality Inventory (Eysenck & Eysenck, 1964) was given to 404 men. A total of 398 men were given all three.

The male nursing students in the sample were significantly more extroverted than the normal population as well as in comparison to female nursing students. The male students were significantly less neurotic than normal populations. Scores on the Mill Hill (Raven, 1962) and Matrices Tests (Raven, 1960) both were expressed in terms of the scores achieved by the general population. Personality scores did not give clues to the men's reactions to the responsibility they were given. In particular, there was no coherent pattern of association between particular personality traits and attitudes to authority, discipline, or working under women.

The main conclusions of Brown and Stones (1972) were summarized as: (a) men appeared to be on the whole suited to nursing and rather more so than comparable groups of female entrants based on test scores; (b) the investigators' general assumptions about the men were confirmed by nursing faculty assessments; (c) there was no close association between personality, intelligence factors, and dropout rates; and (d) the more idealistic reasons for students entering the nursing profession might have been socially conditioned.

Garvin (1976) compared the values of men who were nursing students at Ohio State University with those of female nursing students, college men in general, medical students, teachers, and personnel and guidance workers. The Allport-Vernon-Lindzey Study of Value Scale (1970) was used. Thirty-four male nursing students and 841 female nursing students were part of the total study population. The data revealed that the values of male nursing students were more akin to female students than to male college students. The findings showed that males scored higher than females on theoretical and lower on religious scales. The investigator reasoned that male students were more interested in the discovery of truth and in the critical and empirical ordering of knowledge than were female students. Garvin (1976) concluded that the values male students held could be a useful input into the nursing profession.

Holtzclaw (1981) examined sex-typed perceptions and locus of control as related to men who chose nursing as a profession. Her study was designed to investigate factors that influenced the male nurse's ability to negotiate the role strain and possible status contradictions exerted in a feminine sex-typed profession. Holtzclaw sought to determine if men in nursing differed from those outside the profession in sex-role identity. It was expected that those male nurses who were androgynous would have greater control perceptions about their own identities. A sample of 52 graduate nurses, 26 men and 26 women, was selected randomly from the same university program. The subjects completed a biographical questionnaire and three instruments: the Bem Sex-Role Inventory (Bem, 1982); the Ideal Nurse Survey (Holtzclaw, 1981); and the Rotter I-E Locus of Control Scale (Rotter, Seeman, & Liverant, 1962).

Results of the study did not support the expectation that male nurses were more androgynous than the young nonnurse normative sample. The findings of this study were not consistent with those from earlier studies in which men and women nurses were similar in sex-role identities and more feminine than nonnurse normative samples. Holtzclaw (1981) observed that the research protocols used in earlier studies were bipolar measures that forced a choice between masculine and feminine endorsements. The Bem Sex-Role Inventory (1982) more precisely measured androgynous characteristics. The BEM scale was purported to measure the factors that permit individuals to make better adaptations to a wide range of social situations. Another important factor was that the study was done with university students rather than with those in diploma and associate degree programs. The generalized societal relaxation in college of many sex-role boundaries also might have influenced the perceptual process (Bem & Lenney, 1976). An unexpected finding was the sex-reversed perceptions of the female subjects in the sample. The investigator suggested that the women nurses, like the men nurses, did not view the nursing role as traditionally feminine. The expectation that locus of control would be related to sex-role identity was not supported by the data.

Snavely and Fairhurst (1984) studied the male nursing student as a token. Individuals have been identified as tokens when they entered a job environment with a history of their social category being numerically scarce in a given occupation. The outcomes of being in this state have been described as social isolation, entrapment in stereotypical roles, and being placed under increased pressure to perform more than majority members.

The sample was selected from two midwestern, two-year diploma schools. For one school the sample consisted of 17 males and 176 females; for the other, the sample was 26 males and 147 females. Instruments were used to measure social isolation, upward communication distortion, performance pressure, and communication apprehension. The research failed to support the propositions regarding token dynamics reported in studies of female tokens.

Brown and Stones (1972) chose a much more representative sample than other investigators. Their sample was drawn from a number of schools; thus, some of the parochialism was reduced in its effect. In addition to data accruing from the interrelationships among scores on the standardized test batteries, they gathered assessments from the instructors of the students to ascertain whether the test data were congruent with the real-world phenomena of the instructional setting. As a consequence, their data were more believable.

To reduce spurious male/female dichotomies, Holtzclaw (1981) used the concept of androgyny. This innovative approach provided a means of assessing characteristics that were desirable in nursing practice rather than toiling with male/female polarity, which might have brought more confusion than order to clarification of issues. In designing this approach, she increased the objectivity of viewing the gender role in the profession. It seemed reasonable to assume that such traits as intelligence, career aspirations, empathy, tact, imagination, integrity, and similar desirable professional traits were not sex-linked. The more insight that is attained about these characteristics in both sexes, the less likely will be the distancing of males from females.

SUMMARY AND
DIRECTIONS FOR FUTURE RESEARCH

Holtzclaw (1981, p. 116) capsulated the issue clearly when she stated, "The man in nursing has been faced with elements of myth, conjecture and stigma for much of this country's history." She postulated that much of the emotional coloring came from societal expectations on sex-appropriateness as reflected in social norms for the occupational role. If clarification of the male role in the nursing profession was a goal of the research done so far, then there are major shortcomings in both the research and the outcomes of research.

It seems unnecessary to do more studies that elicit opinion. It is questionable whether these studies have much utility. There are more important studies that have the potential for helping the profession. In the present rapid expansion of knowledge, the methodologies for doing more sophisticated studies are available. Future studies can be used as a means of bringing insight and clarity rather than searching for labeling or stereotypical behaviors. Reliable data on one minority group might produce insights into the experiences of all minority groups and might assist in the growth of the profession. This type of scholarly endeavor might act as one of the buffers against sudden disruptions that occur as consequences of change in the societal environment.

The studies of men in nursing are few in number. This may be due to the relatively limited number of men, especially male nurses who are researchers, in the profession. Furthermore, the studies primarily have been descriptive surveys with questionable study samples. The data about male nurses are meager and may not represent reality. The population of men in the nursing profession is relatively sparse. Hence, studies carefully tailored to sites in which men are sufficient in numbers to yield reliable data are needed.

The studies of record seem broadly to tap the degree of role strain experienced by persons in nontraditional roles rather than: (a) any differences in strength of clinical development; (b) level of organizational stability; (c) career orientation; (d) economic impact; (e) relationships with relevant others in the various health professions; (f) ability to innovate; and (g) similar important areas. Reliable data about behavioral activities and professional lifestyles of male nurses that impact on the profession in one way or another have not been compiled.

To be helpful, the studies of the future should build on the beginnings of Holtzclaw (1981) and Brown and Stones (1972). There is a need to reduce conjecture and stereotypical thinking about men in the profession analogous to that required to reduce stereotypical thinking about the women going into professions dominated by men. Sample sizes have to be much larger to diminish a parochial effect associated with single site studies. In addition, the samples should be composed of enough diversity to make them representative of the populations being studied.

A fruitful research agenda includes: (a) cohort studies over time; (b) controlled field experiments assessing competence in both academic and practice settings; (c) comparative studies of settings in which the presence of men nurses is noticeable with settings with none or only a few men; and (d) the nature and quality of interaction of male nurses with patients as well as physicians as compared with female nurses to ascertain whether or not any differences exist. Further viable research topics are: (a) the structural barriers in both academic and clinical settings that place artificial impediments to the free expression of professional aspirations of both sexes; (b) an inquiry into why approximately 110 men out of the roughly 57,000 male nurses have earned doctoral degrees, compared to approximately 3,500 female nurses out of roughly 1,830,500 who have earned doctoral degrees (American Nurses' Association, 1984); and (c) experiments to introduce nontraditional role choice possibilities to students at the junior high school level and to trace the outcomes of these endeavors. As with all research, unanswered questions provide the incentive for further research. It may be necessary to recruit more men into the profession as the occupational market for women becomes more competitive. It will be useful to have much better data to plan this recruitment. Perhaps nurses may be able to demonstrate to the other professions that competency and other desirable characteristics are not sex-linked and, thus, contribute to the full democratization of all professions.

REFERENCES

Aldag, J., & Christiansen, C. (1967). Personality correlates of male nurses. *Nursing Research, 4*, 375–376.

Allport, G. W., Vernon, P. E., & Lindzey, G. (1970). *Study of values*. Iowa City, IA: Riverside.

American Nurses' Association. (1984). *Directory of nurses with doctoral degrees*. Kansas City, MO: Author.

Bem, S. L. (1982). *Administration and scoring guide for the Bem Sex Role Inventory*. Palo Alto, CA: Consulting Psychologists Press.

Bem, S. L., & Lenney, C. (1976). Sex typing and the avoidance of cross-sex behavior. *Journal of Personality and Social Psychology, 33*, 48–54.

Brown, R. G. S., & Stones, R. H. W. (1972). Personality and intelligence characteristics of male nurses. *International Journal of Nursing Studies, 9*, 167–177.

Bush, P. J. (1976). Male nurse: A challenge to traditional role identities. *Nursing Forum, 4*, 391–405.

Division of Nursing, U.S. Department of Health and Human Services. (1984). (National sample survey of registered nurses). Unpublished data.

Dolan, J. A. (1973). *Nursing in society, a historical perspective*. Philadelphia: Saunders.

Eysenck, H. J., & Eysenck, S. B. G. (1964). *Manual of the Eysenck Personality Inventory*. London: University of London Press.

Fottler, M. D. (1976). Attitudes of female nurses toward male nurses: A study of occupational segregation. *Journal of Health and Social Behavior, 17*, 99–110.

Garvin, B. J. (1976). Values of male nursing students. *Nursing Research, 25*, 352–357.

Greenberg, E., & Levine, B. (1971). Role strain in the man nurse. *Nursing Forum, 10*, 416–430.

Hathaway, S. R., & McKinley, J. C. (1951). *The Minnesota Multiphasic Personality Inventory Manual* (rev. ed.). New York: Psychological Corporation.

Holtzclaw, B. J. (1981). The man in nursing: Relations between sex-type perceptions and locus of control. *Dissertation Abstracts International*, 4202A. (University Microfilms No. 81-16, 752)

Jameson, E. M. (1966). *Trends in nursing history, their social intervention and ethical relationships* (6th ed.). Philadelphia: Saunders.

Kalisch, P. A., & Kalisch, B. J. (1976). *The advance of American nursing*. Boston: Little, Brown.

Kauffman, C. (1976). *Tamers of death, the history of the Alexian Brothers*. New York: Seabury.

Kauffman, C. (1978). *The ministry of healing*. New York: Seabury.

Levine, E. B. (1971). *Hippocrates*. New York: Twane.

Levine, E. B., & Levine, M. E. (1965). Hippocrates, father of nursing, too? *American Journal of Nursing, 65*(12), 86–88.

Mannino, S. F. (1963). The professional man nurse: Why he chose nursing, and other characteristics of men in nursing. *Nursing Research, 12*, 185–187.

McCarragher, J. A. (1984). *Attitudes of nurses toward male nurses: A question of stigma*. Unpublished master's thesis, Case Western Reserve University, Cleveland, OH.

Raven, J. C. (1960). *Guide to standard progressive matrices*. New York: Psychological Corporation.

Raven, J. C. (1962). *Mill Hill Vocabulary Scale* (rev. ed.). London, England: H. K. Lewis.

Rogness, H. (1976). A student surveys his classmates. *Nursing Outlook, 24*, 303–305.

Rotter, J. B., Seeman, M., & Liverant, S. (1962). Internal versus external locus of control of reinforcement: A major variable in behavior therapy. In N. F. Washburne (Ed.), *Decisions, values, and groups*. London: Pergamon.

Schoenmaker, A., & Radosevich, D. M. (1976). Men nursing students: How they perceive their situation. *Nursing Outlook, 24*, 298–303.

Snavely, B. K., & Fairhurst, G. T. (1984). The male nursing student as a token. *Research in Nursing and Health, 7*, 287–294.

Vaz, D. (1968). High school senior boys' attitudes toward nursing as a career. *Nursing Research, 17*, 533–538.

PART V
Other Research

Chapter 10

Women's Health

NANCY FUGATE WOODS
SCHOOL OF NURSING
UNIVERSITY OF WASHINGTON

CONTENTS

Women's health scholarship is concerned with: (a) women's health experiences across the life span; (b) women's health in relation to environment; and (c) the processes of attaining, maintaining, and regaining health as women experience it. It is possible to consider this new scholarship "gyn-ecology" in the truest sense of the word: women's health ecology.

The purpose of this review was to describe contemporary nursing research on women's health. The review was organized to provide an overview of nursing research on women's health for 1980 to 1985; integrative reviews of two areas of women's health research in which significant contributions were made—perimenstrual symptoms, and women's roles and their health; and recommendations for future work.

PROCESS OF REVIEW

Seven journals were examined for the review: *Journal of Obstetric, Gynecologic, and Neonatal Nursing, Nursing Research, Research in Nursing and Health, Western Journal of Nursing Research, Advances in Nursing Science, MCN, The American Journal of Maternal-Child Nursing,* and *Health Care for Women International,* formerly *Issues in Women's Health.* The criteria for inclusion of articles were: (a) The article must have dealt with the topic of women's health as a primary concern, not merely with an incidental use of gender in the analysis; and (b) the article must have reflected a systematic investigation of phenomena with the use of woman as a variable in the purpose, problem statement, or theoretical framework. Excluded were articles on maternal role that included values, attitudes, and behaviors of the mother in relation to the child, as opposed to the influence of pregnancy or parenting on the woman's own experience. Categorical analysis of the articles was performed by coding on the following variables: developmental dimension; wellness–illness dimension; research paradigm; contribution to nursing science and practice; and measurement and methods.

This review was supported in part by a grant, NU 001054, from the Division of Nursing, United States Public Health Service. Acknowledgment is made of the technical assistance of Ms. May Phifer in preparation of the manuscript.

WOMEN'S HEALTH RESEARCH: 1980-1985

Developmental Dimension

The developmental dimension included the categories of young adult, middle adult, older adult, and developmental dimension undifferentiated. Of 83 papers, 69% dealt with young adult women, 15% with women in the middle years, and 3% with older women. Thirteen percent of the papers were focused on women from several age groups, primarily young and middle adults. This distribution reflected societal attitudes toward aging rather than the demographics of the population of the United States. So little attention to middle-aged and elderly women reflected neglect of a major proportion of the population receiving nursing services. Women accounted for about 77% of nursing home occupants, yet little published nursing research existed about this population. Some investigators, exemplified by Griffith's (1983a, 1983b) analysis of women's stressors and coping patterns according to age group, purposefully considered the developmental dimension in relation to women's health. Studies of adolescents' contraceptive practices (Burbach, 1980; Hawkins, Fahey, Kurien, Roberto, & Simon, 1981; Marcy, Brown, & Danielson, 1983), teenage pregnancy (Crockett, 1984a) and dieting experience (Mallick, 1982), menopause (Millette, 1981; Muhlenkamp, Waller, & Bourne, 1983; Uphold & Susman, 1981), elderly women's sexual attitudes (Portnova, Young, & Newman, 1984), depression in the elderly (Newman & Guadiano, 1984), and health in older women (Engle, 1984) represented attention to women's health across the life span.

Wellness-Illness Dimension

The wellness-illness dimension included four categories: well women with health promotion needs; women at risk with prevention or early detection needs; symptomatic women with needs for treatment; and women recovering from a significant illness with needs for rehabilitation. Two-thirds (67%) of the papers dealt with wellness and health promotion, whereas only 19% dealt with women at risk of illness. Studies of the decision to undergo amniocentesis (Cox, Sullivan, & Roghmann, 1984; Davies & Doran, 1982), the process of embarking on a weight loss program (White, 1984), the influence of jogging on self-esteem (Rudy & Estok, 1983), and the practice of breast self-examination (Edwards, 1980; Hallal, 1982; Schlueter, 1982; Sheahan, Lee, & Lewis, 1984) were examples of this orientation. Only 4% of the reports were concerned with women who were ill and 10% with women recovering from illness. Studies of menstrual cycle changes in women experiencing surgery (McKeever & Galloway, 1984), self-concept of those recovering from a mastectomy (Jenkins, 1980), needs of women after mastectomy (Grabau, Rustia, & Lucas, 1984), and sexuality after hysterectomy (Humphries, 1981) illustrated the latter categories. This emphasis reflected the growing interest in health promotion seen in the general nursing research literature. Perhaps the lack of attention to women who were ill also reflected the frequently encountered problem of access to participants who were receiving medical services or were hospitalized.

Research Paradigms

Two paradigms have had a dominant influence on contemporary nursing research methods: the positivist-empiricist, and the historicist. The positivist-empiricist approach is based on an assumption that there is a body of facts or principles to be discovered or understood and that these facts or principles exist independently of any historical or social context. Historicist paradigms in nursing include grounded theory and ethnographic and phenomenologic orientations. They derive from an assumption that science is necessarily historical and that facts and principles are embedded in both historical and cultural contexts (Tinkle & Beaton, 1983). A third paradigm is beginning to influence contemporary nursing research. Feminist research is based on a political ideology, and its goal is political change. Research questions are derived from social problems that are critical to women's lives (Duffy, 1984; P. Klein, 1983; Mies, 1983). An important contribution of feminist research is the development of new interpretations to a field of study (MacPherson, 1983).

Only 39% of the research reports included an emphasis on the context for women's health experiences. Studies of postpartum depression as a culturally induced phenomenon (Tentoni & High, 1980), culturally induced stress during childbearing among Filipino women (Stern, Tilden, & Maxwell, 1980), attitudes toward and use of abortion among Taiwanese women (Wang, 1981), and the relationship between social support and weight loss (Gierszewski, 1983) exemplified this category.

Eighty-three percent of the papers were based on the positivist-empiricist paradigm, and 17% on the historicist paradigm. Only two papers were based on a feminist paradigm. Empiricist-oriented papers included those assessing the strength of relationship between marital adjustment and climacteric symptoms (Uphold & Susman, 1981) and the relationship between anxiety, critical thinking, and information processing during and after breast biopsy (Scott, 1983). A study of uncoupled identity in widows (Saunders, 1981), adjusted control in women's perceptions of their pregnancies (Gara & Tilden, 1984), women's experience in self-help groups (Lipson, 1980), and processes of surviving child abuse (Crockett, 1984b) reflected historicist traditions. The research based on a feminist paradigm included a study of achieving high-level wellness in single-parent families (Duffy, 1984) and a study of misogyny and homicide in women (Campbell, 1981). The distribution of papers across paradigms was not surprising considering the dominant mode of research training and the orientation of most contemporary nursing research texts and academic programs.

Contributions to
Nursing Science and Practice

Contributions to nursing science and practice were coded into three categories: (a) fostering understanding of human health-related experiences; (b) expanding awareness of the interrelationships between humans and their environments in health-related situations, for example, supporting and nonsupporting environments; and (c) contributing to understanding of therapeutic measures to promote health and minimize the negative consequences of illness. In 59% of the research reports investigators extended nursing knowledge of how women adapt to health and illness states. Researchers in only 11% were concerned with the interrelationships between women's health and the environment. Twenty-one percent of the studies were reports of clinical trials. Studies dealing with women's adaptation to health and illness were concerned with contraceptive choices of university women (Ayvazian, 1981; Hawkins et al., 1981), perimenstrual symptom experiences (Brown & Woods, 1984; Coyne, 1983; O'Rourke, 1983a, 1983b; Woods, Most, & Dery, 1982a, 1982b), adaptation to cesarian section (Berry, 1983; Cox & Smith, 1982; Cranley, Hedalh, & Pegg, 1983; Tcheng, 1984; Tilden & Lipson, 1981) and pregnancy (Alley, 1984; Ellis, 1980; Glazer, 1980; Hames, 1980; Rankin & Campbell,

1983; Tilden, 1983, 1984), knowledge and attitudes about menopausal symptoms (La Rocco & Polit, 1980; Millette, 1981; Muhlenkamp et al., 1983); adjustment to cancer (Krouse & Krouse, 1982; Marecki, 1981), depression in the elderly (Newman & Guadiano, 1984), and bereavement (Harris, 1984; Saunders, 1981).

Work on the interrelationships between women and the environment was exemplified by investigations of the influence of multiple role demands on women's health and illness experiences (Woods, 1980, 1985), Northwest Coast Indian women's beliefs about childbirth (Bushnell, 1981), misogyny and homicide of women (Campbell, 1981), relationships of life-change events and social support to emotional disequilibrium in pregnancy (Tilden, 1983), and dysmenorrhea (Jordan & Meckler, 1982).

Most investigations on clinical therapeutics were centered on issues during pregnancy, including fetal position (Andrews, 1981), control of labor pain (Geden, Beck, Hauge, & Pohlman, 1984; Manderino & Bzdek, 1984), treatment of pregnancy edema (Jacobs, McCance, & Stewart, 1982), and postpartum problems such as breast engorgement (Brooten, Brown, Hollingsworth, Tanis, & Donlan, 1983; Dickson & Post, 1981), nipple pain (Fleming, 1984), and adjustment (Rhode & Groenjes-Finke, 1981). Others were studies of new foot supports for pelvic exams (Olson, 1981), effects of antepartal exercises on postpartum regeneration of the pubococcygeal muscle (Henderson, 1983; Hendrickson, 1981), influence of an educational gynecological examination on women's attitudes (Latta & Weismeier, 1982), modeling to increase the use of breast self-examination (Edwards, 1980), bereavement crisis intervention for women (Constantino, 1981), measures to reduce stress (Dorensky, 1984), effects of back massage on levels of arousal (Longworth, 1982), and postoperative bladder conditioning (Williamson, 1982).

Measurement and Methods

Ten percent of the papers were concerned with methods and measures for women's health research. These included two reports dealing with basal body temperature (Cooper & Abrams, 1984; Samples & Abrams, 1984), two with perimenstrual symptoms (Woods, Most, & Dery, 1982a, 1982b), one on stressful life events (Norbeck, 1984), one on measurement of the menopausal hot flash (Voda, Imle, & Atwood,

1980), one on a measure of health (Engel, 1984), and one on locus of control specific to pregnancy (O'Connell, 1983).

In the time period of 1980 to 1985 there were two areas in which nurse investigators made substantial contributions to understanding women's health: perimenstrual symptom experiences, and the relationship of women's roles to their health. A review of these studies, including research published after 1985, follows.

PERIMENSTRUAL SYMPTOMS

During the past 5 years there has been a dramatic increase in research reports in which nurse investigators addressed women's perimenstrual experiences. The content of the reports on perimenstrual symptoms pertained to prevalence, stressful experiences, socialization, physiological correlates, consequences, therapies, and methodological contributions.

Prevalence

In the first survey of a healthy population of women in the United States, Woods, Most, and Dery (1982b, 1982c) found that 30% of women reported perimenstrual symptoms, although for the most part their symptoms were mild. Twelve percent reported severe premenstrual irritability, and 17% reported severe menstrual cramps. Parity and oral contraceptive use were associated with less severe cramping, whereas use of intrauterine devices was associated with more severe cramping. Women with long menstrual cycle lengths and longer and heavier menstrual flows reported more severe perimenstrual symptoms, including water retention, cramps, and negative affect, than did their counterparts with short cycles and less flow. Women who could predict their next menses accurately also had more symptoms of weight gain and backache. In general, older women and employed women reported less severe symptoms than younger women. Black women reported less severe cramping and premenstrual negative affect than white women but more weight gain, swelling, and headache. Women who were well educated and had high incomes generally reported less severe symptoms than those with less education and lower incomes.

Shelley and Anderson (1986) found that premenstrual and menstrual distress was greater in alcoholic than nonalcoholic women. Whether alcoholism promotes symptoms or symptoms promote use of alcohol is not known.

Stressful Experiences

Evidence linking stressful experiences to perimenstrual symptoms included the effects of major life events, such as death of a spouse (Jordan & Meckler, 1982; Woods, Dery, & Most, 1982), and daily hassles such as being stuck in traffic (Woods, Most, & Longnecker, 1985). A generally stressful life context seemed more influential than episodes of stressful experiences in either the premenstruum or menstruum (Woods, Most, & Longnecker, 1985). General indicators of a chronically stressful life context included low income and low education, and both were associated with increased severity of perimenstrual symptoms (Woods, Most, & Dery, 1982b). Jordan and Meckler (1982) found that college students who had experienced the most stressful life events also had the most severe dysmenorrhea. The relationship was accentuated among those with little social support.

In addition to stressors from the social environment, physical stressors seemed to have important effects on the menstrual cycle. Jogging appeared to alter menstrual cycle patterns, with heavy jogging producing scant menses, skipped menses, and irregular cycles. For some women, however, jogging reduced menstrual discomfort and breast pain (Estok & Rudy, 1984). Estok and Rudy (1986) found that scant menstrual flow, irregular menses, and menstrual pattern changes occurred more frequently among marathon runners than among nonmarathon runners. Reduced body fat has been implicated as the cause of menstrual disturbances in women athletes. Ouelette, MacVicar, and Harlan (1986) found that percent body fat was not related to menstrual cycle length. Although collegiate athletes in training had significantly lower body fat (16.5%) than the nonathletes (21%), there was not a significant difference in cycle length. Of interest is the finding that among the women who were 18 to 22 years of age, average cycle length for the athletes was 35.91 ± 13.5 and for the nonathletes 35.15 ± 14.2, considerably longer than estimates based on older populations. Moreover, athletes reported a mean menstrual flow length of 4.8 days compared to 3.5 days reported by the nonathletes.

The experience of nongynecologic surgery altered patterns of menstrual cycles, particularly among adolescents. Nearly 70% of adolescent women experienced early menses following surgery. Among adolescents, those who experienced prolonged anesthesia time had shorter menstrual cycles postoperatively (McKeever & Galloway, 1984).

Some women anticipated stressful experiences with menstruation each month. Coyne (1983) found that women who anticipated but did not necessarily experience perimenstrual symptoms had higher electromyogram (EMG) levels during the luteal phase than did women who did not anticipate perimenstrual symptoms. Coyne's work raised the possibility that attributional processes contributed to perimenstrual symptoms.

Socialization

Kay (1981) explored the meanings of menstruation to Mexican-American women. Using ethnosemantic methods, she obtained an ethnography of menstruation. Women connected menstruation with normal physiology and indicated that menstruation was required for health. Kay found that although the Spanish word for menstruation is "sickness," 58% of the women described it as a biological thing. Cultural rules for coping with menstruation included avoiding exposure to cold, food taboos, resting, sexual taboos, and limiting unnecessary activity. Many saw menstruation as removing toxins.

Williams (1983) found that premenarcheal girls (grades 4 to 6) were confused about the anatomy and physiology of menstruation. They attributed changes in affect to menstruation and endorsed many menstrual taboos related to activity, communication, and concealment of menstruation. Their attitudes toward menstruation were more positive than negative. Havens and Swenson (1986) found that 8th and 10th graders, 80% of whom had begun menstruating, first were informed about menstruation by their mothers. They responded to menarche with surprise, fear, and embarrassment. Nevertheless, their current perceptions of menstruation were that it was normal but inconvenient. Although 89% thought boys needed to be informed about menstruation, only 35% wanted boys to be included in classroom discussions.

Some investigators have examined the influence of menarche on relationships with parents. Danza (1983) found that menarche changed the nature of mother–daughter and father–daughter interactions. Menke (1983) reported that mothers and their adolescent daughters shared similar beliefs and reported similar symptom experiences with menstruation. Stoltzman's work (1986) demonstrated that adolescent girls' menstrual experiences resembled those of their peers more than those of their mothers.

The influence of women's menarcheal experiences on menstruation also has been examined. Woods, Dery, and Most (1983) found that women's recollections of menarcheal experiences had little influence on subsequent menstrual attitudes or symptoms in adult women.

Studying the influence of socialization as a woman on perimenstrual symptoms, Brown and Woods (1986) found that neither sex typing (femininity or masculinity) nor sex role orientation (traditional or nontraditional) was related to women's experiences of symptoms. Women in traditional occupations, however, experienced more severe perimenstrual negative affect symptoms. Woods (1985) found that sex role orientation, along with symptom severity and the disability linked to symptoms, influenced women's attitudes toward menstruation. Women with traditional sex role orientations described menstruation as debilitating.

One aspect of menstrual socialization that may be linked to health and menstrual attitudes is menstrual hygiene practices. Patterson and Hale (1985) described women's self-care for menstruation as "making sure." Menstruation, a continuous phenomenon and not under voluntary control, provided a continuous demand for managing flow. Concealment of menstruation was a menstrual taboo that had survived into the 1980s. Integration of menstrual practices within daily living required attending to current menstrual demands, calculating the timing and type of absorbent used, and juggling time, space, and supplies.

Reame's (1983) work underscored the problem on menstrual hygiene for women with spinal cord injury. Although 60% had reduced vaginal sensation after injury, 72% wore tampons as primary menstrual hygiene products. Duration of tampon wear was greater (9 to 9.5 hours) for women with cervical cord lesions compared to women with lower cord lesions (2.9 hours), probably attributable to the need for assistance with tampon insertion by the women with cervical lesions. Users who wore tampons overnight had significantly more urinary tract infections.

Physiological Correlates

Voda (1980) characterized patterns of progesterone, aldosterone, sodium, and potassium levels in menstruating women performing usual activities of daily living. Aldosterone paralleled the luteal phase rise in progesterone as did urinary potassium. Negative affect and concentration symptoms as well as physical symptoms peaked in the late luteal phase. Weight, ankle, and finger girth fluctuated across the cycle. Progesterone and aldosterone were not correlated with other biochemical, physical, or subjective measures, nor were serum sodium and potassium. Although serum sodium levels were not related significantly to aldosterone levels, urinary potassium levels were. According to Voda's work, the relationship between hormone levels and symptoms has not been delineated clearly.

Graham (1980) found that cognitive behavior did not vary with estrogen levels across the menstrual cycle. Cognitive behavior in the luteal phase exceeded that during the follicular phase and at ovulation. Performance on reading, color naming, and subtraction was better in the luteal phase than at other cycle phases, as were women's activation and ability to inhibit competing stimuli.

Consequences

Perimenstrual symptoms have produced variable outcomes for women, ranging from modest effects on well-being to disruption of daily activities. Woods (1985) found that women with the most severe symptoms were most likely to rest in bed or decrease their activities. The perimenstrual symptoms producing the greatest disability were negative affect symptoms, for example, depression and irritability.

O'Rourke (1983b, 1984) found that perimenstrual symptoms were unrelated to psychological well-being in employed women. In contrast, nonmenstrual symptoms were found to have a negative effect on psychological well-being. These seemingly contrary findings are not difficult to reconcile. Although a small percentage of women have experienced a short-term disruption of usual activities, in general perimenstrual symptoms have been unrelated to general well-being when nonmenstrual symptoms were taken into account. Garling and Roberts (1980) found a very low incidence of work absenteeism in a population of nurses, contradicting the assumption of high menses-related absenteeism in working women.

Perimenstrual symptoms and related disability were found to affect women's attitudes toward menstruation, as did their socialization. Women with the most severe symptoms who experienced the most disability perceived menstruation as most debilitating. Women who ascribed to traditional norms about women's roles in society were more likely to view menstruation as debilitating than were their counterparts with nontraditional norms (Woods, 1985).

Although earlier investigators reported that women with severe symptoms experienced the greatest intrusion in daily living, Brown and Zimmer (1986b) were first to consider the family as well as the personal impact of menstrual symptoms. They found that women with frequently recurring symptoms and the greatest number of symptoms experienced the most disruption in their lives. Men who were partners of women with frequent symptoms and men with less education perceived the most severe life disruption. Men cited family effects of their partners' symptoms to include increased conflict, decreased family cohesion, disrupted communication, decreased family participation in shared activities, withdrawal and decreased contact among family members, and decreased performance of household tasks by the women. Men coped with their partners' symptoms by increasing involvement in household tasks and parenting, seeking and providing support, using anger and avoidance, and getting more involved in work. Men whose partners' lives were most disrupted were the least likely to use these coping strategies.

Therapies

Brown and Zimmer (1986a) studied the help-seeking behavior of women who attended a lecture on premenstrual symptoms. All had sought help previously for their symptoms, with many trying several different types of providers. Nurse practitioners were rated most positively. Only one-third of the women in treatment were satisfied with the help they were receiving, with most feeling they were treated disrespectfully or not taken seriously. Women who perceived the most life disruption associated with the symptoms were most likely to be receiving health care.

Taylor and Bledsoe (1986) found that peer support for women with premenstrual symptoms did not reduce symptom severity or number of symptoms significantly, nor increase social network size or satisfaction. Nevertheless, the women found that the group provided education, emotional support, information that they were not alone with the problem, and people with whom to share problems and advice. As a result, these women found that making necessary lifestyle changes to cope with premenstrual symptoms was easier.

Methods

In addition to the substantive findings, there have been important methodological contributions to this literature. Woods, Most, and Dery (1982c) described three clusters of perimenstrual symptoms occurring in a nonclinical population of women. These included: negative affect, fluid retention, and cramping-pain symptoms. Woods, Most, and Dery (1982b) also discovered that only 16 of the symptoms included on the Menstrual Distress Questionnaire (MDQ) (Moos, 1968) differed significantly across menstrual cycle phase.

A second important methodologic contribution was the discovery of large differences in prevalence estimates of perimenstrual symptoms across two measurement approaches. Use of a retrospective questionnaire (Moos MDQ) elicited higher prevalence of symptoms for the same menstrual cycle than did use of a daily open-ended health diary (Woods, Most, & Dery, 1982a).

Finally, Shaver and Woods (1985) found that the concordance of symptom reports across two contiguous menstrual cycles was low except for backache, headache, cramps, cold sweats, depression, tension, and fatigue. Estimates based on only one menstrual cycle may have underestimated or overestimated the prevalence of symptoms. Moreover, a single menstrual cycle has been inadequate as a baseline or follow-up estimate by which to evaluate nursing therapeutics.

WOMEN'S ROLES, WOMEN'S HEALTH

A second area in which significant contributions have been made in the nursing literature was centered on the influence of women's roles on their health. Investigators have proposed links between the stressors and supports inherent in women's work and family roles to their health. Investigators in other disciplines have focused on the effects of either employment or parenting on women's health. Most nursing studies have been concerned with the constellations of women's roles, for example, employment, parenting, and marriage in relation to health.

Support

Support from a partner has been protective of women's health, and the type of support that was most effective seemed to be contingent on women's roles. Duffy's work (1984) with single-parent, woman-headed households underscored the importance of social support in helping women transcend their options to practice positive health behaviors. Among young married women, support from the spouse was an important deterrent to episodes of illness (Woods, 1980). Moreover, the type of support that was most effective in preventing symptoms of poor mental health was contingent on the woman's constellation of roles. For women who were employed and not parents, task-sharing support was most important. For women who were parents and not employed, both access to a confidant and task-sharing support were important. For women who were employed and parents, having non-traditional gender role norms was most protective, as was having task-sharing support from the spouse and access to a confidant (Woods, 1985). The nature and type of support most protective of health was also contingent on the woman's family context. Norbeck (1985b) found that the influence of social support on perceived job stress of female critical care nurses was contingent on their marital status. Work support, such as the ability to talk about work, relax, or reenergize after work, explained more of the variance in perceived job stress than other types of support for married nurses. Support from relatives explained more of the variance in perceived job stress and psychological symptoms than other types of support for unmarried nurses. Although the work environment may have provided a source of support for women, the recent nursing literature has not been focused on this dimension of employment.

Stressors

Griffith (1983a, 1983b) made an important contribution to knowledge of stressors in women's lives. She identified six primary stressor areas for women: love relationships, personal success, physical health, parent-child relationships, personal time, and social relationships. Stressors varied across age groups. Personal time, physical health, and personal success were major stressors for women 25 to 34 years of age; physical health, personal time, and love relationships for women 35 to 44; and physical health and personal time for women 45 to 54, with the same stressors persisting into the next decade. Younger women in Griffith's study (1983b) reported more physical and emotional symptoms than did women over 35. Griffith attributed this phenomenon to the high expectations of young women in the face of many constraints.

The nursing literature contained evidence linking many aspects of women's roles to stressors and health outcomes. Staats and Staats (1983) compared female and male managers, executives, and professionals, finding that women reported higher levels of stress and stressors; but they were family-related, not job-related. Norbeck (1985a) reported that higher levels of job stress among critical care nurses were related to lower levels of job satisfaction and higher levels of symptoms in a predominantly female sample. Not every element of the work environment that was rated as stressful influenced job satisfaction and produced symptoms. Workload and the amount of physical work, physical set-up of the unit, and communication problems with unit nurses had a negative effect on job satisfaction. Physical set-up of the unit, meeting the psychological needs of the patient, noise level on the unit, equipment and its failure, physical injury to the nurse, and communication problems with unit nurses were associated with psychological symptoms.

Woods found that women who had more children reported more symptoms of poor mental health (1985) but had fewer actual episodes of illness than women with fewer children (1980). She suggested that parenting may be stressful, producing symptoms particularly for women who have three or more children. On the other hand, low compatibility of the sick role with parenting acted as a deterrent to episodes of being ill (Woods, 1980).

Studies of women's experiences as parents revealed that parenting probably affected a woman's health in ways that depended on her familial and social context. Mercer (1985) explored the relationship of maternal gratification to various roles for women of varying ages. She found that 20- to 29-year-old women who were experiencing employment-parenting role strain found parenting less gratifying. Those who had a poor relationship with a partner found the parenting role more gratifying. These relationships were not evident for younger or older women.

Life change after the birth of an infant coupled with a woman's illness during the previous year predicted postpartal illness in mothers of 6-month-old infants. Of interest was the finding that network size was negatively related to intensity and helpfulness of the instrumental support provided. There was no evidence for the buffering effect of support on postpartal illness in the face of great life change. The positive relationship between intensity of support and illness raised the possibility of illness inducing support (Lenz, Parks, Jenkins, & Jarrett, 1986).

McEntee and Rankin (1983) found that employed women attending a conference on stress had different experiences contingent on both marital status and the presence of children. Single, white, divorced women without children had the highest number of mind-body distress disorders and reasons for consulting health providers; single, white, divorced women with children had the lowest frequency of illness-related days spent in bed. Married women with children had the lowest absentee rates. Uphold and Susman (1985) found that the more roles women enacted, the less likely they were to experience climacteric symptoms. Childrearing and the number of hours worked were not related to symptoms, but marital adjustment and active role participation were protective against symptoms. The dimensions of employment and parenting that are stressful have yet to be elucidated. Moreover, the supportive and joyful aspects of parenting have been neglected in the literature, with the exception of Mercer's (1985) work.

Although the marital relationship has been shown to be influential as a source of support, Uphold and Susman (1981) described its stressful properties. Middle-aged women with poor marital adjustment reported the most menopausal symptoms. Moreover, women who cared for an ill spouse were at risk of illness themselves. Sexton and Munro (1985) found that wives of men who had chronic obstructive pulmonary disease (COPD) reported higher subjective stress and lower life satisfaction than women who were married to men without chronic illness. The women married to men with COPD assumed more new responsibilities, relinquished more social activities, rated their health lower, and had less frequent sexual activity as a result of the disease. Moreover, they lived with considerable worry about their husbands.

Although some have assumed that military marriages are stressful, Jacobsen (1986) found that anxiety levels of midlife women who were military spouses were not different from those for women who were not military spouses. Both levels were low, indeed lower than the normative samples.

Coping

Women's coping patterns were found to vary with age. Griffith (1983b) found that younger women were likely to use talking, whereas women over 45 years of age were likely to turn to work and religion. Young women tended to use consumption of food and alcohol most frequently, while women over 45 coped by ignoring the problem. Schank, Thomas, and Young (1981) found that young adult women demonstrated both healthy and unhealthy coping strategies, including eating (49%), sleeping (31%), drinking (12%), ignoring the problem (12%), and taking medications (4%).

Staats and Staats (1983) reported that professional women responded to stress by reporting more illness, medical consultations, work loss, medication use, and mental health consultations than men. These women reported greater incidence of mental problems, stress-related disorders, and family history of stress disorders than did men. They were more self-critical of their appearance and attempted habit change more than men. Men, on the other hand, consumed more alcohol, demonstrated more Type A behavior, and had a greater incidence of hypertension than women.

Health and Illness Behaviors

Nursing research also has included studies of women's primary prevention and illness behaviors. Duffy (1986) found that in female-headed single-parent families, nutrition, rest, exercise, and personal hygiene were the most frequently practiced primary prevention behaviors. Major barriers to their health practices were time, laziness, money, and the need for support. Woods (1986) found that, among young adult married women, vitamin use accounted for over half of universal self-care activities. Illness-related self-care activities included use of over-the-counter medications, alteration of activity, prescription medication, and home remedies, in descending order. The nature of self-care activities was related to the nature of a woman's symptoms.

Methods

Norbeck's (1984) revision of the Sarason Life Event Scale (LES) to include items relevant to women's lives was a significant contribution to the methods for studying women's health. The items included: major difficulties with birth control pills or devices, difficulty finding a job, difficulty finding housing, a change in child care arrangements, conflicts with spouse or partner about parenting, conflicts with child's grandparents (or other important person) about parenting, taking on full responsibility for parenting as a single parent, custody battles with former spouse or partner, and being a victim of a violent act (rape, assault).

Collins and Post (1986) developed an instrument to measure coping responses in employed mothers. Efforts to prevent, avoid, or control emotional distress included: wife's occupational change, husband's occupational change, wife's work flexibility, husband's work flexibility, wife's change in household management, husband's contribution to household management, and strain management and overload management.

AGENDA FOR FUTURE RESEARCH

In 1981 McBride and McBride lamented the lack of attention to women's lived experiences in contemporary women's health research. They found that most studies were conducted from a reductionistic rather than a holistic point of view. They called for an increased emphasis on women's first-person experiences, as embedded in the context of their lives, a rapprochement of subjective and objective methods, and the generation of theoretical frameworks to account for women's health. That same year Dunbar, Patterson, Burton, and Stuckert (1981) demonstrated that only a small proportion of clinical nursing research was devoted to women's health; of that literature, the major proportion emphasized primary or secondary prevention.

A large proportion of the research published between 1980 and 1985 was about young adult women dealing with pregnancy experiences, the menstrual cycle, contraception, and women's changing roles. To complement this work, the research agenda for the 1990s should include greater emphasis on adolescent, middle-aged, and elderly women. Incorporation of theoretical models for understanding women's biological, psychological, and social development across the life span could play an essential part in linking future work about women's health to a body of theory accounting for developmental variation.

There was strength in the areas of health promotion, risk reduction, and illness prevention. Investigators have made significant contributions to understanding the relationship between stress and health in well women, adjustment to pregnancy and delivery, and relationship of multiple factors to breast self-examination and contraceptive use. The research agenda for nursing in the 1990s should maintain the emphasis on health promotion and prevention and promote greater emphasis on knowledge about women who are ill, disabled, or recovering from illness.

There is a beginning effort to understand women's health experiences in the first person singular and in relation to the context in which they live their lives. Although nurse investigators have made a significant contribution to the literature on social support and women's health, the research agenda for nursing should emphasize greater understanding of the physical and social environments that support or damage women's health and the means by which they influence health.

The dominant paradigm guiding women's health research in nursing has been rooted in logical positivism. Future nursing research would benefit from a pluralism of paradigms, with work guided by different research traditions providing complementary perspectives on women's health (Stevenson & Woods, 1986).

There has been impressive work in the area of women's adaptations in health and illness. The future research agenda should include increased emphasis on clinical therapeutics for women, as well as work on the contexts that promote women's health. Clinical trials of nursing therapeutics for women were uncommon. The few published reports did not contain design elements reflecting contemporary standards for controlled clinical trials, including adequate power, random allocation of participants to study groups, assessment of pretreatment equivalence, and assessment of withdrawals after random assignment (Jacobsen & Meininger, 1986).

The dominant methods used in the studies published between 1980 and 1985 were questionnaires and interviews administered on a single occasion; these results were consistent with Jacobsen and Meininger's (1985) findings. Yet the most commonly studied topics, such as adaptation to pregnancy, perimenstrual symptoms and menstrual cycle alterations, menopause, contraception experiences, and adjustment to cancer, are inherently dynamic. Longitudinal designs are needed for studying these phenomena.

Moreover, biological dimensions of the phenomena studied during this period were frequently ignored or measured indirectly. For example, menstrual cycle phase was determined indirectly by the woman's self-report rather than by endocrine markers. A notable exception was Coyne's (1983) use of electromyographic levels as an indicator of stress, reflecting an integration of biological and psychosocial aspects of women's health.

Based on this review, future directions for nursing research should include increased emphasis on holistic understanding of perimenstrual symptom experiences and dynamic study of the phenomenon. Most investigators have focused on menstruation as either a biological or social phenomenon. Holistic understanding of women's experiences with menstruation requires research approaches to foster integration of its biological, psychosocial, and cultural components. Understanding of women's menstrual experiences, in context, would be extended through the use of naturalistic methods that rely on experiential analysis in combination with biological markers of the menstrual cycle. Triangulation of approaches hold promise for future endeavors (Lentz & Woods, 1985; Mitchell, 1986).

The menstrual cycle is inherently a dynamic phenomenon. Its cyclic nature cannot be understood without multiple repeated measures over an extended period of time. Both intraindividual and group patterns can be discerned from serial measurements of phenomena over several cycles. Moreover, the relationship between serial measures of multiple variables can extend knowledge of patterns of human experience, such as the relationship between stressors and symptoms (Lentz & Woods, 1985).

Women with severe symptoms were not satisfied with the health care they received, yet only one published nursing study was a therapeutic trial. Exploration of therapies to reduce severe perimenstrual symptoms and their effects on women's lives should be included in future research agendas.

It was evident that both family and work environments were sources of stress and support for women. Coping and illness behavior patterns were influenced by the constellation of women's roles. Traditional research approaches have helped investigators to achieve a crude picture of the factors influencing women's health but have provided limited evidence to explain how they operate in women's lives. Future research endeavors should be focused on experiential, dynamic analyses of women's lives, including transitions to and from parenthood and employment. Perhaps in women's stories lie the explanations for how work, marriage, and parenting simultaneously are sources of stress and support (R. Klein, 1983; Reinharz, 1983).

REFERENCES

Alley, N. (1984). Morning sickness: The client's perspective. *Journal of Obstetric, Gynecologic, and Neonatal Nursing, 13*, 185–189.

Andrews, C. (1981). Nursing intervention to change a malpositioned fetus. *Advances in Nursing Science, 3*(4), 53–66.

Ayvazian, A. (1981). Contraception choices of female university students. *Journal of Obstetric, Gynecologic, and Neonatal Nursing, 10*, 426–429.

Berry, K. (1983). The body image of a primigravida following caesarean delivery. *Issues in Health Care of Women, 6*, 367–376.

Brooten, D., Brown, L., Hollingsworth, A., Tanis, J., & Donlan, J. (1983). A comparison of four treatments to prevent and control breast pain and engorgement in nonnursing mothers. *Nursing Research, 32*, 225–229.

Brown, M., & Woods, N. (1984). Correlates of dysmenorrhea: A challenge to past stereotypes. *Journal of Obstetric, Gynecologic, and Neonatal Nursing, 13*, 259–267.

Brown, M., & Woods, N. (1986). Sex role orientation, sex typing, occupational traditionalism and perimenstrual symptoms. *Health Care for Women International, 7*, 25–38.

Brown, M., & Zimmer, P. (1986a). Help-seeking for premenstrual symptomatology: A description of women's experiences. *Health Care for Women International, 7*, 173–184.

Brown, M., & Zimmer, P. (1986b). Personal and family impact of premenstrual symptoms. *Journal of Obstetric, Gynecologic, and Neonatal Nursing, 15*, 31–38.

Burbach, C. (1980). Contraception and adolescent pregnancy. *Journal of Obstetric, Gynecologic, and Neonatal Nursing, 9*, 319–323.

Bushnell, J. (1981). Northwest Coast American Indians' beliefs about childbirth. *Issues in Health Care of Women, 3*, 249–261.

Campbell, J. (1981). Misogyny and homicide of women. *Advances in Nursing Science, 3*(2), 67–83.

Collins, C., & Post, L. (1986). An instrument to measure coping responses in employed mothers: Preliminary results. *Research in Nursing and Health, 9*, 309–316.

Constantino, R. (1981). Bereavement crisis intervention for widows in grief and mourning. *Nursing Research, 30*, 351–355.

Cooper, K., & Abrams, R. (1984). Attributes of the oral cavity as a site for basal body temperature measurements. *Journal of Obstetric, Gynecologic, and Neonatal Nursing, 13*, 125–129.

Cox, B., & Smith, E. (1982). The mother's self-esteem after a caesarean delivery. *MCN, The American Journal of Maternal Child Nursing, 7*, 309–314.

Cox, C., Sullivan, J., & Roghmann, K. (1984). A conceptual explanation of risk-reduction behavior and intervention development. *Nursing Research, 33*, 168–173.

Coyne, C. (1983). Muscle tension and its relation to symptoms in the premenstruum. *Research in Nursing and Health, 6*, 199–206.

Cranley, M., Hedalh, K., & Pegg, S. (1983). Women's perceptions of vaginal and Caesarean deliveries. *Nursing Research, 32*, 10–15.

Crockett, M. (1984a). The queen of hell syndrome: Social isolation, teenage pregnancies, and depression. *Health Care for Women International, 5*, 125–143.

Crockett, M. (1984b). Surviving child abuse: Self-reported coping histories of fourteen women. *Health Care for Women International, 5*, 49–75.

Danza, R. (1983). Menarche: Its effects on mother–daughter and father–daughter interactions. In S. Golub (Ed.), *Menarche: The transition from girl to woman* (pp. 99–106). Lexington, MA: Lexington Books.

Davies, B., & Doran, T. (1982). Factors in a woman's decision to undergo genetic amniocentesis for advanced maternal age. *Nursing Research, 31*, 56–59.

Dickson, E., & Post, C. (1981). Breast engorgement in nonnursing mothers following administration of estrogen-containing lactation suppressant medication. *Issues in Health Care of Women, 3*, 71–80.

Dorensky, N. (1984). The effects of a regular aerobic exercise program on selected measures of the stress response. *Health Care for Women International, 5*, 459–462.

Duffy, M. (1984). Transcending options: Creating a milieu for practicing high-level wellness. *Health Care for Women International, 5*, 145–161.

Duffy, M. (1986). Primary prevention behaviors: The female headed, one-parent family. *Research in Nursing and Health, 9*, 115–122.

Dunbar, S., Patterson, E., Burton, C., & Stuckert, G. (1981). Women's health and nursing research. *Advances in Nursing Science, 3*(2), 1–16.

Edwards, V. (1980). Changing breast self-examination behavior. *Nursing Research, 29*, 301–306.

Ellis, D. (1980). Sexual needs and concerns of expectant parents. *Journal of Obstetric, Gynecologic, and Neonatal Nursing, 9*, 306–308.

Engel, N. (1984). On the vicissitudes of health appraisal. *Advances in Nursing Science, 7*(1), 12–23.

Engle, V. (1984). Newman's conceptual framework and the measurement of older adults' health. *Advances in Nursing Science, 7*(1), 24–36.

Estok, P., & Rudy, E. (1984). Intensity of jogging: Relationship with menstrual/reproductive variables. *Journal of Obstetric, Gynecologic, and Neonatal Nursing, 13*, 390–395.

Estok, P., & Rudy, E. (1986). Physical, psychosocial, menstrual changes/risks and additions in the female marathon and nonmarathon runner. *Health Care for Women International, 7*, 187–202.

Fleming, P. (1984). The effects of prenatal nipple conditioning on postpartum nipple pain of breastfeeding. *Health Care of Women International, 5*, 453–457.

Gara, E., & Tilden, V. (1984). Adjusted control: An explanation for women's positive perceptions of their pregnancies. *Issues in Health Care of Women, 5*, 427–436.

Garling, J., & Roberts, S. (1980). An investigation of cyclic distress among staff nurses. In A. Dan, E. Graham, & C. Bucher (Eds.), *The menstrual cycle: Vol. 1. A synthesis of interdisciplinary research* (pp. 305–311). New York: Springer Publishing Company.

Geden, E., Beck, N., Hauge, G., & Pohlman, S. (1984). Self report and psychophysiological effects of five pain-coping strategies. *Nursing Research, 33*, 260–265.

Gierszewski, S. (1983). The relationship of weight loss, locus of control and social support. *Nursing Research, 32*, 43–47.

Glazer, G. (1980). Anxiety levels and concerns among pregnant women. *Research in Nursing and Health, 3*, 107–113.

Grabau, A., Rustia, J., & Lucas, J. (1984). Discrepancies between nursing practices with mastectomy clientele needs. *Issues in Health Care of Women, 5*, 251–260.

Graham, E. (1980). Cognition as related to menstrual cycle phase and estrogen level. In A. Dan, E. Graham, & C. Bucher (Eds.), *The menstrual cycle: Vol. 1. A synthesis of interdisciplinary research* (pp. 190–208). New York: Springer Publishing Company.

Griffith, J. (1983a). Women's stress responses and coping patterns according to age groups. *Issues in Health Care of Women, 6*, 327–340.

Griffith, J. (1983b). Women's stressors according to age groups. *Issues in Health Care of Women, 6*, 311–326.

Hallal, J. (1982). The relationship of health beliefs, health locus of control, and self concept to the practice of breast self-examination in adult women. *Nursing Research, 31*, 137–142.

Hames, C. (1980). Sexual needs and interests of postpartum couples. *Journal of Obstetric, Gynecologic, and Neonatal Nursing, 9*, 313–315.

Harris, C. (1984). Dysfunctional grieving related to childbearing loss: A descriptive study. *Issues in Health Care of Women, 5*, 401–425.

Havens, B., & Swenson, I. (1986). Menstrual perceptions and preparation among female adolescents. *Journal of Obstetric, Gynecologic, and Neonatal Nursing, 15*, 406–411.

Hawkins, J., Fahey, M., Kurien, M., Roberto, D., & Simon, R. (1981). Self-care/health maintenance and contraceptive use, information needs, and knowledge of a selected group of university women. *Issues in Health Care of Women, 3*, 287–305.

Henderson, J. (1983). Effects of a prenatal teaching program on postpartum regeneration of the pubococcygeal muscle. *Journal of Obstetric, Gynecologic, and Neonatal Nursing, 12*, 403–408.

Hendrickson, L. (1981). The frequency of stress incontinence in women before and after the implementation of an exercise program. *Issues in Health Care of Women, 3*, 81–92.

Humphries, P. (1981). Sexual adjustment after a hysterectomy. *Issues in Health Care of Women, 2*, 1–14.

Jacobs, M., McCance, K., & Stewart, M. (1982). External pneumatic intermittent compression for treatment of dependent pregnancy edema. *Nursing Research, 31*, 159–162.

Jacobsen, B., & Meininger, J. (1985). The designs and methods of published nursing research: 1956–1983. *Nursing Research, 34*, 306–312.

Jacobsen, B., & Meininger, J. (1986). Randomized experiments in nursing: The quality of reporting. *Nursing Research, 35,* 379–382.

Jacobsen, J. (1986). A comparison of anxiety levels in midlife women who are military spouses and a group of nonmilitary affiliated women. *Health Care for Women International, 7,* 241–254.

Jenkins, H. (1980). Self concept and mastectomy. *Journal of Obstetric, Gynecologic, and Neonatal Nursing, 9,* 38–42.

Jordan, J., & Meckler, J. (1982). The relationship between life change events, social supports, and dysmenorrhea. *Research in Nursing and Health, 5,* 73–79.

Kay, M. (1981). Meanings of menstruation to Mexican American women. In P. Komnenich, M. McSweeney, J. Noack, & N. Elder (Eds.), *The menstrual cycle: Vol. 2. Research and implications for women's health* (pp. 114–123). New York: Springer Publishing Company.

Klein, P. (1983). Contraceptive use and perceptions of chance and ability of conceiving in women electing abortion. *Journal of Obstetric, Gynecologic, and Neonatal Nursing, 12,* 167–171.

Klein, R. (1983). How to do what we want to do: Thoughts about feminist methodology. In G. Bowles & R. Klein (Eds.), *Theories of women's studies* (pp. 88–104). London: Routledge & Kegan Paul.

Krouse, J., & Krouse, J. (1982). Cancer as crisis: The critical elements of adjustment. *Nursing Research, 31,* 96–101.

La Rocco, S., & Polit, D. (1980). Women's knowledge about the menopause. *Nursing Research, 29,* 10–13.

Latta, W., & Weismeier, E. (1982). Effects of an educational gynecological exam on women's attitudes. *Journal of Obstetric, Gynecologic, and Neonatal Nursing, 11,* 242–245.

Lentz, M., & Woods, N. (1985, October). *Women's health research: Implications for design, measurement, and analysis.* Paper presented at the Invitational Conference on Statistics and Quantitative Methods in Nursing, Cleveland, OH.

Lenz, E., Parks, P., Jenkins, L., & Jarrett, G. (1986). Life change and instrumental support as predictions of illness in mothers of 6 month olds. *Research in Nursing and Health, 9,* 17–24.

Lipson, J. (1980). Consumer activism in two women's self-help groups. *Western Journal of Nursing Research, 2,* 393–405.

Longworth, J. (1982). Psychophysiological effects of slow stroke back massage in normotensive females. *Advances in Nursing Science, 4*(4), 44–61.

MacPherson, K. (1983). Feminist methods: A new paradigm for nursing research. *Advances in Nursing Science, 5*(2), 17–26.

Mallick, J. (1982). Health problems associated with dieting activities of a group of adolescent females. *Western Journal of Nursing Research, 4,* 167–176.

Manderino, M., & Bzdek, V. (1984). Effects of modeling and information on reactions to pain: A childbirth-preparation analogue. *Nursing Research, 33,* 9–14.

Marcy, S., Brown, J., & Danielson, R. (1983). Contraceptive use by adolescent females in relation to knowledge, and to time and method of contraceptive counseling. *Research in Nursing and Health, 6,* 175–182.

Marecki, M. (1981). Need priorities of adrenalectomy patients as perceived by patients, nurses, and physicians. *Journal of Obstetric, Gynecologic, and Neonatal Nursing, 10,* 379–383.

McBride, A., & McBride, W. (1981). Theoretical underpinnings for women's health. *Women & Health, 6*(1–2), 37–55.

McEntee, M., & Rankin, E. (1983). Multiple role demands, mind–body distress disorders, and illness-related absenteeism among business and professional women. *Issues in Health Care of Women, 4*, 177–190.

McKeever, P., & Galloway, S. (1984). Effects of nongynecological surgery on the menstrual cycle. *Nursing Research, 33*, 42–46.

Menke, E. (1983). Menstrual beliefs and experiences of mother–daughter dyads. In S. Golub (Ed.), *Menarche: The transition from girl to woman* (pp. 133–138). Lexington, MA: Lexington Books.

Mercer, R. (1985). The relationship of age and other variables to gratification in mothering. *Health Care for Women International, 6*, 295–308.

Mies, M. (1983). Towards a methodology for feminist research, In G. Bowles & R. Klein (Eds.), *Theories of women's studies* (pp. 117–139). London: Routledge & Kegan Paul.

Millette, B. (1981). Menopause: A survey of attitudes and knowledge. *Issues in Health Care of Women, 3*, 262–276.

Mitchell, E. (1986). Multiple triangulation: A methodology for nursing science. *Advances in Nursing Science, 8*(3), 18–26.

Moos, R. (1968). The development of a menstrual distress questionnaire. *Psychosomatic Medicine, 30*, 853–867.

Muhlenkamp, A., Waller, M., & Bourne, A. (1983). Attitudes toward women in menopause: A vignette approach. *Nursing Research, 32*, 20–23.

Newman, M., & Guadiano, J. (1984). Depression as an explanation for decreased subjective time in the elderly. *Nursing Research, 33*, 137–139.

Norbeck, J. (1984). Modification of life event questionnaires for use with female respondents. *Research in Nursing and Health, 7*, 61–71.

Norbeck, J. (1985a). Perceived job stress, job satisfaction, and psychological symptoms in critical care nursing. *Research in Nursing and Health, 8*, 253–260.

Norbeck, J. (1985b). Types and sources of social support for managing job stress in critical care nursing. *Nursing Research, 34*, 225–230.

O'Connell, M. (1983). Locus of control specific to pregnancy. *Journal of Obstetric, Gynecologic, and Neonatal Nursing, 12*, 161–164.

Olson, B. (1981). Patient comfort during pelvic examination: New foot supports vs. metal stirrups. *Journal of Obstetric, Gynecologic, and Neonatal Nursing, 10*, 104–107.

O'Rourke, M. (1983a). Self-reports of menstrual and nonmenstrual symptomatology in university-employed women. *Journal of Obstetric, Gynecologic, and Neonatal Nursing, 12*, 317–324.

O'Rourke, M. (1983b). Subjective appraisal of psychological well-being and self-reports of menstrual and nonmenstrual symptomatology in employed women. *Nursing Research, 32*, 288–292.

O'Rourke, M. (1984). Indicators of psychological well-being in a sample of employed women: An exploratory study. *Health Care for Women International, 5*, 163–177.

Ouelette, M., MacVicar, M., & Harlan, J. (1986). Relationship between percent body fat and menstrual patterns in athletes and nonathletes. *Nursing Research, 36*, 330–333.

Patterson, E., & Hale, E. (1985). Making sure: Integrating menstrual care practices into activities of daily living. *Advances in Nursing Science, 7*(3), 18–31.

Portnova, M., Young, E., & Newman, M. (1984). Elderly women's attitudes toward sexual activity among their peers. *Issues in Health Care of Women, 5,* 289–298.

Rankin, E., & Campbell, N. (1983). Perception of relationship changes during the third trimester of pregnancy. *Issues in Health Care of Women, 6,* 351–359.

Reame, N. (1983). Menstrual health products, practices, and problems. *Women & Health, 8*(3), 37–52.

Reinharz, S. (1983). Experiential analysis: A contribution to feminist research. In G. Bowles & R. Klein (Eds.), *Theories in women's health* (pp. 162–191). London: Routledge & Kegan Paul.

Rhode, M., & Groenjes-Finke, J. (1981). Evaluations of nurse initiated telephone calls to postpartum women. *Issues in Health Care of Women, 2,* 23–41.

Rudy, E., & Estok, P. (1983). Intensity of jogging: Its relationship to selected physical and psychosocial variables in women. *Western Journal of Nursing Research, 5,* 324–336.

Samples, J., & Abrams, R. (1984). Reliability of urine temperature as a measurement of basal body temperature. *Journal of Obstetric, Gynecologic, and Neonatal Nursing, 13,* 319–323.

Saunders, J. (1981). A process of bereavement resolution: Uncoupled identity. *Western Journal of Nursing Research, 3,* 319–332.

Schank, M., Thomas, B., & Young, M. (1981). Health care practices, problems, and needs of young adult women. *Issues in Health Care of Women, 3,* 231–239.

Schuleter, L. (1982). Knowledge and beliefs about breast cancer and breast self-examination among athletic and nonathletic women. *Nursing Research, 31,* 348–353.

Scott, E. (1983). Anxiety, critical thinking and information processing during and after breast biopsy. *Nursing Research, 32,* 24–28.

Sexton, D., & Munro, B. (1985). Impact of a husband's chronic illness (COPD) on the spouse's life. *Research in Nursing and Health, 8,* 83–90.

Shaver, J., & Woods, N. (1985). Concordance of perimenstrual symptoms across two cycles. *Research in Nursing and Health, 8,* 313–319.

Sheahan, S., Lee, G., & Lewis, S. (1984). Breast self-exams: Are health professionals doing their part? *Issues in Health Care of Women, 5,* 243–250.

Shelley, S., & Anderson, C. (1986). The influence of selected variables on the experience of menstrual distress in alcoholic and nonalcoholic women. *Journal of Obstetric, Gynecologic, and Neonatal Nursing, 15,* 484–491.

Staats, M., & Staats, T. (1983). Differences in stress levels, stressors, and stress responses between managerial and professional males and females on the Stress Vector Analysis—Research Edition. *Issues in Health Care of Women, 5,* 165–176.

Stern, P., Tilden, V., & Maxwell, E. (1980). Culturally induced stress during childbearing: The Filipino-American experience. *Issues in Health Care of Women, 2,* 67–81.

Stevenson, J., & Woods, N. (1986). Nursing science and contemporary science: Emerging paradigms. In G. Sorensen (Ed.), *Setting the agenda for the year 2000: Knowledge development in nursing* (pp. 6–20). Kansas City, MO: American Academy of Nursing.

Stoltzman, S. (1986). Menstrual attitudes, beliefs, and symptom experiences of adolescent females, their peers, and their mothers. *Health Care for Women International, 7,* 97–114.

Taylor, D., & Bledsoe, L. (1986). Peer support, PMS and stress: A pilot study. *Health Care for Women International, 7,* 159–172.

Tcheng, D. (1984). Emotional responses of primary and repeat Caesarean mothers to the Caesarean method of childbirth. *Issues in Health Care of Women, 5,* 323–333.

Tentoni, S., & High, K. (1980). Culturally induced postpartum depression. *Journal of Obstetric, Gynecologic, and Neonatal Nursing, 9,* 246–249.

Tilden, V. (1983). The relation of life stress and social support to emotional disequilibrium during pregnancy. *Research in Nursing and Health, 6,* 167–174.

Tilden, V. (1984). The relation of selected psychosocial variables to single status of adult women during pregnancy. *Nursing Research, 33,* 102–107.

Tilden, V., & Lipson, J. (1981). Caesarean childbirth: Variables affecting psychological impact. *Western Journal of Nursing Research, 3,* 127–141.

Tinkle, M., & Beaton, J. (1983). Toward a new view of nursing science: Implications for nursing research. *Advances in Nursing Science, 5*(2), 27–36.

Uphold, C., & Susman, E. (1981). Self-reported climacteric symptoms as a function of the relationships between marital adjustments and childrearing stage. *Nursing Research, 30,* 84–88.

Uphold, C., & Susman, E. (1985). Child-rearing, marital, recreational and work role integration and climacteric symptoms in midlife women. *Research in Nursing and Health, 8,* 73–81.

Voda, A. (1980). Pattern of progesterone and aldosterone in ovulating women during the menstrual cycle. In A. Dan, E. Graham, & C. Bucher (Eds.), *The menstrual cycle: Vol. 1. A synthesis of interdisciplinary research* (pp. 223–236). New York: Springer Publishing Company.

Voda, A., Imle, M., & Atwood, J. (1980). Quantification of self-report data from two-dimensional body diagrams. *Western Journal of Nursing Research, 2,* 707–729.

Wang, J. (1981). Attitudes toward and use of induced abortion among Taiwanese women. *Issues in Health Care of Women, 3,* 179–202.

White, J. (1984). The process of embarking on a weight control program. *Health Care for Women International, 5,* 77–91.

Williams, L. (1983). Beliefs and attitudes of young girls regarding menstruation. In S. Golub (Ed.), *Menarche: The transition from girl to woman* (pp. 139–148). Lexington, MA: Lexington Books.

Williamson, M. (1982). Reducing post-catheterization bladder dysfunction by reconditioning. *Nursing Research, 31,* 28–30.

Woods, N. (1980). Women's roles and illness episodes: A prospective study. *Research in Nursing and Health, 2,* 137–145.

Woods, N. (1985). Relationship of socialization and stress to perimenstrual symptoms, disability and menstrual attitudes. *Nursing Research, 34,* 145–149.

Woods, N. (1986). Self care practices among young adult married women. *Research in Nursing and Health, 8,* 227–234.

Woods, N., Dery, G., & Most, A. (1982). Life stress and perimenstrual symptoms. *Journal of Human Stress, 5,* 23–31.

Woods, N., Dery, G., & Most, A. (1983). Recollections of menarche, current menstrual attitudes and perimenstrual symptoms. In S. Golub (Ed.), *Men-*

arche: The transition from girl to woman (pp. 87–98). Lexington, MA: Lexington Books.

Woods, N., Most, A., & Dery, G. (1982a). Estimating perimenstrual distress: A comparison of two methods. *Research in Nursing and Health, 5*, 81–91.

Woods, N., Most, A., & Dery, G. (1982b). Prevalence of perimenstrual symptoms. *American Journal of Public Health, 72*, 1257–1264.

Woods, N., Most, A., & Dery, G. (1982c). Toward a construct of perimenstrual distress. *Research in Nursing and Health, 5*, 123–136.

Woods, N., Most, A., & Longnecker, G. (1985). Major life stressors, daily hassles, and perimenstrual symptoms. *Nursing Research, 34*, 263–267.

Chapter 11

Human Information Processing

SISTER CALLISTA ROY
SCHOOL OF NURSING
BOSTON COLLEGE, CHESTNUT HILL, MASSACHUSETTS

CONTENTS

As a practice discipline inquiry in nursing is focused on a person's life processes that promote health, and nursing action's that enhance these processes (American Nurses' Association, Cabinet on Nursing Research, 1985; Donaldson & Crowley, 1978; Roy, 1984). Of all hu-

The author acknowledges the contribution of a postdoctoral fellowship in neuroscience nursing to the shaping of this review. The fellowship was under the direction of Dr. Connie Robinson, Associate Professor, Department of Physiological Nursing, University of California, San Francisco, and was funded by the Robert Wood Johnson Foundation, Clinical Nurse Scholars Program, 1983–1985. Additional funds for related clinical research were awarded to the author from the Biomedical Research Support Grant (S07 RR05604-07) and by the Academic Senate Committee on Research of the University of California, San Francisco, as well as the American Nurses' Foundation.

man life processes, one that holds perhaps the greatest significance for people and their health is information processing. What are the mechanisms by which humans understand the world around them and the information they receive from it? This chapter provides a critical, integrative review of the research in this developing content area of nursing. A brief introduction is focused on an organizing framework for viewing this field of study. The critical review then includes research related to each component of the information-processing model: sensory experience, central processing, and context. Finally, direction is provided for basic research on information processes and for research related to nursing interventions to enhance human information processing.

As the twenty-first century nears, global society commonly is called an information society. Information-processing models and research have their origins in telephone switchboard communication theory, uncertainty-reduction definitions of information, and digital computers as computational and analogic devices (Haber, 1974). These three antecedents to current work were being developed during World War II, but attracted attention immediately after the war. Because of their influence a revolution was initiated in studying the unity of sensation, memory, cognition, and knowledge. By the 1970s, 50 to 100 publications related to information processing were appearing in the research literature each month. During the nearly two decades since, this research has become pivotal to understanding the changes of postindustrial society. A major structural change is that information rapidly is replacing energy as society's main resource. As Martel (1986) noted, information, unlike energy, is infinite and does not disappear. Futurists are postulating that processing of information is the key to society's future.

Nurses in practice, research, and education long have been interested in people as processors of information. The premise that people are viewed as information-processing systems undergirded such nursing activities as health teaching, health promotion, anxiety reduction, and even the development of standards for continuing professional education. Several creators of the major conceptual models for nursing practice have highlighted the significance of this view. Orem (1985) emphasized a repertoire of cognitive, perceptual, and communication skills as power components of self-care agency. Roy and Roberts (1981) offered a model of a cognator subsystem that included perception and information processing, acting together with a regulator subsystem to promote the person's adaptation. Perception, interaction, and transaction were central to King's (1981) open systems model. In 1984, Grier presented an integrative review of research on information processing in nursing practice from the point of view of the collection, organization, use, and storage of information needed for nursing practice. However, there has been little attention in the nursing literature to generalized models of human information processing and to systematic research on this topic.

As used here, the term information processing refers to human cognitive and emotional activity whereby the person takes in and responds to the environment. It includes recognition of the particular circumstances surrounding the interaction of the person with the environment. Information-processing models for the person can be distinguished on the basis of the phase of the process that the investigator selects for study. At the input side of the continuum, there are models that deal with perception, such as visual or auditory stimulation held in memory and then recoded. Another class of models is focused on memory-related information processing and its empirical consequences. Investigators of such models deal with elements such as rehearsal, recognition, acoustic representation of linguistic material, processes that underlie forgetting or memory loss, and retrieval and responding as distinct from storage. Given this focus, little attention is paid to input variables. Rather, the theorists simply recognized that sensory input preceeds storage. The third type of model is focused on problem-solving behavior and on verbal associative learning. Investigators using this approach do not pay much attention to perceptual or memory processes as such, but rather they focus on what the person does with the information that is in the system.

Knowledge for nursing is concerned with the entire process of persons taking in and dealing with the environment within a variety of contexts that affect health. A nursing model of information processing, then, will consider input, central processes, and context (Roy, in press). This framework provides a structure to organize and evaluate the nursing research related to human information processing.

Content for this review was drawn from published nursing research that relates to patient sensory experience, to central cognitive processes, and to the context of the processing experience. The field was defined as research conducted by nurses or reported in the nursing literature that sheds light upon the phenomenon of human information processing or upon nursing intervention to enhance that process. Studies could be focused on any part of the process — sensory input, central processes such as planning and decision making, or on the context of the processing. The qualification was made that processing related to health was the particular interest for nursing research.

Excluded from the review were studies in a content area that has had a separate review in these volumes, such as studies focused specifically on patient teaching/learning (Lindeman, in press). Studies also were excluded that were focused narrowly on the content of the information processed; for example, topics such as the identification of factors in the decision of a woman of advanced maternal age to undergo genetic amniocentesis were not included.

Procedures to access studies meeting the above criteria included: (a) seven computer searches using MEDLARS II for years 1966 to October 1986; (b) hand searches of nursing journals as follows: *Nursing Research*, 1974 to October 1986; *Research in Nursing and Health*, 1978 to May 1986; *Western Journal of Nursing Research*, 1979 to May 1986; and *Advances in Nursing Science*, 1978 to May 1986; (c) hand searches of selected volumes of international journals in the English language; and (d) pursuit of citations in two areas of high relevance, provision of sensory information and the concept of uncertainty. Forty-two studies were identified and considered for review in this chapter.

REVIEW OF LITERATURE
ON PATIENT INFORMATION PROCESSING

This section contains a review of the accumulated knowledge concerning patient information processing as a significant life process. Three subsections include content designated in the previously proposed conceptual framework. Studies related to sensory experience are considered first, followed by those with content giving insight into central cognitive processes, and, finally, those that deal with a broad context for information processing. For each section, both the knowledge contributed by the research and the methodology used are summarized and evaluated.

Sensory Input

At the input stage of human information processing, sensory experience depends upon both external environmental factors and factors internal to the person. Although no systematic approach to studying this array of factors is evident in the literature, input factors of interest to nursing are beginning to be identified. The experience of time, stress, and other input changes, sensory information, and parents' perceptions of their children have been studied in both laboratory and clinical settings.

Time. Tompkins (1980) studied the effect of restricted mobility on judgments of time duration in an attempt to understand the process of adaptation to such restrictions. Building upon an earlier series of studies by Newman (1972, 1976, 1979), she hypothesized that perceived duration was likely to be shortened with a restriction of mobility. In this laboratory study, 64 university student subjects walked at their own preferred tempo under three treatment conditions: walking unrestricted, walking with the right leg restricted, and walking with the left leg restricted. The premises underlying the study were that immobility increased the muscular effort needed, disrupted the learned relationship between movement and time, and made the walking pattern an activity divided into a series of asymmetrical, effortful steps. Mobility restrictions were created by the application of brace immobilizers. The investigator used a stopwatch to estimate time duration. Results indicated that both a one-joint restriction (ankle) and a two-joint restriction (ankle and knee) of either leg significantly shortened perceived duration and significantly decreased cadence. The author noted that the slowing of cadence as a result of restricted mobility has been recognized as a physiological mechanism beneficial to the preservation of system integrity. The change in the rate of subjective time also may have been necessary to preserve system integrity.

Smith (1979) reported on a replication and refinement of an earlier study (Smith, 1975) to test the theoretical propositions that (a) duration experience was related to the processing of environmental events and (b) changes in the load and complexity of auditory information would change temporal experience. A sample of 120 subjects was recruited from a university student population. Four conditions of auditory input were used. The load, that is, amount of information, as well as the complexity of input varied across conditions. Complexity was defined as randomly disordered or specific sequential messages. The subjects received the input during 2 1/2 hours of bed rest in a soundproof room equipped electronically for measurement of estimates of a 40-second time interval. Major findings included that all judgments of time duration were longer than 40 seconds; that is, a shortened temporal duration relative to clock time was found for all subjects. Furthermore, when time "passed slowly" subjects' scores on a rest scale indicated that they felt tired at the end of the period of bed rest. The conditions of complexity affected the findings in the direction of the hypothesis, but the differences noted were not statistically significant. Smith's discussion of the differences between the 1975 and 1979 study samples, and the individual differences within the samples, pointed to the importance of individual responses to time structure. In a recent study, Smith (1986) reported support for the hypotheses that the perception of restfulness was related to auditory input and specifically that harmonic auditory input was effective in promoting restfulness.

Newman's research (1982) on time related to movement included a study of time as an index of expanding consciousness with age. The 85 subjects, aged 60 to 88 years, produced estimates of 40 seconds under two conditions: (a) while sitting quietly, and (b) while walking around a prescribed oval track at their preferred rate of walking. Consciousness was described as the informational capacity of a system and the capacity of the system to respond to stimuli. The measure of consciousness was an index of comparison between subjective time and objective time. Neither the age–time nor the movement–time relationship was confirmed in this sample. Newman applied the index of consciousness ratio to data from earlier studies (Bull, 1973; Newman, 1972, 1976, 1979). The trend toward increasing consciousness with age then was apparent, but not unequivocal. Explanations offered for the discrepancies in results were differences in setting, methodology, culture, and sex. The differences in perceived duration in relation to sex led the investigator to raise questions regarding the associated influence of right-left brain orientation.

To summarize findings from the above studies, in situations of immobility there was generally an experience of time passing slowly. However, the individuality of responses was noted by all investigators. Internal or external structuring of the situation seemed to be a key factor in time perception. Finally, persons who reported time passing slowly also reported feeling more fatigued. These studies were built from one to another and included replications and refinements. One methodological refinement has been the use of electronic timers rather than stopwatches to measure estimates of time duration. Each investigator raised questions about the methodology used and made further suggestions for improvement. The pursuit of robust methods to study a developing concept related to sensory input was particularly apparent here. In addition, Sanders (1986) has developed a tool to measure subjective time experience that included six factors: meaning, fast tempo, slow tempo, attention to death, future orientation, and past orientation. The authors' discussions of the implications of findings provided some interesting insights, but often were more speculative than reflective of actual data presented.

Stress and Other Input Changes.   Perceived stress of hospital events is an important factor in considering how and what people process in situations related to health. Several studies by Volicer (1973, 1974) and associates (Volicer & Bohannon, 1975; Volicer, Isenberg, & Burns, 1977) have provided information on this immediate sensory experience. These investigators developed a method for quantifying the psychosocial stress that resulted from the experience of hospitalization. In an initial series of validity and reliability studies, a list of 49 events related to hospitalization were ranked by medical–surgical patients according to the relative stress involved and the clustering of specific stress factors.

Volicer and Burns (1977) then used hospital stress as an outcome variable and identified predictors of the level of hospital stress. This report included analysis of 468 interviews with short-term medical and surgical patients. Data for medical patients indicated that (a) hospital stress decreased as age increased and as the number of years since the last hospitalization increased; and (b) hospital stress increased as the number of previous hospitalizations increased, as life stress increased, and as estimated pain increased. Correlations for surgical patients provided evidence that predictors of hospital stress in this group included age, sex, life stress, and the estimated pain score. Being younger, female, and having greater life stresses and pain were related to greater hospital stress. Even though much of the variation in level of hospital stress remained unexplained, the investigators considered that the variables identified were potential risk factors and could be assessed by the nurse at the time of the patient's admission. Volicer and Burns (1977) pointed out that more research is needed to determine why these factors are related to hospital stress, that is, to learn more about patients' processing of both prehospitalization experiences and events occurring during hospitalization.

In an exploratory study Scott (1982) aimed to describe the relationships among anxiety, critical thinking, and information processing in 85 women facing breast biopsy. Anxiety was measured by the State-Trait Anxiety Inventory (Spielberger et al., 1980); critical thinking ability was determined by the Watson-Glaser Critical Thinking Appraisal (Watson & Glaser, 1964). Capacity to process information was measured as the difference between a subjective judgment of time and the objective length of the interval (clock time). Measures were taken on two occasions, before the biopsy and 6 to 8 weeks after the individual had been notified that results of the breast biopsy indicated a nonmalignant condition.

Scott drew several conclusions from tests of seven different hypotheses. Critical thinking or general reasoning ability was reduced substantially at the time of hospitalization when compared with 6 to 8 weeks after discharge; that is, at a time when critical decisions were demanded from patients. Anxiety levels of patients prior to knowledge of diagnostic results were extremely high; for example, the group average was above norms for acutely ill psychiatric patients. There was a positive correlation between scores on critical thinking and anxiety, indicating that patients with high anxiety had increasing difficulty in the reasoning process and in decision making. Although judged duration, a measure of information-processing capacity, did not change significantly between the hospital and postdischarge periods, scores did shift in the hypothesized direction.

Other works to be considered in looking at the changes related to the input of information for patients are associated with postcardiotomy delirium. The reader is referred to an early review from the psychiatric literature by Vasquez and Chitwood (1975) for a summary of findings from 22 studies reporting on psychologic patterns after open heart surgery. The authors also summarized the treatments for postcardiotomy delirium that had been studied.

A study of the effects of preoperative nursing intervention on delirium in cardiac surgical patients was done by Owens and Hutelmyer (1982). These investigators tested the hypothesis that patients who are educated preoperatively about the possibility of unusual sensory or cognitive experiences postoperatively will not have such experiences or will feel comfortable or in control of the experiences if they occur. Sixty-four adult cardiac surgical patients admitted consecutively to the study were assigned to either an experimental or a control group. The experimental group was advised of the possibility of unusual experiences, such as loss of memory, inability to concentrate, inability to recognize familiar objects or persons, and possibly seeing or hearing things that could not be explained or were not really there. They were told that the cause of these temporary disturbances was unknown, and that they should tell the staff about any unusual feeling or experience so that the staff could validate their experiences. As determined by interview and chart review, subjects in both experimental and control groups had unusual sensory or cognitive experiences at about the same rate (68%). However, in the experimental group, significantly more patients understood what was happening and were not uncomfortable. The investigators noted that the seven patients who had an intraaortic balloon pump inserted had an unusual experience, adding to the evidence of a physiologic effect on a patient's perceptions of his environment.

In a laboratory study DeVellis, Adams, and DeVellis (1984) looked at the effects of varying contextual information on responses to patient situations. Fifty-seven student nurses responded on audiotape to one of four patient situations. The primary hypothesis was that information about reasons for remaining childless would affect nurses' attitudes and behavior toward the patient. Patient situations reflected different intellectual levels (retarded or nonretarded) and different referral sources (physician-referred or self-referred). Data from the taped interactions and from paper-and-pencil attitude measures provided evidence for the importance of considering the influence of contextual variables on nurses' perceptions of patients and, in turn, on patients' perceptions of nurses as supportive or interested.

The studies in this section were more diffuse in both content and methods than were the studies of time perception. Volicer (1973, 1974) and Associates' (Volicer & Bohannon, 1975; Volicer & Burns, 1977) work has provided a useful list of possible stressful inputs and risk factors for perceiving stress. However, the investigators noted that much of the variation in the level of hospital stress remained unexplained. To understand individual patients interacting with their environments, future researchers need to focus more specifically on how a common set of potentially stressful events is processed differently by different persons. Programs of sequential studies building on the content of this early work and the extension of methods is essential.

In Scott's (1982) research information processing was measured by comparing subjective time judgments with objective clock time. Newman (1982) used this same comparison as a measure of expanding consciousness. Clarity of conceptual and operational definitions of key variables is needed. Measurement of input changes was defined more carefully and controlled in the work by DeVellis et al. (1984), but extrapolations from laboratory to clinical situations were limited by the fact that student nurses were the subjects.

Owens and Hutelmyer (1982) changed one part of the patient input related to cognitive central processing after cardiac surgery; that is, what information the patient had about possible cognitive disturbance. They seemed to have made a difference in the patients' experiences of those events; however, they did not affect the cognitive disturbances themselves. These results highlighted the need to understand further the basic processes involved, including the effect of physiological changes on the sensory and cognitive experiences.

Sensory Information. Studies focused on providing sensory information were a third category at the input phase of human information processing. For more than a decade Johnson, her colleagues, and others have studied the effect of information on emotional responses during threatening situations. This work (Fuller, Endress, & Johnson, 1978; Johnson, 1973, 1975; Johnson & Leventhal, 1974; Johnson & Rice, 1974; Johnson, Kirchoff, & Endress, 1975; Johnson, Leventhal, & Dabbs, 1971; Johnson, Rice, Fuller, & Endress, 1978) initially focused on the theoretical hypothesis that congruency between expected and experienced physical sensation results in a reduction of emotional responses during a threatening procedure. When pulse rate, general behavior, and self-reports were used as indexes of distress, sensation information was more effective in reducing distress during aversive procedures than were other types of information. Significant positive correlations between preprocedure fear and distress measures resulted in the investigators identifying fear as an individual difference variable affecting processing of information.

Using a measure of anxiety proneness to control for individual variations in responding to stressful situations, Hartfield and Cason (1981) conducted a quasi-experimental study to extend Johnson's findings. Twenty-four hospitalized patients scheduled for barium enemas were assigned to one of three information conditions: sensation information, procedure information, or no information. The investigators restated Johnson's hypothesis in terms of both state and trait anxiety and examined the treatment effects on cognition, while controlling for the influence of acquired dispositions or trait anxiety. Subjects who received sensation information reported less anxiety than did subjects who received no information or procedure information. However, contrary to findings in earlier studies, the data indicated that no information tended to be better than procedure information, but not significantly so. The investigators suggested that the cognitions produced by the procedure information affected anxiety quite differently from those produced by the sensation information. They further noted that a knowledge of both is necessary for a nurse to identify the preprocedure interventions of most benefit to the patient.

In another extension of the sensory information hypothesis, Hill (1982) used a four-condition experimental design with patients randomly assigned to: (a) behavioral instructions; (b) sensory information; (c) both behavioral instructions and sensory information; or (d) general information. Behavioral instructions were based on Seligman's (1975) theory of means for patients to reduce perceptions of helplessness. The sensory information intervention was based on Johnson's (1975) approach of focusing on patients' subjective experiences of threatening events. The subjects were 40 patients scheduled for their first unilateral cataract surgical experience. The dependent variables included self-report measures of anxiety and depression, ambulation, hospital days to discharge, and first time ventured from home after discharge. Findings indicated that neither behavioral instructions nor sensory information had a significant effect on any of the dependent variables. However, the combination of behavioral and cognitive control intervention was related significantly to a reduction in the number of days after discharge before patients ventured from their homes. Methodological limitations included the small sample size and the lack of conceptual clarity and valid and reliable indicators of the personal control construct.

Ziemer (1983) added information on coping strategies to procedure information and sensory information in a 3-group intervention study. Based on concepts from the Neuman Systems Model (Neuman, 1982), it was assumed that the individual would use information to strengthen resistance to the impact of a stress event. The subjects, 111 patients undergoing abdominal surgery, were assigned randomly to receive (a) procedure information, (b) procedure information and sensation information, or (c) procedure and sensation information plus information on selected coping strategies. There was no evidence that the type of information increased the reported frequency of coping behaviors or that such behaviors in turn were related to improved outcomes. The investigator concluded that although many studies have identified benefits of providing information to patients before surgery, the mediating factor responsible for these positive outcomes has not been documented.

Sime and Libera (1985) designed a study to look at sensory information, state and trait anxiety, and self-instruction aimed at providing cognitive control by facilitating different reappraisals of the threatening event. Dental surgery was used as the stress situation, that is, the period during which the patient is in the dentist's chair. Patients (113) undergoing gingivectomy were assigned randomly to one of four information groups. There was an interaction effect between treatment conditions and the level of state anxiety. High state anxiety subjects showed the most favorable responses to treatment and benefited more from either sensation information or self-instruction than from a combination of both interventions. The investigators noted the unexpected finding that low state anxiety subjects reported a reduction in positive statements about self with sensation information alone or in combination with self instruction. Suggesting that low state anxiety subjects may best be left untreated, Sime and Libera (1985) pointed out that it would be important to distinguish between trait and state anxiety conditions in selecting a treatment strategy for the reduction of threat-based reactions.

In a recent study, Johnson, Christman, and Stitt (1985) aimed to clarify the relationships between means of exerting control and coping with surgery by investigating the distinct functions of coping. In a sample of 121 black and 47 white patients who had undergone a hysterectomy, a randomized 3-factor design was used to evaluate the short- and long-term effects of interventions that provided different means of exerting personal control over postoperative experiences. The distinct functions of coping related to regulating the emotional response and regulating goal-directed responses. On the first factor, subjects either did or did not receive a description of the experience in concrete sensory terms. Levels of the second factor were instruction in a cognitive coping strategy, a behavior coping strategy, or no instruction. The third factor included experimental or control information about the posthospital experience.

The results showed that sensory information increased patients' perception of their ability to deal with the experience and decreased their perceptions of the difficulty associated with the experience. The investigators noted a perplexing absence of main effects for concrete sensory information during hospitalization. There was, however, support for the processes through which such information was expected to facilitate coping. The behavioral coping technique was associated with reports of better physical recovery during hospitalization, but longer hospitalization. Posthospitalization recovery data, collected by packets of data sheets mailed at 2, 4, and 12 weeks, showed negative effects for both coping techniques. The authors suggested that the interventions could have undermined the patients' confidence in their existing abilities to cope.

Results of the 13 studies that were focused on providing sensory information as a way of reducing emotional responses to threatening procedures have begun to clarify this phenomenon. As each investigator built on previous work, it was noted that the process seemed to involve more than a congruency between expected and experienced physical sensations. Other constructs identified as important were fear, state and trait anxiety, cognitive and personal control, and coping strategies. This work illustrated the complexity of any patient's processing of the environment and the need for sequential programs of research that could continue to extend and refine the characterization of these processes.

Parents' Perceptions.   Three studies were designed to test interventions to affect parents' perceptions of their newborns (Anderson, 1981; Hall, 1980; Perry, 1983). Hall conducted her work on the assumption that a mother's perception of her infant during the early weeks of life was important to the development of a strong healthy bond between the two. Thirty first-time mothers between the ages of 18 and 30 years were assigned randomly to either a control or an experimental group. Experimental subjects received structured, informative teaching concerning infant behavior in areas such as feeding, sleeping, spitting and vomiting, elimination, and predictability. A significant positive change in parents' perception of their infants was found for the experimental group, but not for the control group. Hall concluded that the findings of this study suggest that nurses can, through teaching, promote a healthier maternal–infant bond by improving mothers' perceptions of their infants.

Anderson's study (1981) was designed to explore further the impact of early professional intervention in the development of a reciprocal relationship between mother and child. Thirty primiparous mothers and their newborn infants were assigned randomly to one of three treatment procedures. The Brazelton Neonatal Behavioral Assessment Scale (1973) was used to establish equivalency of neonates among the three teaching groups. In the control group, the mothers received no immediate feedback on their infants. This group was offered only a class on infant furnishings. Mothers in one experimental group received only an explanation of the performance of their infant on the behavioral assessment. In the second experimental group, the mothers observed the investigator performing the examination, saw both the testing stimuli and the baby's responses, and had an ongoing discussion of the assessment. Reciprocity in mother–infant interactions was assessed by a separate investigator during a feeding observation 24 to 48 hours after delivery and again at 10 to 12 days postpartum. Items on the observation tool were clustered to provide maternal, infant, and interactive scores. All three groups manifested a significant increase in scores on each of the three subscales. The investigator noted several extraneous variables that could have contributed to the increase in the mothers' reciprocity scores at posttest. In contrast, changes on the infant subscale showed a different pattern. It seemed that providing mothers with either observational or verbal information about the behavioral characteristics of their infants was responsible for a significant increase in scores on the infant cluster.

Perry (1983) looked at both parents' perceptions of their newborn following structured interactions. The design of the study was descriptive as well as experimental. For 57 married couples and their normal, term, first-born infants, infant behavior was measured twice, after birth and at 1 week. Mothers' and fathers' perceptions of their infants were measured at three different times, after birth, at 1 week, and at 1 month. No relationship was found between infant behavior and parental perception. These same subjects were assigned randomly to one of three treatment groups, differing according to the parent who participated in the structured interaction: mother–infant, father–infant, both parents–infant, or to a control group. The investigator first assessed the infant; then the infant was brought to the subjects in the three treatment groups for assessment. The parental assessment was used to acquaint them with the behavior of their infants. The procedure was repeated in the home at 1 week, and a copy of the instrument was left for the parents to complete when the infant was 1 month old. When treatment effects upon parents were measured, the structured interaction differentially affected perception scores of mothers at 1 week. Perceptions of mothers and fathers achieved some congruence over time. Further analysis showed that seven other variables contributed more to variance in the mothers' than in the fathers' perceptions.

These three investigators have shown that nursing intervention can influence other persons' perceptions positively. Stated simply, one can structure what the person looks at and thereby affect what the person sees. This is an important finding for the continuing evolvement of the nursing role related to input for human information processing. A promising line of research with medical–surgical patients can be mentioned here. Janson-Bjerklie, Carrieri, and Hudes (1986) used a model that proposes a dynamic interplay of many types of variables to identify physical sensations described by persons with dyspnea. They noted that it was the symptom of dyspnea, rather than the disease category, that had the greatest effect on the quality and frequency of sensations reported.

In the studies discussed in relation to the input stage of human information processing, researchers provided some beginning knowledge. Some methodological strengths and weaknesses were noted. Replication and extension of studies were used in the work about time, hospital stress events, sensory information, and parents' perceptions of their infants. This was more successful when concepts were developed clearly and related closely to the measurement tools. The need for adequate outcome measures of the dependent variable was noted repeatedly. Some of these studies were limited by nonrandom assignment of subjects, inadequate control groups, and inadequate longitudinal measures. The studies cited represented both laboratory and clinical research, but they reflected the need for better integration of the two. In several cases the interpretations of data tended to be speculative, and new possible explanatory variables were suggested with each study. The lack of definitive designs to test given hypotheses seemed to be related to the early stage of development of this field of inquiry.

Central Processes of
Thinking and Decision Making

The studies of central cognitive components of patient information processing considered in this review are divided into studies of causal thinking and decision making. It might be noted that the parallel research literature in the field of psychology is directed toward discrete content areas such as memory, learning, motivation, and creative thinking. The nursing research literature, however, reflects efforts to understand the totality of patient situations. With this clinical focus under conditions quite different from those used in other psychosocial research, nurse scholars are contributing further to the understanding of these cognitive processing phenomena.

Causality and Attribution. DuCette and Keane (1984) used an attributional analysis to study why patients undergoing thoracic surgery thought they had their disease and were recovering at an adequate or inadequate rate from the surgery. Ninety subjects were interviewed about 6 days after surgery. Responses were scored using a system of coding attribution by the dimensions of locus, stability, and control. In general, the patients' responses reflected the three-dimensional structure of a theory proposed by Weiner (1979) to account for students' attribution of causality for success or failure in the classroom.

The one major theoretical difference between the patient sample and the previously reported student samples was that the locus dimension seemed to have a different definition in regard to health. Specifically, all internal attributions by patients (for example, bad habits) were controllable, whereas all external ones (for example, outside influences) were uncontrollable.

When attributions were related to recovery, the results presented an ambiguous and somewhat confusing picture. The four factors used to assess recovery were pulmonary, infection, activity status, and a general outcome measure. There was no consistent indication that the use of internal and controllable attributions was more characteristic of patients making better recoveries. Because diametrically opposite attributions characterized patients making good recoveries, the investigators proposed that, theoretically, for a patient, any explanation was better than no answer at all. This finding was consistent with the central premise of attribution theory, that people attempt to attach causes to effects in order to understand and thereby control their world. However, attribution theorists also have contended that attributional thinking was essentially rational and that people sought to find the real cause of events. For many patients in this sample, the attributions held about the cause of their disease did not provide much understanding and were not completely rational. The investigator acknowledged the limitation of generalizing from findings in one patient group. Furthermore, the question might be raised as to whether the correlation between no attribution and poor recovery simply reflected that the person who was not making a good recovery also did not feel like making thoughtful responses to the interviewer's questions. Theories developed in other contexts may not apply to hospitalized patients' processing of their experiences.

In another study, Lowery, Jacobsen, and Murphy (1983) used an attribution analysis to ascertain: (a) to what extent arthritic patients constructed causes for their condition; (b) how the patients' explanations of causes fit with causes given in school achievement situations; and (c) whether the attributions could be linked to patients' general health status measures. Fifty-five rheumatoid arthritic men being treated at a Veterans Administration clinic constituted the sample. Instruments completed by each patient included the Multiple Affect Adjective Checklist (Zuckerman & Lubin, 1965), the recovery index, and an attributions interview schedule. In cross-tabulations of the responses, 72% of the attributions for cause of disease clustered among three cells: (a) external locus, stable, and uncontrollable; for example, impending old age; (b) internal locus, intermediate stability, and controllable; for example, did not take proper care of myself; and (c) internal locus, stable, and uncontrollable; for example, hereditary.

The investigators highlighted the interesting contrasts of their results with the data derived largely from academic settings. Illness situations may have evoked noncausal thinking; patients' responses may have been modified to meet causal theories proposed by physicians, friends, or the media. Some conditions of the three-dimensional attribution theory may have been possible only theoretically in illness situations; for example, it may not have been possible to have a disease process whose cause was external, unstable, and controllable. The external and uncontrollable ascriptions of suffering may have helped people to maintain a positive view of themselves. The results of this study called into question the issue of the efficacy of feelings of personal control. The investigators suggested a need for further testing of the assumption about causal attributions combined with testing of possible cognitive alternatives to causal thinking.

Rudy (1980) also examined causal explanations, but without employing attributional theory. Interviews were conducted with 50 patients following a first-time myocardial infarction (MI) and 50 spouses or significant others during the acute (in hospital) and convalescent phases (at home) of the patients' illness. The purposes of the research were to determine lay persons' explanations about the cause of an MI, whether or not these explanations differed at the acute and convalescent phases, and whether or not the patients' and spouses' explanations differed from each others' and from current professional knowledge. Data indicated that tension was the most frequent cause given for the heart attack at both data-collection times. Although 50% of the patient-spouse pairs disagreed regarding the cause of illness on both occasions, the implications of this finding for rehabilitation were not clear. In general, neither patients with an identifiable medical risk factor nor their spouses named that risk factor as an explanation for the heart attack. However, a high percentage of patients changed their smoking, diet, and exercise behavior without linking those behaviors causally to their diagnosis. The investigator noted that patients and spouses seemed to engage in a perceptual interpretive process whereby a succession of causal explanations was explored and evaluated, but this process had no sense of urgency or of necessity. The frequent identification of tension as a cause was interpreted as a way to decrease feelings of self-blame and to externalize the cause.

Researchers dealt with decision making as a central cognitive process in two studies. Edwardson (1983) explored the decision-making process of physicians and parents in choosing between hospital and home care for children in the terminal phase of cancer. Subjects were a cohort of families who were treated by the physicians involved in a project where home care was an alternative to hospitalization. Results of discriminant function analysis showed that four variables predicted the type of terminal care: (a) number of monitoring activities used in the last week before death, (b) length of hospitalization for the child, (c) distance between the family home and the treatment hospital, and (d) the physician's usual practice. These four variables accounted for 54% of the variability.

Edwardson (1983) offered the interpretation that physician influence outweighed nonmedical reasons for choosing the care option. However, in contrast to this finding, parents saw the physician as having little influence over their choice. They reported that they were most influenced by their child's and their own desires and beliefs about their ability to provide care. These findings reflected a complex decision process. The investigator reported that both physicians and parents indicated that they had tried to read each other's nonverbal messages during discussions of the child's treatment. She proposed that the parents' decision making may have been a two-stage decision process. The physician seemed to have been the major influence until the decision to stop treatment was made; then if treatment failed and home care was a possibility, parents may have considered the second decision as their own based on their beliefs and ability to provide care.

Brien, Haverfield, and Shanteau (1983) studied the processes used by 44 Lamaze-prepared couples in selecting an obstetrician from four perspectives: (a) evaluation of the aspects or issues considered; (b) comparison of evaluations made before and after childbirth; (c) examinations of any differences in husband and wife evaluations; and (d) consideration of how parents would make future selections. There was a consistent concern for choosing an obstetrician who was able to communicate with patients. In making their decision, parents placed an emphasis on issues that had evolved out of the Lamaze preparation. A strong emphasis on the role of the office nursing staff in parents' decisions was reflected in the before–after comparison. The general trend for husbands and wives was similar. Although the investigators provided little interpretation related to decision processes, the findings seemed to reflect the conclusion of Edwardson (1983) that these decision-making processes are complex and may differ at different points of health care service.

The five studies related to central cognitive processes of patients dealing with their environment include reports of inconclusive results. In general, the researchers indicate that patients do seem to try to give reasons for their illnesses and progress in getting well. However, these explanations are not the same as those reported in earlier studies for success or failure in academic situations. Patients' explanations may be arrived at over time without urgency, may not be rational or causal, and are likely to be external or uncontrollable. Externalizing illness may serve the useful function of decreasing self-blame. Giving no reason may correlate with negative outcomes of health status, but has not been a direct link in the studies reviewed. Rather, not being able to state a reason for illness may have been a joint link to another factor, such as the effect of not feeling well on a person's ability to do causal reasoning.

Contextual Factors for
Human Information Processing

In several studies researchers dealt with the context in which information processing took place. These works included both those contextual conditions internal to the patient and those in the environment. Fontes (1983) explored the relationship of cognitive style and interpersonal needs to the eudaemonistic model of health. Cognitive style was measured by the Group Embedded Figures Test (Witkin, Altman, Raskin, & Karp, 1971). The subjects were 163 healthy adults. There was some relationship in the predicted direction between moderation in both cognitive style and interpersonal needs and eudaemonistic health. However, the hypotheses of these relationships were not supported statistically. The investigators questioned the idea promoted in the literature that moderation and balance are correlates of health. She recommended looking at a dynamic range of these phenomena.

In a prospective study of 34 burn patients, Blank and Perry (1984) described emotional responses, thought content, and defensive operations during delirium. These processes were examined to determine which might correlate with and predict postdelirium psychological outcome. The seven patients who had severe symptoms, that is, depression or stress disorders, showed significantly more preoccupation with their trauma and injury, had greater anxiety and fear, and differed in their use of defensive operations from patients who did not have these symptoms. The processing used by this group was referred to as intrusion, whereas the group that fared better used avoidance. A preinjury activity-dominant coping style was more predictive of a poor outcome than was premorbid psychopathology. Results were interpreted to suggest that patients might benefit from psychotic processes, such as halluci-nations, delusions, disorientation, displacement, and depersonaliza-tion. As the delirium resolved, those patients gradually were able to acknowledge and integrate the overwhelming experience. Viewing de-lirium primarily as an organic disorder may be questionable in light of these findings.

Mishel's work (1981, 1983, 1984) on the perceptual variable of uncertainty was relevant to the discussion of contextual correlates of information processing. Her early work was focused on measurement of uncertainty, which related to being unable to assign definite values to objects and events or to predict outcomes accurately. She proposed that, in illness, the characteristics of uncertainty may reside in the nature of the stimulus, the characteristics of the perceiver, or in an interaction between stimulus and perceiver in relation to four general classes of illness-treatment events. Patient situations have been replete with ambiguity, lack of clarity, lack of information, and unpredict-ability. Mishel (1983) then reported a study to examine uncertainty as a major perceptual variable influencing parents' experiences during their child's illness. Only the relationship between the multi-attributed ambiguity factor and seriousness of illness was of substantive signifi-cance. She noted that this outcome seemed to result from the concep-tual difficulty in explaining how parents seek a stable understanding of the illness and its implications. Unpredictability might be preferred over a negative predictability. Lack of information might function as a constraint against judged seriousness and might moderate an evalua-tion of the gravity of the situation.

In a later study, Mishel (1984) used a sample of 100 patients with a medical diagnosis to study the relationship of uncertainty to percep-tion of stress. The investigator postulated an explanatory model in which uncertainty was the major intervening variable in linking to stress the exogenous variables of seriousness of illness, education, age, and prior hospitalization. A patient's level of perceived uncertainty was related strongly to ratings of hospital stress measured by Volicer and Bohannon's (1975) Hospital Stress Rating Scale. Only multiat-tributed ambiguity and age were identified as significant predictors of stress when the other variables were controlled. Calculation of both direct and indirect effects increased the percent of explained variance in stress to 49%, thus indicating good initial strength of the model, even though much of the variation in stress remained unexplained. The investigator suggested that decreasing the heterogeneity of the medical diagnoses of the sample might have helped to clarify the relationships being studied. Furthermore, she noted that this work emphasized the importance of nursing intervention techniques to influence the patient's cognitive processes.

The final contextual correlate to be considered was social structure and process as studied by Kishi (1983), who investigated patterns of verbal communication between the health care provider and the client in well-baby clinics and the relationship of those patterns to clients' recall of health information. Data were analyzed from 68 direct observations of client–provider interactions. The theoretical notion that higher indirect influence, more teacher questions, more student questions, and more relative student talk would lead to higher learning was not supported by this study. In explaining the findings, the investigator noted the significant differences between the classroom situation and clinic health teaching. Furthermore, differences were noted between the communication patterns of white mothers and black mothers.

In summary, only a tentative beginning knowledge was found about contextual factors for human information processing. No specific conclusions could be drawn from a single study about patient cognitive style as part of the context of cognitive processing related to health. For severely burned patients, however, an activity-dominant coping style seemed to provide a negative context for dealing with the illness. In her work on uncertainty, Mishel has clarified that concept in several patient situations and has developed tools to measure it. Furthermore, uncertainty has been related to hospital stress. Efforts to relate social structure and process to patients' information processing showed that communication patterns were not the same in health care as in classroom teaching. The findings of many of these studies were contrary to predictions.

CONCLUSIONS AND
DIRECTIONS FOR FUTURE RESEARCH

This review of nursing research has been focused on the highly significant human life process of information processing. The beginnings of some accumulated knowledge related to each component of information processing have been pointed out at the end of each subsection. However, considering the early stage of systematic study of this topic, it seems appropriate to offer some general, though tentative, conclusions related to the current state of nursing knowledge related to human information processing:

1. Time, uncertainty, and sensory information are highly relevant and promising variables for the study of patients' information processing.
2. People who are given the same type of information process the information differently based on the internal and external contexts.
3. Models taken from other disciplines and settings may not be applicable to information processing in many patient situations.
4. Noncausal thinking and other changes of thought processes may serve a useful purpose in threatening patient situations.
5. Attempts to change a person's processing style may be detrimental in some patient situations.
6. Information processing may reflect general principles of system integrity that have physiological or behavioral bases.
7. Patient decision making is likely a stepwise process that varies within the stages of the patient experience.

Based on the current state of knowledge and the critique of the research reviewed, the following recommendations are made to nurse researchers in regard to future studies on patient information processing.

1. Develop and operationalize an information-processing model based on the discipline's holistic view of person and health.
2. Conduct systematic programs of research that deal with the key variables within the model.
3. Design and implement coordinated laboratory and clinical studies of the basic processes of patient information processing.
4. Review related areas of research, such as health teaching, compliance, and coping, to identify knowledge relevant to an understanding of patient information processing.
5. Plan a systematic approach to research on nursing interventions to enhance each component of patient information processing to promote health.
6. Facilitate collaborative efforts to integrate physiological and behavioral aspects of patient information-processing research.
7. Promote the refinement and replication of study designs that prove most productive in exploring this developing field.

As the information society moves into the twenty-first century, nurses will be concerned increasingly with how patients process information and thereby create their own health experiences. Contributions of nursing research toward understanding this phenomenon have been examined in this chapter. As yet, the research has been unfocused, but these beginning efforts provided both the motivation and direction to shape the future work of individual investigators and programs of research. Loomis (1985) reported that 25.8% of 250 clinical nursing research dissertations from 25 nursing doctoral programs between the years 1976 and 1982 dealt with cognitive human response systems. Lenz (1984) presented a six-step process model of information-seeking as a component of client decisions and health behavior. Kogan and Betrus (1984) used an information processing model to develop a nursing mode of therapeutic influence. These were hopeful signs that the scholars and practitioners within the profession will meet the challenge of developing knowledge in this vital area.

REFERENCES

American Nurses' Association, Cabinet on Nursing Research. (1985). *Directions for nursing research: Toward the twenty-first century*. Kansas City, MO: Author.

Anderson, C. J. (1981). Enhancing reciprocity between mother and neonate. *Nursing Research, 30*, 89–93.

Blank, K., & Perry, S. (1984). Relationship of psychological processes during delirium to outcome. *American Journal of Psychiatry, 141*, 843–847.

Brazelton, T. B. (1973). *Neonatal behavioral assessment scale*. Philadelphia: Lippincott.

Brien, M., Haverfield, N., & Shanteau, J. (1983). How Lamaze-prepared expectant parents select obstetricians. *Research in Nursing and Health, 6*, 143–150.

Bull, D. (1973). *Effects of aging on temporal experience*. Unpublished doctoral dissertation, Purdue University, Lafayette, IN.

DeVellis, B. M., Adams, J. L., & DeVellis, R. F. (1984). Effects of information on patient stereotyping. *Research in Nursing and Health, 7*, 237–244.

Donaldson, S., & Crowley, D. (1978). The discipline of nursing. *Nursing Outlook, 2*(6), 113–120.

DuCette, J., & Keane, A. (1984). "Why me?": An attributional analysis of a major illness. *Research in Nursing and Health, 7*, 257–264.

Edwardson, S. R. (1983). The choice between hospital and home care for terminally ill children. *Nursing Research, 32*, 29–34.

Fontes, H. M. (1983). An exploration of the relationships between cognitive style, interpersonal needs, and the eudaimonistic model of health. *Nursing Research, 32,* 92–96.

Fuller, S., Endress, M. P., & Johnson, J. E. (1978). The effects of cognitive and behavioral control on coping with an aversive health examination. *Journal of Human Stress, 4*(4), 18–25.

Grier, M. R. (1984). Information processing in nursing practice. *Annual Review of Nursing Research, 2,* 265–287.

Haber, R. N. (1974). Information processing. In E. C. Carterette & M. P. Friedman (Eds.), *Handbook of Perception* (Vol. 1, pp. 313–333). New York: Academic Press.

Hall, L. A. (1980). Effect of teaching on primiparas' perceptions of their newborn. *Nursing Research, 29,* 317–321.

Hartfield, M. J., & Cason, C. L. (1981). Effect of information on emotional responses during barium enema. *Nursing Research, 30,* 151–155.

Hill, B. J. (1982). Sensory information, behavioral instructions and coping with sensory alteration surgery. *Nursing Research, 31,* 17–21.

Janson-Bjerklie, S., Carrieri, V. K., & Hudes, M. (1986). The sensations of pulmonary dyspnea. *Nursing Research, 35,* 154–159.

Johnson, J. E. (1973). Effects of accurate expectations about sensations on the sensory and distress components of pain. *Journal of Personality and Social Psychology, 27,* 261–275.

Johnson, J. E. (1975). Stress reduction through sensation information. In I. G. Sarason & C. D. Spielberger (Eds.), *Stress and anxiety* (Vol. 2, pp. 356–362). New York: Halsted Press.

Johnson, J. E., Christman, N. J., & Stitt, C. (1985). Personal control interventions: Short- and long-term effects on surgical patients. *Research in Nursing and Health, 8,* 131–145.

Johnson, J. E., Kirchoff, K., & Endress, M. P. (1975). Altering children's distress behavior during orthopedic cast removal. *Nursing Research, 24,* 404–410.

Johnson, J. E., & Leventhal, H. (1974). The effects of accurate expectations and behavioral instructions on reactions during a noxious medical examination. *Journal of Personality and Social Psychology, 29,* 710–718.

Johnson, J. E., Leventhal, H., & Dabbs, J. (1971). Contribution of emotional and instrumental response processes in adaptation to surgery. *Journal of Personality and Social Psychology, 20,* 55–64.

Johnson, J. E., & Rice, V. (1974). Sensory and distress components of pain: Implications for the study of clinical pain. *Nursing Research, 23,* 203–209.

Johnson, J. E., Rice, V. H., Fuller, S. H., & Endress, M. P. (1978). Sensory information, instruction in a coping strategy and recovery from surgery. *Research in Nursing and Health, 1,* 4–17.

King, I. (1981). *A theory for nursing.* New York: Wiley.

Kishi, K. I. (1983). Communication patterns of health teaching and information recall. *Nursing Research, 32,* 230–235.

Kogan, H. N., & Betrus, P. A. (1984). Self-management: A nursing mode of therapeutic influence. *Advances in Nursing Science, 6*(3), 55–71.

Lenz, E. R. (1984). Information seeking: A component of client decision and health behavior. *Advances in Nursing Science, 6,* 59–72.

Loomis, M. E. (1985). Emerging content in nursing: An analysis of dissertation abstracts and titles: 1976–1982. *Nursing Research, 34,* 113–116.

Lowery, B. J., Jacobsen, B. S., & Murphy, B. B. (1983). An exploratory investigation of causal thinking of arthritics. *Nursing Research, 32,* 157–162.

Martel, L. (1986). *Mastering change: The key to business success*. New York: Simon and Schuster.

Mishel, M. H. (1981). The measurement of uncertainty in illness. *Nursing Research, 30*, 258–263.

Mishel, M. H. (1983). Parents' perception of uncertainty concerning their hospitalized child. *Nursing Research, 32*, 324–330.

Mishel, M. H. (1984). Perceived uncertainty and stress in illness. *Research in Nursing and Health, 7*, 163–171.

Neuman, B. (1982). *The Neuman Systems Model: Application to nursing education and practice*. East Norwalk, CT: Appleton-Century-Crofts.

Newman, M. A. (1972). Time estimation in relation to gait tempo. *Perceptual and Motor Skills, 34*, 359–366.

Newman, M. A. (1976). Movement tempo and the experience of time. *Nursing Research, 25*, 273–279.

Newman, M. A. (1979). *Theory development in nursing*. Philadelphia: F. A. Davis.

Newman, M. A. (1982). Time as an index of expanding consciousness with age. *Nursing Research, 31*, 290–293.

Orem, D. E. (1985). *Nursing: Concepts of practice* (3rd ed.). New York: McGraw-Hill.

Owens, J. F., & Hutelmyer, C. M. (1982). The effect of preoperative intervention on delirium in cardiac surgical patients. *Nursing Research, 31*, 60–62.

Perry, S. E. (1983). Parents' perceptions of their newborn following structured interactions. *Nursing Research, 32*, 208–212.

Roy, C. (1984). *Introduction to nursing: An adaptation model*. Englewood Cliffs, NJ: Prentice Hall.

Roy, C. (in press). Altered cognition: An information processing approach. In P. Mitchell, L. Hodges, M. Muwaswes, & C. Walleck (Eds.), *Neuroscience Nursing: Phenomena and Practice*. East Norwalk, CT: Appleton-Lange.

Roy, C., & Roberts, S. (1981). *Theory construction in nursing: An adaptation model*. Englewood Cliffs, NJ: Prentice Hall.

Rudy, E. B. (1980). Patients' and spouses' causal explanations of myocardial infarction. *Nursing Research, 29*, 352–356.

Sanders, S. A. (1986). Development of a tool to measure subjective time experience. *Nursing Research, 35*, 178–182.

Scott, D. W. (1982). Anxiety, critical thinking and information processing during and after breast biopsy. *Nursing Research, 32*, 24–28.

Seligman, M. E. (1975). *Helplessness: On depression, development and death* (Psychology Series). San Francisco: W. H. Freeman.

Sime, A. M., & Libera, M. B. (1985). Sensation information, self-instruction and response to dental surgery. *Nursing Health, 8*, 41–47.

Smith, M. J. (1975). Changes in judgment of duration with different patterns of auditory information for individuals confined to bed. *Nursing Research, 24*, 93–98.

Smith, M. J. (1979). Duration experience for bed-confined subjects: A replication and refinement. *Nursing Research, 28*, 139–144.

Smith, M. J. (1986). Human-environment process: A test of Rogers' principle of integrality. *Advances in Nursing Science, 9*(1), 21–28.

Spielberger, C. D., et al. (1980). *The STAI manual*. Palo Alto, CA: Consulting Psychologists Press.

Tompkins, E. S. (1980). Effect of restricted mobility and dominance on perceived duration. *Nursing Research, 29*, 333–338.

OTHER RESEARCH

Vasquez, E., & Chitwood, W. R. (1975). Postcardiotomy delirium: An overview. *International Journal of Psychiatry in Medicine, 6*, 373–383.

Volicer, B. J. (1973). Perceived stress levels of events associated with the experience of hospitalization: Development and testing of a measurement tool. *Nursing Research, 22*, 491–497.

Volicer, B. J. (1974). Patients' perceptions of stressful events associated with hospitalization. *Nursing Research, 23*, 235–238.

Volicer, B. J., & Bohannon, M. W. (1975). Hospital stress rating scale. *Nursing Research, 24*, 352–359.

Volicer, B. J., & Burns, M. W. (1977). Preexisting correlates of hospital stress. *Nursing Research, 26*, 408–415.

Volicer, B. J., Isenberg, M. A., & Burns, M. W. (1977). Medical–surgical differences in hospital stress factors. *Journal of Human Stress, 3*, 3–13.

Watson, G., & Glaser, E. M. (1964). *Manual for Forms YM and ZM: Watson-Glaser Critical Thinking Appraisal.* New York: Harcourt, Brace, & World.

Weiner, B. (1979). A theory of motivation for some classroom experiences. *Journal of Educational Psychology, 71*, 3–25.

Witkin, H. A., Altman, T. K., Raskin, E., & Karp, S. A. (1971). *A manual for the embedded figures test.* Palo Alto, CA: Consulting Psychologists Press.

Ziemer, M. M. (1983). Effects of information on postsurgical coping. *Nursing Research, 32*, 282–287.

Zuckerman, M., & Lubin, B. (1965). *Manual for the multiple affect adjective checklist.* San Diego: Educational and Testing Service.

Chapter 12

Nursing Research
in the Philippines

PHOEBE DAUZ WILLIAMS
COLLEGE OF NURSING
UNIVERSITY OF FLORIDA

CONTENTS

This chapter includes two major sections. The first is a review of studies in the following areas: education, nursing service administration, community health nursing, maternity nursing, psychiatric nursing, medical–surgical nursing, and pediatric nursing. The second is devoted to evaluation and recommendations.

Historically, Williams (1980b) surveyed studies done by nurses in the Philippines between 1935 and 1979 to identify the areas of knowledge most and least commonly studied. The survey showed a heavy emphasis on studies in nursing education (37%) and nursing service administration (40%). Only 16% of studies were done in patient care and 7% in related research. Much of the research was limited in scope: the immediate aim seemed to be the generation of answers to specific problems in the researchers' work settings. Many of the studies were done to satisfy the requirements of a graduate degree. A majority of the studies were performed using nonexperimental approaches

263

and descriptive methods of data analysis. However, there were several methodological studies and studies using experimental designs. Overall, compared to earlier studies, the research designs used have become stronger in the late 1970s and 1980s. Nurse researchers also have been able to compete for funding from national and international sources.

REVIEW OF STUDIES

Sources used in identifying studies for inclusion in this review were: (a) articles published up to 1985 in three journals, the *UPCN Journal, ANPHI Papers*, and the *Philippine Journal of Nursing*; (b) *Nursing Research in the Philippines: A Sourcebook* (Williams, 1980a); (c) the *UPCN Research Bulletin: 1980–1983*; (d) abstracts of theses and dissertations done in the Philippines between 1980 and 1985; and (e) a MEDLINE search of studies done on nursing in the Philippines in the 1970s and 1980s. Eighty original reports of research and 350 abstracts were screened. Selection for inclusion was based on strength of the research design, including related aspects such as sampling, sample size, control of variables, and data analysis.

Nursing studies reviewed in this chapter are divided into three general categories: studies in nursing education, studies in nursing service administration, and studies in patient care. Studies in nursing education deal with the quality of education that nursing students receive following admission to a program and the management of such a program. Studies in nursing service administration deal with nursing resources (kinds, numbers, and the functions of nurses) and the management of the delivery of nursing services. Studies in patient care deal with modes of direct care to patients in primary, secondary, and tertiary health care settings. The major goal of investigators in this group of studies has been the design of better modalities of care through an increased understanding of patient responses and behavior dynamics in health and illness. Five subsections on patient care include community health nursing, maternity nursing, psychiatric nursing, medical–surgical nursing, and pediatric nursing.

Many of the studies included herein are not generally available. For this reason, each study is described in some detail prior to a critique of the study.

Education

Five studies are included in this category. An assessment was done of 14 government schools of nursing (Salmin, 1983), their human and physical resources, and community service activities. Data were obtained by questionnaires, interviews, and observations from 187 respondents (20 nurse administrators and 167 teachers) selected by purposive sampling. The sample was 83.5% of the target population. Descriptive analysis showed that the typical nurse administrator in education was 50 to 51 years old, married, female, had at least a master's degree in nursing, and was upgrading toward a doctoral degree. She taught an average of 6 hours per week and received between 1,000 and 1,399 pesos per month. (In 1983, the exchange rate was 1 : 15, so this would be $67 to $93 in U.S. currency). The typical teacher was 34 to 35 years old, married, female, and a baccalaureate graduate with credits towards a master's degree. She had a rank of instructor and taught an average of 6 hours in the classroom and 20 to 25 hours in the clinical area, and had two to three other assignments, for example, committees. She received a monthly salary of between 700 to 799 pesos plus fringe benefits including living allowance, insurance, and retirement benefits. No recent study of private schools of nursing was available.

The relationships between criteria for student selection, academic achievement, and graduate performance were studied by Tungpalan (1981) and replicated by Lara and Boquiren (1983) in another setting. Tungpalan studied graduating classes of 1973 and 1974 ($N = 52$; 73% return rate) 1 to 2 years after graduation. She found that scores on the college admission test were related significantly to achievement at the College of Arts and Sciences and that College of Nursing grade averages were related significantly to average grades in general education courses and to board examination grades. The grade in practicum was the best predictor of on-the-job performance as rated by the employer.

Using similar variables and methods to evaluate graduates of 1980 ($N = 151$), Lara and Boquiren (1983) found that the college admission test scores were related significantly to weighted grade averages at the College of Nursing and that the College of Nursing grades were correlated highly with weighted grade averages in general education courses and with board examination ratings. Selected admissions based on standardized tests and weighted grade averages on general education courses were recommended by the investigators in both studies. Maximizing clinical, especially practicum, experiences also was recommended.

The effects of coping skills training on nursing students' reactions to a stressful situation was studied by Lantican (1981) and replicated by Lantican and Merritt (1983). A pretest–posttest control group design with pretreatment matching and random assignment to groups was used in the 1983 study; a posttest-only control group design with random assignment to groups was used in the 1981 study. Similar coping skills training methods were used in the two studies. Debriefing of subjects after the study was done by the investigators. Observational and self-report outcome measures were used. In both studies it was found that the Spielberger State-Trait Anxiety Inventory state scale scores of the experimental group were significantly lower (Spielberger, Gorsuch, & Lushene, 1970). An observational anxiety scale independently rated by two "blind" observers (interrater $r = .90$) during the first and second 10 minutes of the stress situation also showed significantly lower scores for the experimental group in both studies. The design, implementation, and analysis of the two studies were rigorous. The sizes of the samples of the two studies, however, were small, 14 and 20 respectively, with equal distribution into both groups. There was no attrition in the first study; five subjects dropped out of the second study. Based on the results, the teaching of stress management strategies to nursing students and practicing nurses was recommended.

Nursing Service Administration

Three descriptive studies are included in this category. A week-long, 3-shift time activity study of 85 nursing personnel in six units (four medical and surgical, one pediatric, and one obstetric) of a 960-bed public general hospital has been done [University of the Philippines College of Nursing (UPCN), 1980]. Results showed that head nurses, staff nurses, and nursing attendants spent 54%, 63%, and 31% of their time, respectively, in patient-centered activities. They spent 25%, 15%, and 54%, respectively, in unit-centered activities, and 5%, 2%, and 0.5% in personnel-centered activities. The remaining time was spent in other-centered activities. Observer reliability in this study was maintained through intensive training and monitoring. Trained nurse observers recorded activities every 15 minutes of an average of eight personnel; they worked at most for 4 hours to prevent fatigue.

Evangelista (1983) studied the factors affecting anxiety levels and attitudes toward death and dying of 217 nurses at four hospitals in two southern cities. Among the factors that significantly affected level of death anxiety were frequency of caring for the dying, nursing position held, area of work, level of nursing education, religiosity, and death experience involving immediate family members. The respondents also indicated that 47% had participated in seminars on abortion, 39% on life-sustaining treatments, 35% on death and dying, and 24% on euthanasia; 93% said they would welcome a continuing education offering on death and dying.

A survey of the salary scales and fringe benefits of nurses in the private sector was done (UPCN, 1976). Respondents were 1,802 nurses working in 115 agencies such as hospitals, schools of nursing, doctors' clinics, and industrial establishments. There was a 67% return of questionnaires. Among the findings were: (a) the mean salary of private duty nurses was the highest among 11 groups; staff nurses had the lowest, and clinical instructors the second lowest; (b) industrial nurses, college instructors, and school nurses ranked among the first three with the most fringe benefits, and staff nurses the least; (c) nurses in urban areas had better pay and more fringe benefits than nurses in rural areas. A related larger study was done 10 years earlier (Sotejo & Sabas, 1966) on the salary and work conditions of nurses working in privately owned hospitals, industrial firms, educational institutions, public health agencies, and on private duty. Though 10 years apart, the two studies identified similar problems, particularly related to salary and working conditions. These factors also were reported as the "pull" factors that encouraged migration in a study by Asperilla (1971) on the mobility of Filipino nurses.

A conceptual framework for the study of stress and coping among nurses was developed by Tungpalan (1983), and exploratory studies have been done of nurses' responses to specific stressors such as an intensive care unit (Miranda, 1981) and dying patients in a cancer unit (Banisa, 1983). In these two studies researchers used a survey approach; both were limited by the small sample sizes used.

Patient Care

Community Health Nursing.   Six studies are included in this category. Lara (1985) evaluated the impact of a demonstration project, funded by the International Development Research Center (IDRC), on the use of a mobile nursing clinic to provide primary health care services to three communities in the highlands of Benquet province. Staffed mainly by nurses who provided medium-range health care similar to that provided by nurse practitioners in the United States, the aim of the project was to establish an empirical basis for comparison with the existing health care system. The existing system utilized mainly midwives with 2-year college education who did routine care and referred cases to a doctor. A total of 338 visits were made by the mobile clinic over the 3-year period from 1979 to 1981. A total of 26,678 patients was seen; in many cases this was the first contact of a patient with a professional health worker. Community participation was promoted by involving community leaders and training volunteer health workers who helped identify health needs of the community and monitor the implementation of health care measures. Among the findings of the project were: (a) Nurses, with the help of a medical technician, were capable of diagnosing and treating most health problems, and the need for referral to a physician rarely arose. (b) The most prevalent illnesses encountered were upper respiratory tract infections and gastrointestinal diseases, most of which were preventable in nature. (c) The main community health problem was unsanitary environmental conditions. (d) The population tended to be young, with many in the high-risk groups under 5 and of childbearing age. (e) The respondents in the communities initially saw the mobile clinic as a source of free medicines and as a source of cure for existing illnesses. (f) The preventive, promotive, and rehabilitative aspects of health care then were appreciated gradually. (g) The volunteer health workers quickly developed the motivation and capability to identify and report community health problems and initiate and monitor intervention measures. (g) The community petitioned for a continuation of the mobile clinic beyond its demonstration phase. Funding of the project was renewed through 1987.

A primary health care nursing clinic was established in 1978 by the University of the Philippines College of Nursing in barrio Bagong Silangan, Quezon City (Barrameda, 1981). The main goal was to demonstrate the role of such a clinic in total community development toward self-direction, self-reliance, and self-support. During the 5 years of the project, faculty members, students, and a full-time professional nurse staffed the clinic assisted by community health volunteers in training. Clinic functions covered a range of preventive–promotive, curative–rehabilitative, and family care services. Some achievements of the project included (a) the training of unit leaders to identify community problems and to organize and communicate their needs, and (b) mobilizing city government to provide pumps for drinking water and sanitary public toilets. Labor was supplied by the community. Twenty-one volunteers were trained; indigenous resources were developed; an herb garden was grown; and community health volunteers and families were taught to prepare herbs for common ailments such as diarrhea and cough. The preparation of protein concentrates also was taught, using powdered beans, shrimps, and anchovies; this was used as supplementary food for infants and older malnourished children. At the end of 5 years an evaluation of the project was done. Trained health volunteers provided adequate first-level health care. Effective linkages with the city health department and local government were established.

Barrameda (1980) measured the health status of an indigenous tribe, the Tinguians, in the remote highlands of Abra province using a function level scale and a symptom and problem scale developed by Patrick, Bush, and Chen (1973). Rigorous data collection was done in three phases. First, a socioeconomic survey was done of the 68 households comprising the village (barrio). Second, ethnographic interviews were done to obtain the peoples' perceptions of health and illness, daily activities, work cycles, and medical histories. Third, the two scales were administered. Systematic sampling was done using every third family on the list provided by the village leader. A total of 150 individuals from the 20 families chosen were interviewed and examined. Results showed that 72% of the subjects were functioning at Level 29, that is, performed major and other activities, traveled freely, and walked freely. However, the symptom scale did not validate the function level scale. For instance, the people went about their chores even while ill. Productivity was low. The below-subsistence economy, based mainly on agriculture and hunting, could be explained partly by the primitive farming methods used. In turn, the poverty bred ill health. The implications were that any attempt at improving the people's health status must be coupled with efforts to increase farm yields. Research results were used successfully to seek agricultural assistance and resources for establishing a community-based health program.

A study was done by Cruz (1980) of the help-seeking behavior of residents in an urban community. The community setting had several private clinics and public health centers, two large hospitals, and several practicing indigenous health workers (e.g., herbolarios). A total of 213 respondents was obtained by multistage sampling. Housewives were interviewed regarding family health history and practices. Data analysis showed that low education, low socioeconomic status, transience of residence, and a rural orientation were associated significantly with (a) greater use of indigenous health workers and public health centers, (b) use of herbs and over-the-counter consultation for drug prescriptions, and (c) nonseeking of preventive health checkups.

Recio, Abarquez, Dohm, and Kuan (1979) conducted a survey of the perceptions of health and illness and patterns of health care interventions among Filipinos. A sample size of 2,000, divided proportionately among all 13 regions (including Metro-Manila), were interviewed. Among the findings of the study were: (a) In general, there was high consistency in perceived common diseases and patterns of health care across the 13 regions. (b) A majority of the respondents claimed to be healthy because they felt no pains or discomforts and were able to perform their social roles. (c) Change of weather was viewed as the main threat to health and beyond one's control. Thus, when the cool or wet weather turned hot or dry, gastrointestinal ailments were expected to occur. When hot or dry weather turned cold or wet, colds, fever, or influenza were expected to occur. (d) The reported sequence of responses to illness was: First recourses were home remedies including patent medicines; then, medical consultation was sought at the rural health unit; and if both failed, indigenous health practitioners were sought.

Layo (1978) conducted a study on the determinants of Philippine morbidity patterns. A randomly selected national sample of 3,000 heads of household was interviewed. Multiple regressions showed that: (a) Age was the highest predictor of morbidity, particularly the number of family members over 64 years old; (b) two environmental variables, quality of drainage and quality of ventilation, were the second best predictors; (c) traditional health beliefs and health knowledge had lesser effects on morbidity; and (d) level of education beyond the elementary grades had a slight negative effect on morbidity.

Maternity Nursing. Five studies are included in this category. Recio and Corcega (1979) assessed the acceptability of two injectable contraceptives, the DMPA (depomedrexy-progesterone acetate-depoprovera) injected every 3 months and the NET-DEN (norethistherone denanthate) injected every 2 months, based on satisfaction with the contraceptive and on continued use over a 6-month period. Subjects ($N = 120$) were drawn from volunteers, with random assignment and equal distribution to each of the two groups. They were interviewed before treatment and during each return visit. Results showed that: (a) There were 80% continuers for the two methods. (b) More than 50% of the subjects reported side effects during the first 2 to 3 months of use, with the DMPA users giving more complaints, particularly the cessation of bleeding. The NET-DEN users complained more of nausea, headache, and weight gain. (c) Given the choice of 3-, 6-, and 12-month intervals for injectable contraceptives, women who participated in order to space pregnancies preferred the 3- or 6-month intervals; women who wanted to stop pregnancies preferred the 12-month interval. Two other studies on the acceptability of contraceptives have been done by Recio (1983a, 1983b), funded by the World Health Organization.

The attitudes of 100 postpartum mothers in a provincial hospital toward tubal ligation were studied by Reorizo (1978). Data analysis showed that 86% of the women agreed to tubal ligation. Higher educational attainment of husband and wife, family size of 3 to 6 children, and older maternal age were related positively to acceptance of tubal ligation.

A survey of the beliefs and practices of rural mothers during pregnancy and childbirth was done by Crispino and Bailon (1970). Random selection of 93 families from a household listing of 136 families for 12 of 13 villages in Bay, Laguna comprised the sample. The findings were: (a) The initial prenatal checkup occurred in the second or third trimester of pregnancy for 50% of the mothers. (b) Certain foods were avoided by 37% of mothers prenatally and 74% postnatally, with the list including specific vegetables, fish, meat, and fruits. (c) A cloth belt (bigkis) was worn by 80% of the mothers prenatally and 92% postnatally. (d) Home delivery was preferred by most, and the indigenous midwife (hilot) was the preferred attendant. (e) "Soub," a crude form of perineal heat, was used by 74%. (f) Abdominal massage was done daily by a hilot on 91% of the mothers for a week to 10 days after delivery. (g) Ambulation was done within a day after delivery by 88%. (h) The colostrum was not given to the baby by 75%, and 66% gave the baby bitter melon (ampalaya) juice as a purgative prior to initial infant feeding. (i) Breastfeeding was done by 80%; condensed milk was preferred over evaporated milk by those who preferred to bottle feed.

A survey of the needs of primigravidas in an urban area was done by Kimseng (1980). Women with normal pregnancies ($N = 136$) registered in four health centers comprised the sample. Level of knowledge about prenatal care and infant care was positively related to maternal education, age, socioeconomic status, and marital status. About 65% preferred hospital delivery; most of those who preferred home delivery said they would call for a health center provider or a licensed midwife. However, more than half did not know of the necessary preparations for a home delivery. The majority chose to breastfeed the baby; working mothers said they would either mix-feed or bottle-feed to be able to resume work after delivery.

Quial (1976) studied the relationship between fathers' involvement in caregiving activities of the newborn and the development of fathering behaviors. Thirty fathers were chosen by purposive sampling and randomly distributed to an experimental and a control group. Lecture demonstrations on the care of the newborn (bathing, feeding, burping) were given to the experimental group during the postpartum period. Compared to the experimental group fathers, most control group fathers believed that care of the newborn was the mother's role. Some fathers in the experimental group approached the infant initially by touching the infants with their fingertips as described by Rubin (1967). These fathers also held the baby more than fathers in the control group and indicated that they were going to assist the mother in several caregiving tasks.

Psychiatric Nursing. Two studies are described in this category. Santos (1976) studied the health maintenance and adjustment to the family and community of 102 adult patients discharged from an urban public hospital for the mentally ill. The subjects were chosen by purposive sampling. Interviews showed that the majority of family members had positive attitudes and that a positive attitude was related significantly to adjustment of subjects as measured by productivity scores. The majority of subjects resumed responsibility in family affairs within 1 month of discharge; 79% of those who had jobs before illness also resumed work within the first month. During the first and the second follow-up home visits, 60% and 52% respectively reported that they had returned for medical supervision. Herb doctors were consulted by most prior to hospitalization, and by the second follow-up visit 56% had gone back to the herb doctor.

The conceptions of and reactions to mental illness by lay people in a southern university community were studied by survey (Ponteñila, 1979). A total of 160 urban and rural households were selected by cluster and random sampling. Household heads were interviewed. The results gave evidence that public awareness of mental health services in this community was high and that the services most preferred for the treatment of mental illness were ranked in the following order: psychiatrist, mental hospital, mental hygiene clinic, and herb doctor. Psychotherapy was perceived as the best treatment of mental illness; the next choices were shock therapy, drugs, and spiritual offering. The perceived causes of mental illness were varied and included physical, environmental, hereditary, and interpersonal factors; supernatural causes were less popular. The mentally ill person was described as sloppy-looking, addicted to drugs, nervous, and speaking a strange language. Some believed that the mentally ill were dangerously unpredictable.

Medical-Surgical Nursing. Three studies are included in this category. A three-phase study was done with patients who had malignant neoplasms of the uterus and breast (Williams et al., 1983). Phase I was a survey of beliefs, attitudes, and behaviors of 63 posthysterectomy and 42 postmastectomy patients attending the outpatient clinic of a large public hospital in 1979. Family members also were interviewed. Findings were used to design Phase II.

Phase II was a posttest control group design. Sixty subjects (30 mastectomy and 30 hysterectomy, equally subdivided into experimental and control groups) were selected by purposive sampling from patients at a large public hospital. Both groups statistically were comparable as to age, marital status, education, and type of surgery within each of the two surgical groups. Other means were used to obtain control of variables. One trained nurse administered the structured preoperative teaching on early ambulation, discharge planning, and postoperative rehabilitation to all the experimental subjects. Each subject was observed for a total of 5 hours on postoperative days 1 and 2. Performance of ambulation tasks, such as dangling of legs, sitting up, and walking, were rated. Two trained observers observed each patient simultaneously but independently. Interobserver reliability was high.

Data analyses showed that: (a) Significantly more patients in the group given preoperative instructions required neither prompting nor assistance in the initiation and completion of the tasks compared to the uninstructed group. Most patients in the uninstructed group did not initiate or complete the tasks despite prompting and physical assistance from the nurse. (b) The mastectomy group tended to report more difficulties or problems compared to the hysterectomy group. It is important to note that because of the open-ward set-up of the study setting, systematic variance between both conditions could not be maximized (Kerlinger, 1973) with random assignment to groups. Confounding (mixing) of treated and untreated subjects was very likely. Therefore, control subjects were first observed until the desired sample sizes were obtained. Then the experimental conditions were applied. With this approach, history was a threat to the internal validity of the study (Cook & Campbell, 1979).

During the return-to-clinic phase (III), only 40 subjects were available. Among the mastectomy patients, 10 were in the experimental group and 10 in the control group. Among the hysterectomy patients, 10 were in each group. In this phase, two nurse observers were trained to collect data. Instruments used were the Self-Care Rating Scale and the Complications Checklist (which were devised for the study). T-test analyses showed that both the instructed postmastectomy and posthysterectomy groups performed self-care activities at home significantly better than and more frequently than the uninstructed group. The instructed postmastectomy subjects reported a lesser number of preventable complications than the uninstructed group. No remarkable differences were seen in the incidence of preventable complications between the instructed and uninstructed posthysterectomy patients (Gloria, 1984).

Caña (1980) also did a study of the effects of preoperative instruction about early ambulation on patients' postoperative performance of selected perambulation tasks. A posttest control design was used. Fifty patients were selected by purposive sampling from patients of a public hospital. For reasons similar to those in the preceding study, data collection for the control group was done before the experimental group. Both groups were comparable on a number of sociodemographic and other variables at the start of the study. Only one trained nurse administered the instrument measuring the independent variable. Nursing students were trained as observers and observed subjects in pairs simultaneously but independently. A high degree of reliability in the use of the scale was obtained. Outcome measures were taken between the 8th and 12th hours after surgery. Three perambulation tasks, deep breathing, leg exercise, and turning to sides, were rated. Quality of performance was based on four criteria: time interval of first performance, prompting required, assistance required, and frequency of performance. T-test analyses showed the experimental group had significantly higher mean levels of performance on all three perambulation tasks.

Finally, Luna (1969) studied the effects of varied types of nursing approaches on pain behavior of 24 females and 16 males after surgery at a private hospital. Subjects were chosen by purposive sampling with a consecutive order of assignment to eight study groups in a $2 \times 2 \times 2$ factorial design. The independent variable was preoperative support, which consisted of structured teaching, postoperative reinforcement, and nurse visits. One outcome measure was overt pain behaviors as measured on a scale that included the following: complaints of pain; degree of restlessness; and degree of fist-clenching, teeth-grinding, frowning, and grimacing. Analgesic use was another outcome measure. Only one nurse administered the study treatment. Trained observers collected data, with a high degree of reliability, every 2 hours during the first 12 postoperative hours and once in the morning of the first two postoperative days. Using analysis of variance, a significant main effect of preoperative support and interaction effects of preoperative support and postoperative nurse visits on overt pain behaviors was obtained. A small trend toward lesser use of analgesics also was seen among patients who received preoperative support.

Pediatric Nursing. Clusters of studies were evident among those reviewed in this section. The researchers focused on developmental assessment, development and care of high-risk newborns, developmental disabilities, family coping, preparation of children for surgery, play interviews, school-age children's concepts of the body and illness, and death and dying.

A restandardization of the Denver Developmental Screening Test (DDST) (Frankenburg, Fandal, & Dodds, 1970) was done in the Philippines in 1977 to 1980 by Williams (1984). The subjects were 6,006 children between the ages of 2 weeks and 6¹/₂ years from 4,846 households of six municipalities of Metro-Manila. The test was renamed the Metro-Manila Developmental Screening Test (MMDST). A combination multistage, cluster (with implicit stratification), systematic, and quota sampling was used. Some of the original DDST materials and methods were modified; these are described elsewhere (Williams, 1984). Interrater reliability, test–retest reliability, and mother–tester reliability were calculated. Total agreement on all three ranged between 96% and 97%. Concurrent validity ($r = .97$) was obtained (Layug, 1980) using the Gesell test. Probit analysis was done of the normative data obtained to establish the ages at which 25%, 50%, 75%, and 90% of the sample passed each of the 105 test items. On the basis of these results, a test form similar to the DDST was made. Discriminant analysis using the 45 variables showed four clusters of factors that were associated significantly with children's performance. These were a substitute caregiver variable cluster, a mother variable cluster, a child-situational variable cluster, and an age variable cluster.

Other investigators have determined significant variables related to children's performance on a developmental screening test. Andaya (1978), testing 566 children aged 13 months to 6 years, found that upper- and middle-class children had significantly less number of delays than lower-class children and that three behavior sectors showed these differences: language, fine motor-adaptive, and gross motor. Bacalzo (1979) tested 221 rural and 222 urban children aged 13 months to 6 years (127 with normal weights and 316 with weights below the 10th percentile of standards). She found that 20% of the behaviors compared were performed significantly earlier by urban children, and that 26% of the behaviors compared were performed significantly earlier by children with normal weights. Decena (1978) tested 103 boys and 97 girls with heart disease, ages ranging from 18 days to 6 years, in the clinics of two public hospitals. She found that compared to norms the children weighed significantly less, but their heights were normal. The children also were delayed significantly in the gross motor section of the DDST. Williams and Williams (1985b), comparing 340 children with weights below the 10th percentile who were excluded from the standardization study, reported that the children had almost three times as many questionable and abnormal performances as the normative children. Florencio, Lacuesta-Manalo, and Goco (1983), comparing the MMDST performance of children before and after participating in a comprehensive rehabilitation program for severely malnourished children, reported an average of nine delays upon admission to the program to one delay upon discharge.

Finally, the Metro-Manila norms were compared with DDST norms developed in four other locales, Denver, the Netherlands, Japan, Okinawa (Williams & Williams, 1987), and results were discussed in light of Philippine childrearing practices. An MMDST manual has been published (Williams, 1985) and test kits produced by the University of the Philippines College of Nursing. The school has been conducting training for nurses in the use of the tool in primary health care. Further predictive validation of the tool should be undertaken by nurses similar to one done earlier (Williams, 1984). Madrazo and Williams (1985) also recommended modification of the early identification model for developmental screening to better suit conditions in low-income developing countries.

Pacis (1982), Dial (1981), Porter (1972), Williams and Williams (1985a), and Fuentes (1981) focused their studies on the development and care of high-risk and normal infants. Because unusual life support measures were not available in the Philippines, high-risk survivors in these studies were in effect larger prematures.

Pacis (1982) compared 41 normal and 42 at-risk infants at birth, 1 month, and 3 months as to weight, length, and behavior development as measured by the MMDST. Risk infants had a score of 42 and normal infants 69 on the Maternal-Child Health Care Index (Nesbit & Aubry, 1969), as modified by Puertollano (1978) and validated by Williams (1980d). Data analysis showed that at birth there was no significant difference between normal and at-risk babies in both weight (2.91 compared to 2.86 kg) and length (48.5 compared to 48.1 cm). At 1 month, normal babies were significantly heavier but were the same height as high-risk babies. At 3 months normal babies were significantly heavier and longer than the high-risk babies. Three infants in the risk group and one in the normal group died in the course of the study. Thirty-five items of the MMDST were administered at 1 and 3 months postbirth. Performance at 1 month on two test sectors was significantly different between the two groups, but not on the 3rd-month assessment. Thus, at 1 month, 36% of high-risk babies compared to 12% of the normal group failed all items administered in the personal–social sector. In the gross motor sector, 21% of high-risk babies failed all items while all the normal babies passed the items administered.

Fuentes (1981) compared maternal caregiving during the first 2 to 3 months for high-risk ($n = 30$, 15 preterm and 15 small for gestational age) and term ($n = 30$) infants in a southern city. The infants were chosen by purposive sampling of hospital registries, and the mothers were interviewed at home. All the high-risk infants weighed over 1800 grams except three between 1361 and 1389 grams. Data analysis showed that birth condition did not affect significantly the extent of maternal caregiving activities or of maternal attitudes as measured by the Paternal Attitude Research Inventory (Shaeffer & Bell, 1958). Both groups of mothers held similar concepts relative to infant feeding, daily care, infant crying, and mother–infant interaction. However, mothers of high-risk babies often used health care services for well-baby checkups while mothers of term babies used the clinic more often for sick-baby consultations. It appeared that the risk status of the infants was emphasized to mothers upon hospital discharge, with encouragement to seek regular checkups.

In a replication of an earlier study (Porter, 1967) on 94 infants between 4 and 40 weeks of age, Porter (1972) reported significantly greater gains in weight and length and in motor, adaptive, language, and personal–social behaviors on the Gesell test among infants who received a physical-physiological activity program daily at home for 2 months in comparison with control infants. The two groups were matched for age and gender. The study was done in a southern Philippine community.

Dial (1981) studied the effects of developmental stimulation in a newborn nursery and at home for 8 weeks on growth and development of preterm infants. Purposive sampling was done; the infants had birth weights between 3.8 and 5 pounds, gestational ages between 36 and 38 weeks, no birth complications, and were born in the same hospital. Multimodal stimulation was given to the experimental group ($n = 19$) and none to the control group ($n = 15$). There were no initial differences between the two groups in Apgar score, weight, length, Dubowitz score, and days in the hospital. One nurse gave all the interventions. Another

was trained to collect the outcome measures in the 8th week. No significant differences in weight and length were found. Behavioral development as measured by the MMDST (Williams, 1984), however, was significantly different. That is, nine control group infants had three delays
each compared to only one experimental group infant with one delay.
Differences occurred on all except the language sectors.

Williams and Williams (1985a) studied 911 children with histories
of perinatal risk events: birth weights less than 2,500 grams, age of
gestation less than 37 weeks, and instrumental delivery. They aimed to
determine the variables that characterize normal and abnormal or questionable performance on the MMDST. Children's ages ranged between
2 weeks and $6^{1}/_{2}$ years with 53% male and 47% female. In addition to
MMDST performance, data on 34 variables were used in discriminant
analysis. Thirteen variables with significant discriminant function coefficients formed five clusters: a child situational variable cluster, health variable cluster, mother variable cluster, socioeconomic variable cluster, and
age variable cluster. In a related study, Williams, Dial, and Williams (1986)
also showed that compared to the normative sample for the MMDST, the
high-risk children had five times more abnormal performances.

Two studies on the rearing of handicapped children were available
(Madrazo, 1982; Quimbo, 1979). Quimbo studied the rearing of 120
children attending a rehabilitation clinic for cerebral palsy. The children
ranged in age from infancy to adolescence. Mothers were interviewed.
Among the findings were: (a) Parental initial concerns were focused on
developmental delays in crawling and rolling to prone position. (b) The
task of teaching the children activities of daily living was the mother's.
(c) Relationships with maternal and paternal relatives were generally
pleasant. Chi-square analyses of sociodemographic variables and parental attitudes as measured by the Parental Attitude Research Inventory (Shaeffer & Bell, 1958) showed that the female child was more likely
than the male to be overprotected, that the eldest or only child was
treated with more leniency than the middle or youngest child, and that
lower-class parents with manual or service type jobs and with lower
education (elementary level or less) were more likely to foster depen-
dence, to overprotect, and to discipline punitively.

Madrazo (1982) compared the rearing of deaf ($n = 28$), mentally
retarded ($n = 19$), and normal children ($n = 50$) by means of maternal
interviews. Results showed that the age ranges at which deafness or
mental retardation (MR) were detected was 7 months to $5^{1}/_{2}$ years, and
birth (Down's Syndrome) to 7 years, respectively. The earliest signs

recalled by mothers of deaf children were: lack of response to sounds, lack of startle, weak cry, and nonimitation of sounds produced by the mothers. The earliest signs recalled by mothers of mentally retarded children were: lack of head control, inability to crawl or walk at expected ages, and poor motor coordination. Among the deaf, diagnosis was ascertained usually between the ages of 7 months and 3 years. Except for the child with Down's Syndrome, the MR children generally were diagnosed later. Significantly more deaf than normal children were able to wash, feed, and dress themselves between 3 and 6 years of age. Bowel and bladder control were achieved before age 3 by both the deaf and normal groups and after age 3 by the MR group. These findings were discussed with reference to the early identification of disease or disability model (Madrazo & Williams, 1985).

Family coping with children's chronic illness was the subject of the Lorenzo (1981) study. Fifty-seven mothers of cardiac patients and 43 mothers of children with neurological illnesses were interviewed regarding changes in family roles and changes in activities of siblings following illness onset. The ill children were located in pediatric wards ($n = 11$) and outpatient departments ($n = 89$) of three public hospitals and one private hospital in metropolitan Manila. Data analysis showed a significant increase in household chores and decrease in school and social activities of siblings. Decrease in social activities of adolescent siblings was significantly greater than those of school-age siblings and of siblings of neurology patients more than siblings of cardiac patients. More than 50% of the children with neurological conditions had seizure disorders, the care of whom seemed to be delegated to siblings. However, mothers of cardiac patients reported a decrease of caretaking of their other children because of the care needs of the ill child (46% had rheumatic heart disease). Female siblings were delegated more caretaking responsibilities than male siblings. Fifty-six percent of the families were nuclear; in extended families, mothers and mothers-in-law also helped with caretaking tasks. All social activities of the family, except church activities, decreased after illness onset; husband–wife relationships were reported not to be adversely affected.

Two studies have been done on the preparation of children for surgery (Tayko, 1980; Williams, 1980c). Tayko compared the effects of two methods of preparation for surgery of preschool children aged 3 to 6.8 years at a large public hospital. Method 1 ($n = 7$) was a story followed by a 30-minute play session; Method 2 ($n = 9$) was the story only. A control group ($n = 10$) was not given any treatment. Postoperative behavior was measured by the Global Mood Scale (Torrance, 1968). A modified 3-group posttest design was used. Because the clinic waiting room was one large open space, the study treatments could not be done simultaneously. Instead, the treatments were rotated on a weekly basis. Only one person administered all the treatments. Observers were trained to use the Global Mood Scale; their percentage agreement ranged between 97 and 100%. Two observers then collected data independently and simultaneously. Data analysis showed that subjects receiving Method 1 demonstrated significantly less upset behavior before induction of anesthesia and in the recovery room compared to those receiving Method 2 and the control groups. Subjects receiving Method 2 also were significantly less upset in the recovery room compared to those in the control group. The findings support the use of play methods to communicate with preschool children, as demonstrated earlier by Erickson (1958) and replicated by Garrucho (1977).

A similar design and methods were used by Williams (1980c) on 36 children, 7 to 12 years old, scheduled for elective surgery in the same hospital during the same time period as the Tayko study (1980). Ten children were in Method 1, 11 in Method 2, and 15 in the control group. Subjects in the three groups were similar in age, sex ratio, and place of residence. Father's education and mother's education of the control subjects were higher than the experimental groups; control subjects also had a higher proportion of simple surgeries. Despite these latter biases, however, the results gave evidence that children in the experimental group showed significantly less upset behavior in the recovery room. Method 2 (story only) was as effective as Method 1. The greater verbal capabilities at this age level may have influenced the findings. Cultural practices were discussed in relation to hospitalization of children for surgery.

Tamba (1984) and Atuel (1980) studied children's concepts and reactions to death and dying by using similar structured interview schedules and projective test pictures. Tamba (1984) compared responses of hospitalized children ($n = 65$) with acute, chronic, and fatal illness and nonhospitalized ones ($n = 49$). Waechter's (1968) method was used to score the projective test responses. Twenty percent of the coded stories were recoded independently by another coder. High reliability coefficients were obtained. Analysis of variance and multiple t-test comparisons showed a main effect of illness condition: Children with fatal illness used mutilation imagery, whereas the other three groups used death imagery most often. Well children also used separation imagery significantly more often than hospitalized children. Concepts of death were classified into four phases (Waechter, 1968): (a) a relative ignorance of the meaning of death; (b) denial of death; (c) death is final but functions are attributed to the dead; and (d) death is final with cessation of life functions. The study produced evidence of a clear age progression from the first to the fourth phase; however, no clear chronological age division was observed. In addition to the age factor, previous experience with death in the family or neighborhood significantly affected level of conceptual development. Age, sex, socioeconomic status (SES), religion, and place of residence significantly affected fear level. Older and male children were more fearful, as well as children in lower SES levels, Catholics, and rural children. Parallel results with Waechter (1968) and Melear (1972) were obtained.

Atuel (1980) used similar methods to study children's reactions to the death of a sibling. School-age children ($N = 73$) with siblings who had died within a year at the time of data collection were located through the registries of four public and one private hospital and the civil registries of five municipalities. The children were then visited in their homes. Findings showed that the nature of death and age of dead sibling significantly affected fear level as elicited by the projective test; those whose siblings were older and had died of a chronic illness reported higher fear levels than other children. School grades of the children were significantly lower immediately following the death of the sibling. Time interval since death, age of sibling, and socioeconomic status significantly affected the level of grief; a lower level was seen with a longer time interval since death, higher SES, and a younger sibling.

Williams (1983) studied the concepts of body organs and illness of children in grade levels 1, 3, and 5; 229 were well children and 130 were hospitalized children. The schoolchildren were drawn from 4 public schools: two located in metropolitan Manila, one with an innovative and the other with a regular curriculum, and two schools in communities located 25 and 400 kilometers, respectively, north of Manila. Nineteen to twenty children were chosen randomly from each class sampled. The 130 hospitalized children were drawn purposively from two public and one semiprivate hospitals in Manila. All of the hospitals admitted patients from all parts of the country. Smith's (1973) interview methods were replicated. High intrarater and interrater reliability in scoring the responses was obtained. "Blind" rating of protocols was done. Among the findings were: (a) the hospitalized children knew significantly more about illness, but not about internal body parts, than well children; (b) four variables significantly influenced knowledge of body parts and of illness: grade level, father's and mother's education, and gender; (c) place of residence and mother's occupation significantly affected the scores only of well children (in favor of the urban child with a working mother, that is, income-generating); (d) the five most commonly identified body parts by the 359 children were bones, intestines, heart, brain, and blood vessels; (e) hospitalized children often cited germs and contagion or described how an injury was brought about; well children cited natural phenomena as causes of illness, such as exposure to heat, cold, dew, or wind and also cited folk medical treatments. This last finding reflected adults' concepts of illness as reported by Recio et al. (1979). When the raw data from children in the innovative curriculum were compared with Smith's (1973) raw data, no statistically significant differences in body and illness scores were seen (Williams, 1978). When the children of the four public schools were compared, those from the innovative curriculum scored significantly higher than the others; the children from the rural school farthest from Manila scored lowest (Williams, 1977a). Finally, a third study (Williams, 1977b) provides evidence that the third graders of the innovative program knew as much as third-year high school students of the farther rural community studied.

EVALUATION AND RECOMMENDATIONS

Issues of design, replication, dissemination, utilization of findings, research content analysis, and funding for nursing research are addressed in this section. Some research included in this review was descriptive in nature. In descriptive research, an investigator attempts to determine the distribution of certain events and attributes. Done on a national scale, like the studies done by Salmin (1983) and the UPCN (1976), the data from these studies could form a rational basis for nursing action related to the economic and social welfare of Filipino nurses (PNA, 1978). The recent demonstration projects in primary health care (Barrameda, 1980; Lara, 1985) also provide descriptive data on outcome measures that could support new thrusts in community health care and nurses' roles in such innovations.

Descriptive research also has value in hypothesis generation. In a review of nursing studies done in the Philippines between 1935 and 1979, however, Williams (1980b) has noted the predominance of small-scale descriptive studies and limited explanatory research. A recommendation was made for more research that would test hypotheses generated by the many descriptive studies. The need for stringent control in research design was stressed. This control could be achieved in several ways, including the active manipulation of treatment variables, use of control groups, and statistical control of errors and extraneous variables.

Compromises in research design are seen in the clinical research included in this review. The most common reason for nonuse of randomization was the open ward environment of most hospitals in which confounding of treatment and control group conditions was very real. Thus, consideration of internal validity involved weighing the effects of history against that of confounding of treatment effects. Some investigators used weekly rotation of treatments as a compromise (Tayko, 1980; Williams, 1980c). Others used static group design, having the control group dealt with before the experimental group. As additional control, initial equivalence between groups was tested statistically (Caña, 1980; Dial, 1981; Williams et al., 1983); and trained observers kept blind of treatment conditions observed independently and simultaneously (Caña, 1980; Tayko, 1980; Williams, 1980c; Williams et al., 1983). Randomized controlled studies remained the ideal whenever possible, nevertheless (Lantican & Merritt, 1983; Luna, 1969; Porter, 1972).

In addition to recommendations about strong research design, the need for more replication studies is essential. Repeated study of the same research question in different settings using different samples or populations and conducted by different investigators helps to establish the generalizability of research findings. Replication rarely means exact duplication of a research study; researchers usually change the operational definition of certain variables or procedures in a planned way (Shelley, 1984). Individual nurse researchers with a program of research in a specific area utilize this approach (Johnson & Rice, 1974; Rice & Johnson, 1984). Cluster studies done by several investigators that focus on various aspects of a specific concept in a planned way also accomplish the same objective. Examples of these clusters are studies on the development and care of risk and normal newborns (Dial, 1981; Fuentes, 1981; Pacis, 1982; Williams, Dial, & Williams, 1986); studies on developmental assessment (Andaya, 1978; Bacalzo, 1979; Williams, 1984; Williams & Williams, 1987); families and children with developmental disabilities (Madrazo, 1982; Quimbo, 1979); preparation of children for surgery (Tayko, 1980; Williams, 1980c); children's concepts of death and dying and of body organs and illness (Atuel, 1980; Tamba, 1984; Williams, 1977a, 1977b, 1978). These approaches are only beginning to become evident in the nursing studies being done currently in the Philippines. Because research utilization in nursing necessitates replicated findings (Stetler, 1984), this trend needs support and encouragement.

If nursing research is to function as the bridge to excellence in practice, interchange and collaboration between researchers and clinicians are essential (Mercer, 1984). This practice helps to ensure clinical relevance and evaluation of nursing studies. Again, beginning efforts in this direction in certain settings, for example, the University of the Philippines, are evident. Transdisciplinary research collaboration also has been supported. The National Science Development Board has funded research into five costly diseases, with researchers from the College of Medicine focusing on biomedical aspects and researchers from the College of Nursing focusing on social science aspects of the same diseases. Undoubtedly, research of this magnitude entails efficient management; in this case the University Office of Research Coordination handles the job. Dissemination of results of this research effort is due soon. Nursing input has been utilized in past training and research projects (Campos, 1975).

Dissemination of research findings is an essential component of the research process. This can be achieved in several ways. Presentation of research findings to peers at local, regional, national, and international forums ensures timely sharing of current research. Publication of research entails a greater time lag from the completion of a project. However, it reaches a larger group of practitioners and also allows a detailed printed report of research, which then serves to guide succeeding studies.

Several nursing groups actively have supported dissemination of research findings. These include the Academy of Nursing in the Philippines, which started a journal, *The ANPHI Papers*, in 1966. The University of the Philippines College of Nursing in 1983 also initiated the *UPCN Journal* to aid in the dissemination of nursing research and theoretical papers. The Philippine Nurses' Association also publishes research reports in the *Philippine Journal of Nursing*. More researchers need to publish their studies in international journals, to share knowledge with a wider circle of peers. Exchange rates to the dollar, however, have been forbidding, especially when one thinks of several revisions before a report gets into print. Because salaries are low the mailing costs become prohibitive. Assistance from international sources may help remedy the problem. Continued participation in cross-cultural research needs enhancement.

Nursing research results have been disseminated to the public, along with results of research from other disciplines, by the National Science Development Board, University of the Philippines Integrated Research Program. Avenues used included not only the publication of books (Williams, 1983) and articles but also a public-oriented magazine that presents content in comic-book format (Recio, 1980; Williams, 1981). The magazine has been popular with science and social studies teachers in public high schools throughout the country. Linkage with other media is another avenue for dissemination of research results. Along with researchers from other disciplines, nurses (e.g., Cruz, 1980; Recio et al., 1979; Williams, 1980c, 1983, 1984) present and discuss results of research periodically with reporters for national newspapers, who in turn feature these researchers in their papers. Traveling research symposia to the various provinces have also been done to reach an audience of professionals (mostly teachers) and lay people (mostly farmers). Interesting dialogues have ensued following "So what?" questions posed. The entire model of research dissemination needs funds and efficient coordination; nevertheless, it is a good model. Nurse researchers fully appreciate the totality of the research process after having participated in the above program.

Nurse researchers have successfully competed for funds from the National Science Development Board (Recio et al., 1979; Williams, 1984). Recently, they have also been successful in obtaining funds from international agencies (Lantican & Corcega, 1986; Lara, 1985). Funding from private sources, such as drug companies, has also been successfully solicited, for example, for research with a physiopharmacology base (Lantican, 1980). All these are viable alternative sources of funds for nursing research that future researchers could compete for, in addition to sources offered by various nursing organizations.

Finally, the process of content analysis of nursing studies initiated earlier (Williams, 1980a) needs to be done periodically. This serves to define areas of need as well as areas of knowledge that have gained greater generalizability through replication. Emerging nursing content and theory thus can be identified. In contrast to the earlier review that identified nursing education and administration as the major focus of studies done by nurses between 1935 and 1979, there has been a noticeable refocusing of research efforts on patient care at all levels. The demonstration projects on the delivery of nursing care at the primary health care level are noteworthy. Although this service has been done by nurses for many years, this is the first attempt to test systematically the nurse practitioner model of care. Geographical, financial, cultural, and functional accessibility of care (World Health Organization, 1978) is a major goal. Research at the secondary and tertiary health care levels across specialty areas also is noteworthy. All these are encouraging trends worthy of perpetuation by Philippine nurses.

REFERENCES

Andaya, E. C. (1978). *Social class differentials in the performance on the Denver Developmental Screening Test of preschoolers in selected areas of greater Manila.* Unpublished master's thesis, University of the Philippines, Quezon City.

Asperilla, P. F. (1971). *The mobility of Filipino nurses.* Unpublished doctoral dissertation, Teacher's College, Columbia University, New York, NY.

Atuel, T. M. (1980). *Determinants of Filipino children's responses to the death of a sibling.* Unpublished master's thesis, University of the Philippines, Quezon City.

Bacalzo, F. T. (1979). *State of nutrition and type of community as determinants of performance of preschoolers on the Denver Developmental Screening Test.* Unpublished master's thesis, University of the Philippines, Quezon City.

Banisa, R. P. (1983). Reactions of nurses toward the care of dying patients in a selected cancer unit. *UPCN Journal, 1*(2), 28–33.

Barrameda, M. C. (1980). Measuring health status in a Tinguian community. In P. D. Williams (Ed.), *Nursing research in the Philippines: A sourcebook* (pp. 134–145). Quezon City, Philippines: JMC Press.

Barrameda, M. C. (1981). The community environment. In P. D. Williams & L. B. Tangpalan (Eds.), *Fundamentals of nursing* (pp. 215–222). Quezon City, Philippines: JMC Press.

Campos, P. C. (1975). *Comprehensive community health.* Quezon City, Philippines: National Science Development Board and University of the Philippines.

Caña, R. P. (1980). Effects of preoperative instruction about early ambulation on patients' post-operative performance of selected perambulation tasks. In P. D. Williams (Ed.), *Nursing research in the Philippines: A sourcebook* (pp. 34–43). Quezon City, Philippines: JMC Press.

Cook, T. D., & Campbell, D. T. (1979). *Quasi-experimentation: Design and analysis issues for field settings.* Boston: Houghton Mifflin.

Crispino, J. B., & Bailon, S. G. (1970). A survey of beliefs and practices during pregnancy and childbirth in Bay Laguna. *ANPHI Papers, 5*(2), 5–14.

Cruz, E. B. (1980). A comparative study of help-seeking behavior in an urban community. In P. D. Williams (Ed.), *Nursing research in the Philippines: A sourcebook* (pp. 125–133). Quezon City, Philippines: JMC Press.

Decena, A. Z. (1978). Effects of heart disease on the growth and development of Filipino children ages 0–6 years. Unpublished master's thesis, University of the Philippines College of Nursing, Quezon City.

Dial, M. N. (1981). *The effects of developmental stimulation intervention on the growth and development of preterm infants.* Unpublished master's thesis, University of the Philippines, Quezon City.

Erickson, F. H. (1958). Play interviews for four-year-old hospitalized children. *Monographs for the Society for Research in Child Development, 23*(Serial No. 69).

Evangelista, T. M. (1983). *Anxieties and attitudes of nurses toward death and dying in selected hospitals in Davao and Iligan cities.* Unpublished master's thesis, University of the Philippines, Manila.

Florencio, C., Lacuesta-Manalo, R., & Goco, M. (1983). *Dynamics of rehabilitating severely malnourished children in a nutri-ward and nutri-cottage.* University of the Philippines–Ministry of Health, Quezon City.

Frankenburg, W. K., Fandall, A., & Dodds, J. (1970). *Denver Developmental Screening Test manual* (rev. ed). Denver: University of Colorado Press.

Fuentes, N. A. (1981). *A comparative study of mothers' caretaking roles and activities in relation to risk and normal infants.* Unpublished master's thesis, University of the Philippines, Quezon City.

Garrucho, R. E. (1977). *Reactions of hospitalized Filipino preschoolers to intrusive procedures as reflected in their play behavior.* Unpublished master's thesis, University of the Philippines, Quezon City.

Gloria, M. D. (1984). Long-term effects of preoperative teaching and postoperative rehabilitation on postoperative adjustment of mastectomy and hysterectomy patients. *UPCN Journal, 2,* 14–19.

Johnson, J., & Rice, V. H. (1974). Sensory and distress components of pain: Implications for the study of clinical pain. *Nursing Research, 23,* 203–209.

Kerlinger, F. N. (1973). *Foundations of behavioral research* (2nd ed.). New York: Holt, Rinehart, and Winston.

Kimseng, I. G. (1980). Maternal needs of primigravidae in certain areas of the city of Manila. In P. D. Williams (Ed.), *Nursing research in the Philippines: A sourcebook* (pp. 56–59). Quezon City, Philippines: JMC Press.

Lantican, L. S. (1980). *Effects of ferrous sulfate on carbon monoxide toxicity, brightness discrimination and reversal learning in mice.* Unpublished doctoral dissertation, University of the Philippines, Quezon City.

Lantican, L. S. (1981). Effects of coping skills training on nursing students' reactions to a stressful situation. *ANPHI Papers, 16*(3,4), 2–20.

Lantican, L., & Corcega, T. (1986). *Alternative training strategies for Barangay health workers in primary health care.* Unpublished document, College of Nursing, University of the Philippines, Manila.

Lantican, L. S., & Merritt, B. F. (1983). Stress management training for nursing students: An experimental analysis. *UPCN Journal, 1*(2), 4–17.

Lara, J. B. (1985). The mobile nursing clinic: A model health care facility for providing primary health care services to selected communities in Benguet Province, Northern Luzon, Philippines. *Philippine Journal of Nursing, 55*(1), 3–5.

Lara, J. B., & Boquiren, C. F. (1983). Correlation between measures of student selection, academic achievement and board examination performance. *ANPHI Papers, 8*(1,2), 9–20.

Layo, L. L. (1978). Determinants of Philippine mortality patterns. *Nutrisyon, 3*(2), 16–28.

Layug, E. M. (1980). *Concurrent validity of the Denver Development Screening*

Test, Metro-Manila version. Unpublished master's thesis, University of the Philippines, Quezon City.

Lorenzo, F. D. (1981). *Long term illness in children: Its effects on patterns of behavior of siblings and on family roles*. Unpublished master's thesis, University of the Philippines, Quezon City.

Luna, H. Q. (1969). The effects of varied types of nursing approaches on pain behavior after surgery. *ANPHI Papers, 6*(3,4), 7-9.

Madrazo, C. V. (1982). Mothering of deaf and mentally retarded children: A comparison of maternal attitudes, child rearing practices and child behavior. *ANPHI Papers, 17*(1,2), 3-11.

Madrazo, C. V., & Williams, P. D. (1985). Early identification of the child at risk — A Philippine perspective. In W. K. Frankenburg, R. Emde, & J. Sullivan (Eds.), *Children at risk: An international perspective* (pp. 309-316). New York: Plenum.

Melear, J. D. (1972). *Children's conceptions of death*. Unpublished doctoral dissertation, University of Northern Colorado, Greeley.

Mercer, R. T. (1984). Nursing research: The bridge to excellence in practice. *Image, 16*(2), 47-51.

Miranda, E. F. (1981). Stressful situations and coping mechanisms of intensive care unit nurses of X hospital. *ANPHI Papers, 16*(3,4), 21-28.

National League of Nursing. (1977). *Community health nursing services in the Philippine Ministry of Health* (5th ed.). Manila, Philippines.

Nesbit, R., & Aubry, R. (1969). High risk obstetrics II. Values of semi-objective grading system in identifying the vulnerable group. *American Journal of Obstetrics and Gynecology, 103*, 972-985.

Pacis, C. R. (1982). Serial comparison of normal and risk babies in terms of six indicators. *ANPHI Papers, 17*(1,2), 18-19.

Patrick, D., Bush, J., & Chen, M. (1973). Toward an operational definition of health. *Journal of Health and Social Behavior, 14*, 6-23.

Philippine Nurses' Association (PNA). (1978). Declaration on the economic and social welfare of Filipino nurses. *Philippine Journal of Nursing, 68*(3).

Ponteñila, E. (1979). *Conceptions and reactions to mental illness by the public of Dumaguete City*. Unpublished master's thesis, University of the Philippines, Quezon City.

Porter, L. S. (1967). *Physical-physiological activity and infants' growth and development*. Unpublished doctoral dissertation, New York University, New York.

Porter, L. S. (1972). The impact of physical-physiological activity on infants' growth and development. *Nursing Research, 21*, 210-219.

Puertollano, N. (1978). A modified maternal child health care index. In *Report on the national consultation on maternal mortality and perinatal mortality*. Manila, Philippines: Ministry of Health.

Quial, M. G. (1976). *The relationship between paternal involvement in caretaking activities of the newborn and the development of paternal behavior*. Unpublished master's thesis, Silliman University, Dumaguete City, Philippines.

Quimbo, C. B. (1979). *The child with cerebral palsy: His effects on parental attitudes and childrearing practices*. Unpublished master's thesis, University of the Philippines, Quezon City.

Recio, D. (1980). Ivatan medical practices. In *Socio-Technological Bulletin*. Quezon City, Philippines: National Science Development Board.

Recio, D. M. (1983a). Acceptability of paper pill vs. oral tablet among women undergoing clinical trial. In *UPCN Research Bulletin (1980–1983)* (p. 15). Manila: University of the Philippines, College of Nursing.

Recio, D. M. (1983b). Free choice of three types of contraceptives among women in rural Philippines. In *UPCN Research Bulletin (1980–1983)* (p. 14). Manila: University of the Philippines, College of Nursing.

Recio, D. M., Abarquez, L., Dohm, D., & Kuan, L. (1979). *Perceptions of health and illness and patterns of health care intervention in relation to improving the quality of life of the Filipino.* Quezon City, Philippines: National Science Development Board and University of the Philippines.

Recio, D. M., & Corcega, T. (1979). Acceptability of the 2–3 monthly injectable contraceptives in clinical trial. In P. D. Williams (Ed.), *Nursing research in the Philippines: A sourcebook* (p. 302). Quezon City, Philippines: JMC Press.

Reorizo, C. I. (1978). *The attitudes of post-partum mothers toward tubal ligation.* Unpublished master's thesis, Philippine Women's University, Manila.

Rice, V. H., & Johnson, J. (1984). Preadmission self-instruction booklets, post-admission exercise performance and teaching time. *Nursing Research, 33,* 147–151.

Rubin, R. (1967). Attainment of the maternal role, processes. *Nursing Research, 16,* 237–245.

Salmin, D. B. (1983). An assessment of government schools and colleges of nursing in the Philippines: 1980–1981. *Philippine Journal of Nursing, 53*(2), 23–31.

Santos, J. J. (1976). *A study of patients discharged from a national mental hospital into the Greater Manila area, their health maintenance and adjustment to the family and community.* Unpublished doctoral dissertation, Johns Hopkins University, Baltimore.

Shaeffer, E. S., & Bell, R. Q. (1958). Development of a parental attitude research instrument. *Child Development, 29,* 339–361.

Shelley, S. I. (1984). *Research methods in nursing and health.* Boston: Little, Brown.

Smith, E. (1973). *School-age children's concepts of body organs and illness.* Unpublished doctoral dissertation, University of Pittsburgh, Pittsburgh, PA.

Sotejo, J. V., & Sabas, L. (1966). Salary and work conditions of nurses in the Philippines. *ANPHI Papers, 1*(4), 14–40.

Spielberger C. D., Gorsuch, R. L., & Lushene, R. E. (1970). *Manual for the state-trait anxiety inventory.* Palo Alto, CA: Consulting Psychologists Press.

Stetler, C. B. (1984). *Nursing research in a service setting.* New York: Prentice-Hall.

Tamba, M. (1984). Factors influencing Filipino children's concepts and affective responses to death. *UPCN Journal, 2,* 3–11.

Tayko, N. P. (1980). Effects of two methods of pre-operative preparation of preschool children. In P. D. Williams (Ed.), *Nursing research in the Philippines: A sourcebook* (pp. 27–33). Quezon City, Philippines: JMC Press.

Torrance, J. (1968). *Children's reactions to intramuscular injections: A comparative study of needle and jet injections.* Cleveland, OH: Case Western Reserve University Press.

Tungpalan, L. B. (1981). The relationship between measures of student selection, academic achievement and graduate performance. *ANPHI Papers, 16*(1,2), 3–26.

Tungpalan, L. B. (1983). Stress in nursing. *UPCN Journal, 1*(2), 18–27.

University of the Philippines College of Nursing. (1976). A study of the salaries and work conditions of nurses in the private sector. *ANPHI Papers, 11*(1,2), 2-40.

University of the Philippines College of Nursing. (1980). A study of activities of head nurses, staff nurses, nursing attendants and nursing students in selected units of a general hospital. In P. D. Williams (Ed.), *Nursing research in the Philippines: A sourcebook* (pp. 93-103). Quezon City, Philippines: JMC Press.

University of the Philippines College of Nursing. (1983, March). The UP College of Nursing teaching program. *UPCN Journal, 1a*, 35-36.

Waechter, E. H. (1968). *Death anxiety in children with fatal illness.* Unpublished doctoral dissertation, Stanford University, Palo Alto, CA.

Williams, P. D. (1977a). A comparison of concepts of body organs and illness of children from a laboratory school to that of children from three public schools. *ANPHI Papers, 12*(1), 2-11.

Williams, P. D. (1977b). A comparison of concepts of body organs and illness of children from five levels of schooling in one rural community. *Philippine Journal of Pediatrics, 26*(2), 10-14.

Williams, P. D. (1978). A comparison of Philippine and American children's concepts of body organs and illness in relation to five variables. *International Journal of Nursing Studies, 15*, 193-202.

Williams, P. D. (1980a). Clinical nursing research: The focus of nursing research in the Philippines in the 1980's. In P. D. Williams (Ed.), *Nursing research in the Philippines: A sourcebook* (pp. 199-204). Quezon City, Philippines: JMC Press.

Williams, P. D. (1980b). *Nursing research in the Philippines: A sourcebook.* Quezon City, Philippines: JMC Press.

Williams, P. D. (1980c). Preparation of school age children for surgery: A program of preventive pediatrics. *International Journal of Nursing Studies, 17*, 107-119.

Williams, P. D. (1980d). The risk approach to maternal-child health care. In P. D. Williams, *Nursing research in the Philippines: A sourcebook* (pp. 60-68). Quezon City, Philippines: JMC Press.

Williams, P. D. (1981). Filipino children's concepts of body organs and illness. In *Socio-Technological Bulletin.* Quezon City, Philippines: National Science Development Board and University of the Philippines.

Williams, P. D. (1983). *Filipino children's concepts of body organs and illness.* Quezon City, Philippines: National Science Development Board and University of the Philippines Office of Research Coordination.

Williams, P. D. (1984). The Metro-Manila Developmental Screening Test: A normative study. *Nursing Research, 33*, 208-212.

Williams, P. D. (1985). *The Metro-Manila Developmental Screening Test: Manual.* Quezon City, Philippines: University of the Philippines College of Nursing.

Williams, P. D., Dial, M. N., & Williams, A. R. (1986). Children at risk: Perinatal events, developmental delays and the effects of a developmental stimulation program. *International Journal of Nursing Studies, 23*, 21-38.

Williams, P. D., Valderrama, D. M., Pascoquin, L. G., Saavedra, L. D., Gloria, M. D., de la Rama, D. T., Ferry, T. C., Abaquin, C. M., & Zaldivar, S. B. (1983). *Nursing care and rehabilitation in malignant neoplasms of the uterus and breast, Phases I-II.* Quezon City, Philippines: University of the Philippines College of Nursing.

Williams, P. D., & Williams, A. R. (1985a). Factors affecting development of risk children. *Journal of Pediatric Psychology, 10*, 77–86.

Williams, P. D., & Williams, A. R. (1985b, November). *Low nutritional levels and child development in the Philippines.* Paper presented at the Fifth Annual Research Conference of the Southern Council for Collegiate Education of Nurses, Orlando, Florida.

Williams, P. D., & Williams, A. R. (1987). DDST norms: A cross-cultural comparison. *Journal of Pediatric Psychology, 12*, 39–57.

World Health Organization (WHO). (1978). *Alma Ata conference on primary health care.* Geneva: World Health Organization.

Index

Contents of Previous Volumes

VOLUME II

VOLUME V

ORDER FORM

Save 10% on Volume 7 with this coupon.

___Check here to order the ANNUAL REVIEW OF NURSING RESEARCH, Volume 7, 1989 at a 10% discount. You will receive an invoice requesting pre-payment.

Save 10% on all future volumes with a continuation order

___Check here to place your continuation order for the ANNUAL REVIEW OF NURSING RESEARCH. You will receive a pre-payment invoice with a 10% discount upon publication of each new volume, beginning with Volume 7, 1989. You may pay for prompt shipment or cancel with no obligation.

Name _____

Institution _____

Address _____

City/State/Zip _____

Examination copies for possible course adoption are available to instructors "on approval" only. Write on institutional letterhead, noting course, level, present text, and expected enrollment (Include $2.50 for postage and handling). Prices slightly higher overseas. Prices subject to change.

Mail this coupon to:
SPRINGER PUBLISHING COMPANY
536 Broadway, New York, N.Y. 10012